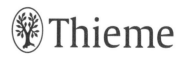

Problems in Periorbital Surgery

A Repair Manual

Foad Nahai, MD, FACS, FRCS (HON)
Maurice. J Jurkiewicz Chair in Plastic Surgery
Professor of Surgery
Emory University School of Medicine
Atlanta, Georgia

Ted H. Wojno, MD
James and Shirley Kuse Professor of Ophthalmology
Director
Oculoplastic and Orbital Surgery
Department of Ophthalmology
Emory University School of Medicine
Atlanta, Georgia

276 illustrations

Thieme
New York • Stuttgart • Delhi • Rio de Janeiro

Managing Editor: Elizabeth Palumbo
Developmental Editor: Judith Tomat
Director, Editorial Services: Mary Jo Casey
Production Editor: Torsten Scheihagen
International Production Director: Andreas Schabert
Editorial Director: Sue Hodgson
International Marketing Director: Fiona Henderson
International Sales Director: Louisa Turrell
Director of Institutional Sales: Adam Bernacki
Senior Vice President and Chief Operating Officer: Sarah Vanderbilt
President: Brian D. Scanlan
Illustrations: Amanda Tomasikiewicz, CMI, and Bill Winn
Printer: King Printing

Library of Congress Cataloging-in-Publication Data

Names: Nahai, Foad, 1943- editor. | Wojno, Ted H., editor.
Title: Problems in periorbital surgery : a repair manual / [edited by] Foad Nahai, Ted H. Wojno.
Description: New York : Thieme, [2019] | Includes bibliographical references and index. |
Identifiers: LCCN 2018041465 (print) | LCCN 2018041933 (ebook) | ISBN 9781626237704 (ebook) | ISBN 9781626237087 (hardback) | ISBN 9781626237704 (eISBN)
Subjects: | MESH: Blepharoplasty—adverse effects | Reconstructive Surgical Procedures | Eyelids—surgery | Rejuvenation | Dermal Fillers—adverse effects | Case Reports
Classification: LCC RD119.5.E94 (ebook) | LCC RD119.5.E94 (print) | NLM WW 205 | DDC 617.7/710592—dc23
LC record available at https://lccn.loc.gov/2018041465

Important note: Medicine is an ever-changing science undergoing continual development. Research and clinical experience are continually expanding our knowledge, in particular our knowledge of proper treatment and drug therapy. Insofar as this book mentions any dosage or application, readers may rest assured that the authors, editors, and publishers have made every effort to ensure that such references are in accordance with **the state of knowledge at the time of production of the book.**

Nevertheless, this does not involve, imply, or express any guarantee or responsibility on the part of the publishers in respect to any dosage instructions and forms of applications stated in the book. **Every user is requested to examine carefully** the manufacturers' leaflets accompanying each drug and to check, if necessary in consultation with a physician or specialist, whether the dosage schedules mentioned therein or the contraindications stated by the manufacturers differ from the statements made in the present book. Such examination is particularly important with drugs that are either rarely used or have been newly released on the market. Every dosage schedule or every form of application used is entirely at the user's own risk and responsibility. The authors and publishers request every user to report to the publishers any discrepancies or inaccuracies noticed. If errors in this work are found after publication, errata will be posted at www.thieme.com on the product description page.

Some of the product names, patents, and registered designs referred to in this book are in fact registered trademarks or proprietary names even though specific reference to this fact is not always made in the text. Therefore, the appearance of a name without designation as proprietary is not to be construed as a representation by the publisher that it is in the public domain.

Thieme Publishers New York
333 Seventh Avenue, New York, NY 10001 USA
+1 800 782 3488, customerservice@thieme.com

Thieme Publishers Stuttgart
Rüdigerstrasse 14, 70469 Stuttgart, Germany
+49 [0]711 8931 421, customerservice@thieme.de

Thieme Publishers Delhi
A-12, Second Floor, Sector-2, Noida-201301
Uttar Pradesh, India
+91 120 45 566 00, customerservice@thieme.in

Thieme Publishers Rio de Janeiro, Thieme Publicações Ltda.
Edifício Rodolpho de Paoli, 25º andar
Av. Nilo Peçanha, 50 – Sala 2508
Rio de Janeiro 20020-906 Brasil
+55 21 3172-2297 / +55 21 3172-1896

Cover design: Thieme Publishing Group
Typesetting by DiTech Process Solutions

Printed in the United States by King Printing   5 4 3 2 1

ISBN 978-1-62623-708-7

Also available as an e-book:
eISBN 978-1-62623-770-4

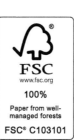

FSC
www.fsc.org
100%
Paper from well-managed forests
FSC® C103101

Contents

Video Contents

Preface

A few years ago, Dr. Nahai was invited to write a chapter for *Problems in Breast Surgery: A Repair Manual* to be published by Quality Medical Publishing (QMP) and edited by Jack Fisher and Neal Handel. Soon after accepting to do so, Karen Berger, CEO of QMP, approached Dr. Nahai and asked if there was any interest in editing a similar book on complications related to blepharoplasty.

Sonny McCord, a good friend and a mentor to both Dr. Nahai and Dr. Wojno, had recently retired. For 15 years, he and Dr. Nahai had practiced together at Paces Plastic Surgery. We felt such a book would be a wonderful and fitting tribute to Sonny whose career was devoted to teaching others not only how "to do it better" but also how to make it safe and prevent and take care of complications. Sonny has trained tens of fellows and residents over his long and illustrious career. Through his many publications and lectures worldwide, he has reached and educated thousands more. At Paces Plastic Surgery alone, he mentored over 35 fellows and equipped them well, not only to feel comfortable around the eyelids but also with the knowledge and skills to deal with untoward outcomes. We reached out to those residents and fellows, as well as leaders in the field of oculoplastic surgery who were close friends of Sonny, and invited them to contribute to this book honoring and celebrating Sonny's long and productive career. The response was enthusiastic and this work is a collection of their contributions.

The meteoric rise of injectables and noninvasive or minimally invasive treatments has led to a paradigm shift in facial rejuvenation, and periorbital rejuvenation is no exception. As rejuvenation of the eyelids and periorbital area is no longer solely in the surgical domain, we have invited experts in nonsurgical treatments to contribute to the book as well.

The case series approach to the discussion of complications and unfavorable results was introduced in the volume mentioned earlier by Drs. Fisher and Handel. It is our intent and hope that our readers will recognize similar cases from their own practices. Some of the more common complications, such as lid retraction, have several chapters discussing differing approaches to the same problem. This was intentional, as we realize that there is no single best approach for dealing with lid retraction. We do not believe in a "one-size-fits-all" approach and encourage individualization of treatment based on the evaluation of each patient and circumstances unique to each case and each individual surgeon familiarity with specific techniques. We include an e-book version with each print copy for convenient reference, and the book is also published with 10 videos.

We are very excited about this volume and trust the novel approach will prove useful to all who consult it. This book is not only intended for our surgical colleagues in Oculoplastic, Facial Plastics, and Plastic Surgery but for all physicians involved in surgical and nonsurgical rejuvenation of the face and periorbital area.

Foad Nahai, MD, FACS, FRCS (HON)
Ted H. Wojno, MD

Acknowledgments

We are indebted to our friends, colleagues, and associates who have made this book possible.

We acknowledge the contributors who willingly joined us in this tribute to our mentor, Sonny McCord, who was also directly or indirectly a mentor to them.

The physicians of the Emory Aesthetic Center— Felmont Eaves, MD, Vincent Zubowicz, MD, Anita Sethna, MD, and Gabrielle Miotto, MD—for their support and encouragement. The staff—in particular my assistant Maggie Burke and nurses Jennifer Ellerbe, Ashlee Spence, and Caroline Carothers—for their assistance.

The physicians and staff of the Emory Department of Ophthalmology, especially the always reliable and always cheerful Brent Hayek, MD, and H. Joon Kim, MD.

We are grateful to the two gifted medical illustrators Brenda Bunch and Bill Winn for the excellent and clear illustrations, which enhance the book. Sue Hodgson, Judith Tomat, and the entire team at Thieme for their encouragement, unfailing support, and hard work in seeing this project to fruition.

To Shahnaz Nahai for her unconditional support throughout Foad's career.

Contributors

Andrew Anzeljc, MD
Oculoplastics Fellow
Section of Oculoplastic and Reconstructive Surgery
Emory University
Atlanta, Georgia

Ryan Scot Burke, MD
Resident Physician
Division of Plastic Surgery
Emory University
Decatur, Georgia

Alison B. Callahan, MD
Assistant Professor
New England Eye Center
Tufts Medical Center
Boston, Massachusetts

William Pai-Dei Chen, MD
Clinical Professor of Ophthalmology
Department of Ophthalmology
UCLA School of Medicine
Irvine, California

Mark A. Codner, MD
Clinical Assistant Professor
Plastic Surgery
Emory University
Atlanta, Georgia

Michael A. Connor, MD
Ophthalmic Plastic and Reconstructive Surgeon
Oculoplastic and Orbital Consultants
Palm Beach Gardens, Florida

Raymond Scott Douglas, MD
Professor of Ophthalmology
Cedars Sinai Medical Center
Los Angeles, California

Francesco M. Egro, MBChB, MSc, MRCS
Plastic Surgery Resident
Department of Plastic Surgery
University of Pittsburgh Medical Center
Pittsburgh, Pennsylvania

Joseph A. Eviatar, MD, FACS
Director of Aesthetic Medicine
Omni Aesthetic MD
New York, New York

Jack A. Friedland, MD, FACS
Clinical Professor of Surgery (Plastic Surgery)
University of Arizona College of Medicine, Phoenix
Associate Professor Plastic Surgery
Mayo Medical School
Paradise Valley, Arizona

Sri Gore, MD
Surgeon
Great Ormond Street Hospital
Chelsea and Westminster Hospital
London, United Kingdom

Brent Hayek, MD
Associate Professor of Ophthalmology
Section of Oculoplastic and Reconstructive Surgery
Emory University
Atlanta, Georgia

T. Roderick Hester Jr.
Retired
Division of Plastic Surgery
Emory University
Atlanta, Georgia

Elizabeth B. Jelks, MD
Adjunct Staff
Department of Plastic Surgery
Lenox Hill Hospital
New York, New York

Glenn W. Jelks, MD
Associate Professor Hansorg Wyss
Department of Plastic Surgery
Associate Professor
Department of Ophthalmology
New York University Medical Center
New York, New York

Naresh Joshi, MD
Consultant Oculoplastic Surgeon
Chelsea and Westminster Hospital
London, United Kingdom

Sergei Kalsow, MD
Cosmetic and Reconstructive Plastic Surgeon
Private Practice
New York, New York

Denise S. Kim, MD
Clinical Instructor
Department of Ophthalmology and Visual Sciences
University of Michigan Medical School
W.K. Kellogg Eye Center
Ann Arbor, Michigan

H. Joon Kim, MD
Assistant Professor of Ophthalmology
Emory Eye Center
Emory University School of Medicine
Atlanta, Georgia

Richard D. Lisman, MD, FACS
Professor of Ophthalmology
NYU School of Medicine
Director of Ophthalmic Plastic Surgery
Institute for Reconstructive Plastic Surgery (NYU)
NYU Medical Center
Manhattan Eye and Ear Hospital
NYU Medical Center
New York, New York

Michelle Barbara Locke, MD
Senior Lecturer in Surgery
Department of Surgery
Faculty of Medicine and Health Science
University of Auckland
Consultant Plastic Surgery
Counties Manukau District Health Board
Auckland, New Zealand

Mark R. Magnusson, MBBS, FRACS (Plast)
Plastic Surgeon
Private Practice
President
Australasian Society of Aesthetic Plastic Surgeons
Toowoomba, Australia

Guy G. Massry, MD
Clinical Professor of Ophthalmology
Ophthalmic Plastic and Reconstructive Surgery
Keck School of Medicine of University of Southern
    California
Beverly Hills, California

Clinton McCord, MD
Retired Oculoplastic Surgeon

Juan Diego Mejia, MD
Private Practice
Medellin, Colombia

Brian Mikolasko, MD
Physician
Montefiore Medical Center/Albert Einstein College of
    Medicine
Icahn School of Medicine at Mount Sinai
New York Eye and Ear Infirmary of Mount Sinai
New York, New York

Gabriele Cáceres Miotto, MD, MEd
Assistant Professor of Surgery
Division of Plastic and Reconstructive Surgery
Emory University School of Medicine
Atlanta, Georgia

Farzad R. Nahai, MD
Clinical Assistant Professor
Plastic Surgery
Emory University School of Medicine
The Center for Plastic Surgery at MetroDerm
Atlanta, Georgia

Foad Nahai, MD, FACS, FRCS (HON)
Maurice. J Jurkiewicz Chair in Plastic Surgery
Professor of Surgery
Emory University School of Medicine
Atlanta, Georgia

**Tim Papadopoulos, BSc, MBBS, FRACS (Gen), FRACS
(Plast)**
Cosmetic Plastic Surgeon
Private Practice
Pyrmont, Australia

Michael Patipa, MD
Oculoplastic Surgeon
Oculoplastic and Orbital Consultants – Retired
North Palm Beach

Carisa K. Petris, MD, PhD
Assistant Professor of Clinical Ophthalmology
Eye and Vision Care
University of Missouri
Columbia, Missouri

Kathleen F. Petro, MD
Resident
Emory Eye Center
Emory University
Atlanta, Georgia

Allan M. Putterman, MD
Professor of Ophthalmology
Codirector Oculofacial Plastic Surgery
University of Illinois College of Medicine
Chicago, Illinois

Dirk Richter, MD, PhD
Specialist, Plastic and Aesthetic Surgery
Department of Plastic Surgery
Dreifaltigkeits-Hospital Wesseling
Wesseling, Germany

Jose Rodríguez-Feliz, MD
Private Practice
Voluntary Clinical Faculty
FIU Herbert Wertheim College of Medicine
Miami, Florida

Richard L. Scawn, MD
Consultant Oculoplastic Surgeon
Chelsea and Westminster Hospital
London, United Kingdom
Wycombe Hospital
Buckinghamshire NHS Trust
Buckinghamshire, United Kingdom

Nina Schwaiger, MD
Specialist, Plastic and Aesthetic Surgery
Department of Plastic Surgery
Dreifaltigkeits-Hospital Wesseling
Wesseling, Germany

Hisham Seify, MD, PhD, FACS
Assistant Clinical Professor
Department of Plastic Surgery
UCLA
Newport Beach, California

Hema Sundaram, MA(Hons), MA, MD, FAAD
Founding Director
Dermatology, Cosmetic & Laser Surgery
Rockville, Maryland

Patrick Tenbrink, MD
Physician
Department of Urology
University of Maryland Medical Center
Baltimore, Maryland

Oren Tepper, MD
Director of Aesthetic Surgery
Director of Craniofacial Surgery
Assistant Professor of Plastic Surgery
Montefiore Medical Center
Albert Einstein College of Medicine
Bronx, New York

Ted H. Wojno, MD
James and Shirley Kuse Professor of Ophthalmology
Director
Oculoplastic and Orbital Surgery
Department of Ophthalmology
Emory University School of Medicine
Atlanta, Georgia

Part I

Clinical Overview

I

1 Management of Complications of Aesthetic Eyelid Procedures

Foad Nahai and Ted H. Wojno

Summary
Complications are inevitable in any surgery. We list the common complications likely to be encountered in eyelid surgery that will be discussed in the following chapters.

Keywords: Bleeding, infection, visual loss, diplopia, eyelid malposition

1.1 Introduction

Despite the rise of injectables, which have had a profound effect on facial rejuvenation including the periorbital area, blepharoplasty remains a popular procedure. According to the annual procedural statistics compiled by the American Society for Aesthetic Plastic Surgery, blepharoplasty is the fifth most popular procedure in women and third most popular in men.

Although facial rejuvenation is no longer solely in the surgical domain, we feel that the results of surgical procedures are longer lasting and more cost effective in the long run, with results that surpass those of nonsurgical procedures. Noninvasive procedures including injectables have proven safe, effective, and, at least in the short term, less expensive than surgery. These are office procedures with minimal down time and limited morbidity. Complications related to nonsurgical procedures are included in this text.

Complications following blepharoplasty may be as minor as a noticeable scar or as devastating as visual loss or anything in between. Most of the complications in between are related to lid malposition and its consequences. Typically, the complications are obvious and clearly visible, but, occasionally, despite an acceptable or good aesthetic result, eyelid dysfunction leads to exposure problems and symptoms. Even mild alteration in eyelid position and function following surgery may result in symptoms.

Complications following Blepharoplasty

Unfavorable Aesthetic Results

- Unacceptable scar.
- Residual skin access.
- Overresection or underresection of fat.
- Overresection or underresection of orbicularis oculi muscle
- Changes in eye shape.
- Eyelid symmetry.
- Overinjection of fat.

Functional Problems

- Chemosis.
- Hematoma.
- Exposure problems.
- Infection.

- Lid retraction.
- Ptosis of the upper eyelid.
- Muscle palsy (most commonly the inferior oblique muscle).
- Loss of vision.
- Paresthesias of the eyelid.
- Refractive changes.

(Adapted from Nahai F, ed. The Art of Aesthetic Surgery: Principles and Techniques. 2nd ed. New York, NY: Thieme; 2010.)

Complications can occur early or late, and are either unfavorable aesthetic results or functional problems. The two categories are not mutually exclusive and may have to be dealt with simultaneously.

Early complications include bleeding, corneal abrasions, chemosis, infection, wound healing issues, and, extremely rarely, skin loss. The majority of late complications are related to lid retraction and its many consequences including dry eye, exposure problems, ectropion, and eyelid fissure changes.

Early and Late Complications

Early Complications

- Bleeding
- Visual loss
- Infection
- Chemosis
- Corneal abrasion
- Corneal exposure
- Dry eye

Late Complications

- Lid retraction
- Ptosis
- Dry eye
- Exposure problems
- Lagophthalmos
- Lid malposition

1.2 Bleeding

Postoperative bleeding, if unrecognized or untreated, will lead to devastating consequences, including visual loss, lid retraction, and skin slough. The bleeding may occur within the orbit or in the lid itself. Intraorbital hemorrhage leading to a retrobulbar hematoma compressing the central retinal artery or optic nerve is a true vision-threatening emergency. Immediate measures, as described in Chapter 3, may avert permanent visual loss. Bleeding into the eyelids, if untreated, may result in skin loss. Unresolved hematoma in the middle lamella will lead to scarring and lid retraction.

1.3 Infection

Given the robust blood supply to the lids and orbit, infection is fortunately a rare complication. It is most often manifested as a cellulitis of the eyelids in the immediate postoperative period. Since eyelid surgery often includes opening of the orbital septum, any wound infection can more easily spread to the orbit and result in orbital cellulitis or frank abscess formation. Given the rise in antibiotic resistance in the general population, culture of any suspected infection is prudent, followed by appropriate oral or intravenous therapy.

1.4 Visual Loss

Fortunately, visual loss is extremely rare (3.3 cases per 100,000), but appropriately it is the most feared consequence. Visual loss may be caused by retrobulbar hemorrhage occluding the central retinal artery or embolism following filler or fat injections. Extremely rarely, perforating globe injuries may lead to visual loss.

1.5 Ocular Motility Disorders

Diplopia is another infrequent complication of eyelid surgery and is usually due to injury to one or more of the extraocular muscles or, more rarely, one of the oculomotor nerves. This can occur from direct trauma from instrumentation or overzealous use of cautery. The inferior oblique muscle is most prone to injury given its relatively superficial position between the nasal and central fat pockets. Complaints of diplopia in the first few hours after eyelid surgery are virtually always secondary to spread of injected local anesthetics to the extraocular muscles and motor nerves, which resolve quickly with the return of normal sensation.

2 Evaluation of the Eyelid

Foad Nahai and Ted H. Wojno

Summary
The preoperative evaluation is essential to determine the needs of the patient and suitability for aesthetic surgery. We propose a simple patient questionnaire to assist in gathering information and a check list of important points to be covered in the evaluation.

Keywords: preoperative evaluation, eyelid evaluation

2.1 Introduction

Performing complication-free aesthetic surgical and nonsurgical procedures (and, for that matter, all medical and surgical treatments) is an ideal but unattainable goal. Nevertheless, it is a worthy pursuit to which we are all committed.

Thorough preoperative planning, careful surgical execution, and attentive postoperative management can minimize true complications or results that simply fail to meet patient expectations.

2.2 Preoperative Evaluation

This should include a thorough history as it relates not only to the eyelids but also to the patient's general health, as outlined in ▶ Fig. 2.1. An assessment of the patient's expectations and the surgeon's understanding of them are essential and will help in avoiding postoperative disappointment despite a successful, complication-free procedure. Video imaging and review of pre- and postoperative images is an important part of this process.

A thorough examination, as outlined in ▶ Fig. 2.2 and the accompanying video must be undertaken. This is an essential part of procedure planning, predicting expected outcomes, and assessment of risk.

A full presentation of possible complications and management must be discussed as part of the informed consent process. Patients must be made aware of all complications including those threatening vision.

We believe that, thorough preoperative evaluation, appropriate surgical planning and skilled execution of the procedure are essential. Pre- and postoperative management should include educating patients about the importance of their role in care and compliance. Adherence to these principles will significantly reduce the risk of complications and unfavorable outcomes and enhance patient satisfaction.

If, despite our best efforts, complications arise, we trust that this volume will assist the surgeon in addressing them.

EMORY
AESTHETIC CENTER

Welcome to the Emory Aesthetic Center! Please help us take the best care for you by providing us with the following important health information.
Thank you!

Name: _____ Date: _____

Phone number: _____ Date of last eye exam: _____

Name of Eye Care Physician:
_____

Yes   **No**   At your last eye exam, were you told you have any problems with your eyes?

If yes, please explain: _____

Yes   **No**   Do you wear contact lenses (hard or soft) or glasses?

Yes   **No**   Have you sustained any injuries to the eyes or eyelids?

If yes, please explain: _____

Yes   **No**   Do you have any cornea conditions?

If yes, please explain: _____

Yes   **No**   Have you previously had surgery on your eyes or eyelids? If yes, please provide the name of your surgeon and type of surgery:
_____
_____

Yes   **No**   Are your eyes sensitive to light?

Yes   **No**   Do you feel that your eyes or eyelids swell excessively?

Yes   **No**   Do you experience frequent irritation or "allergies" of the eyes or eyelids?

Yes   **No**   Do you currently or have you previously taken any medications or drops for the eyes?
If yes, please explain: _____

Yes   **No**   Are you bothered by "dry eyes"?

If yes, have you been tested for dry eyes? _____
If yes, please explain: _____

Yes   **No**   Do your eyes tear or "water" spontaneously (without emotional stimulation)?

Yes   **No**   Have you had Lasik surgery or Radial Keratotomy on your eyes?

Yes   **No**   Do you now or have you ever had any visual problems with one or both eyes?

Yes   No   Do you or has anyone in your family suffered from eye problems or diseases such as cataracts, glaucoma, macular degeneration, thyroid problems or Graves' Disease?

If the answer to any of these questions is yes, please indicate and explain:_____

_____

Please be advised that despite filling out this survey and disclosing all relevant medical information to your plastic surgeon, you still may need to obtain medical clearance from your ophthalmologist prior to any surgical procedure.

Thank you for taking the time to complete this survey. By doing so, it will allow your doctor to better assess and suggest the best possible treatment option for your individual case. By signing below, you certify that the information contained in this document has been filled out to the best of your ability and is accurate.

Signature: _____   Date: _____

Fig. 2.1 Preoperative evaluation questionnaire.

Eyelid Evaluation

General Evaluation :

Evaluation of Entire Face. *Blepharoplasty alone be sufficient or will the patient require*

Other procedure for an optimal result?

Symmetry of Eyelids and Brow

Brow position in relation to the upper lid. Brow Ptosis

Lower Lid, Lid Cheek Junction, Tear Trough

Skin Quality Skin Quantity

Orbicularis Muscle

Fat Compartments

Lid Position: Upper Lid position in relationship to the cornea PTOSIS or Lid Retraction

Lower Lid Position Scleral show

Lid Tone

Lateral Canthal Position, *at, above or below the medial canthus*

Eye Prominence   Hertel Measurements

Lid Tone   Snap Test

Distraction Test

Schirmers Test   Individualised based onhistory of dry eyes

Visual Acuity   (On an individual Basis)

Visual Field   (On an individual Basis)

Fig. 2.2 Examination checklist.

3 General: Clinical Overview

Ted H. Wojno

Loss of vision and/or double vision is a devastating complication of ocular and periocular surgery and disease. Often, the patient fails to make a complete recovery once this ensues. This can be a life-changing event for the individual, and even small amounts of visual impairment can lead to loss of normal functioning, with major consequences on activities of daily living and employment. If the loss is secondary to surgery, the physician is likewise impacted emotionally and often legally. Needless to say, such problems should be recognized and handled as promptly as possible, enlisting the help of other specialties if needed.

In keeping with the old axiom that "An ounce of prevention is worth a pound of cure," I always include "loss of vision, double vision, and need for further surgery" on my surgical consents for both major and minor procedures. Additionally, I verbally stress these potential risks to the patient. Patients will often display a significant degree of surprise when I mention this since they usually do not consider that these major complications can occur. They are usually reassured upon learning that these are indeed rare events and that I will do everything possible to mitigate the risks of the surgery. In 34 years of practice, I have had only one patient change his or her mind at the time of surgery because of this. We also discuss these complications at the time of the initial office visit to be as certain as possible that the patient is fully informed.

The following chapters will discuss these events and their management.

4 Retrobulbar Hemorrhage

Denise S. Kim

Summary

Retrobulbar hemorrhage is an infrequent but acutely vision-threatening complication of periorbital and orbital surgery in which hemorrhage in the retrobulbar space causes orbital compartment syndrome.

Keywords: retrobulbar hemorrhage, retrobulbar hematoma, orbital compartment syndrome, canthotomy, cantholysis, vision loss

4.1 Patient History Leading to the Specific Problem

The patient is a 59-year-old white woman who presented with a history of left posterior orbital mass of undiagnosed etiology, referred for biopsy with the oculoplastics service. Preoperative vision in the left eye was 20/25 and extraocular movements were full. A left orbitotomy was performed under general anesthesia, and specimens of soft tissue and bone were obtained. The remainder of the surgical case was uneventful. During initiation of awakening from general anesthesia, the patient was witnessed to have a significant gag reflex with Valsalva. She subsequently developed immediate clinical signs of left retrobulbar hemorrhage including tense periorbital ecchymoses and 360° bullous subconjunctival hemorrhage (▶Fig. 4.1).

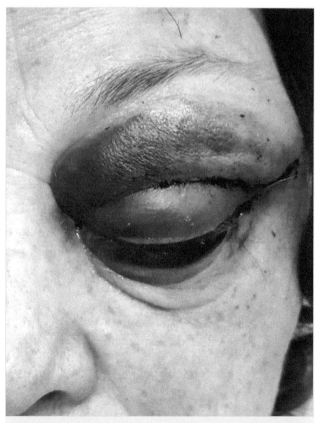

Fig. 4.1 Retrobulbar hemorrhage causing diffuse periorbital ecchymoses and bullous subconjunctival hemorrhage.

4.2 Anatomic Description of the Patient's Current Status

Hemorrhage in the retrobulbar space may lead to a compartment syndrome as the hematoma fills the rigid bony orbit and pushes the globe anteriorly (proptosis) to the maximum extent the eyelids will allow. Further hemorrhage within the confined space of the orbit will then compress the orbital contents, which may rapidly lead to an ischemic optic neuropathy, central retinal artery occlusion, or central retinal vein occlusion, all of which may cause permanent vision loss.

4.3 Recommended Solution to the Problem

Immediately release sutures closing the incision in order to reopen the orbital compartment and relieve intracompartmental pressure.

If this is insufficient to relieve the compartment syndrome, perform a lateral canthotomy with inferior cantholysis, with additional superior cantholysis as needed.
- Re-establish general anesthesia.
- Explore the surgical wound to identify source of hemorrhage.
- Obtain hemostasis.
- Consider replacing incision closure only if the eyelids are soft and mobile and concern for redevelopment of orbital compartment syndrome is low.
- If the patient presents postoperatively with a retrobulbar hemorrhage and orbital compartment syndrome, perform a lateral canthotomy and cantholysis to relieve the intraorbital pressure.

4.4 Technique

The Prolene sutures closing the skin incision, the Vicryl sutures closing orbicularis muscle, and the Vicryl sutures closing the periosteum were immediately cut and released. With release of the previously placed sutures, the periorbital tissues became less tense and the eyelids became more freely mobile over the globe. General anesthesia was resumed and the patient was reprepped in the standard fashion for oculoplastic surgery. The surgical wound was explored and the source of bleeding was identified. Hemostasis was achieved with a combination of bipolar cautery and Avitene. Closure of the periosteum, orbicularis, and skin was replaced.

In alternative presentations, retrobulbar hemorrhage causing a compartment syndrome may be addressed with a canthotomy and cantholysis at the lateral canthus, the outer angle of the eyelids (▶ Fig. 4.2). One may consider cleaning the surgical site and injecting local anesthetic to the subcutaneous tissue of the lateral canthus; however, these steps may be bypassed in certain scenarios given the emergent nature of the problem.

The lateral canthotomy is performed using the available scissors to cut horizontally from the angle of the lateral canthus to the lateral orbital rim, approximately 1 cm (▶ Fig. 4.3).

Grasp the lower lid laterally with toothed forceps and distract the lid away from the globe—it will still feel tethered in place due to the attachment of the inferior crus of the lateral canthal tendon (▶ Fig. 4.4).

Use the closed blades of the scissors to strum the tissue still tethering the lateral lower lid to the orbital rim near the globe—this represents the inferior crus of the lateral canthal tendon which should be cut (▶ Fig. 4.5).

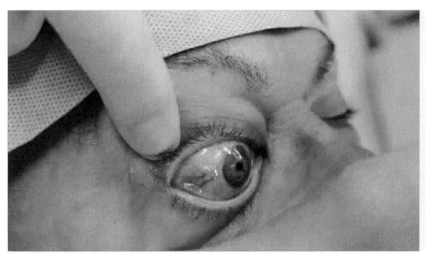

Fig. 4.2 The lateral canthus.

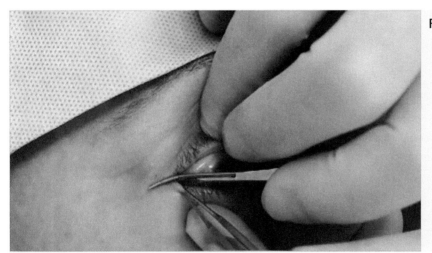

Fig. 4.3 Lateral canthotomy.

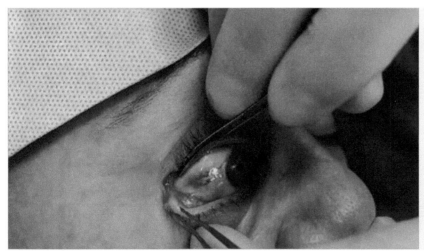

Fig. 4.4 Demonstrating that the lower lid remains tethered to the orbital rim.

Once the inferior crus is identified, inferior cantholysis is performed by an approximately 1-cm cut from the cut edge of the lower lid in an inferoposterior direction (▶ Fig. 4.6).

Upon successful inferior cantholysis, the lower lid should be freely mobile and no longer adherent to the orbital rim (▶ Fig. 4.7).

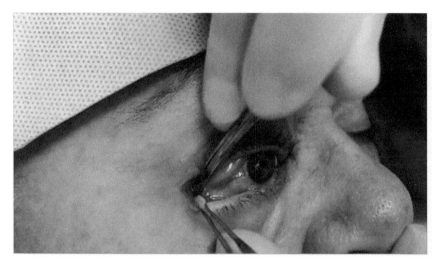

Fig. 4.5 Strumming the inferior crus of the lateral canthal tendon.

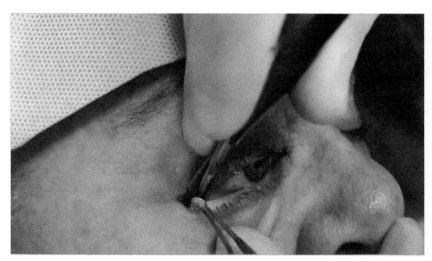

Fig. 4.6 Inferior cantholysis

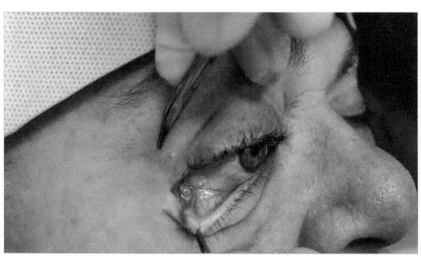

Fig. 4.7 Demonstrating that the lower lid has been released and is freely mobile.

At this point, if the upper lid is noted to be tense and tight against the globe and there remains concern for an orbital compartment syndrome, a superior cantholysis may be performed. Grasp the upper lid laterally with toothed forceps and distract the lid away from the globe. Use the closed blades of the scissors to strum the superior crus which tethers the lateral upper lid to the orbital rim. Superior cantholysis is performed by an approximately 1-cm cut from the cut edge of the upper lid in a superoposterior direction. Upon successful superior cantholysis, the upper lid should be freely mobile and no longer adherent to the orbital rim.

4.5 Postoperative Photographs and Critical Evaluation of Results

Successful management of intraoperative or postoperative retrobulbar hemorrhage is defined by timely relief of the compartmental syndrome. In this case, the retrobulbar hemorrhage was noted immediately and intervention was swift (▶ Fig. 4.8).

At her 2-week postoperative check, vision in the left eye was 20/30 and there was no relative afferent pupillary defect. Residual extraocular movement deficits were noted in all directions but were improving. Periorbital ecchymoses and subconjunctival hemorrhage were still present but improving. The patient was subsequently lost to follow-up.

4.6 Teaching Points

- Retrobulbar hemorrhage is a rare but emergent intra- or postoperative complication of periorbital and orbital surgeries.
- Expanding hemorrhage within the confined space of the orbit can cause an orbital compartment syndrome with decreased perfusion to the optic nerve and/or retina leading to permanent vision loss if not addressed.
- The orbital compartment can be relieved by releasing the surgical closure or by performing lateral canthotomy and cantholysis.
- Swift intervention may lead to excellent postoperative outcomes.

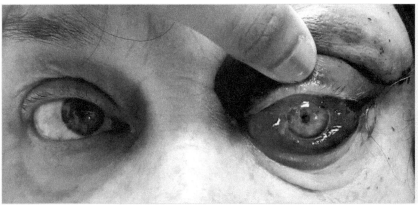

Fig. 4.8 Post-operative day 1. This photo demonstrates easy mobilization of the left upper lid, indicating absence of a compartment syndrome. Bullous subconjunctival hemorrhage and periorbital ecchymoses are persistent, typically for several weeks.

Suggested Reading

[1] Ballard SR, Enzenauer RW, O'Donnell T, Fleming JC, Risk G, Waite AN. Emergency lateral canthotomy and cantholysis: a simple procedure to preserve vision from sight threatening orbital hemorrhage. J Spec Oper Med. 2009; 9(3):26–32

[2] Cruz AA, Andó A, Monteiro CA, Elias J, Jr. Delayed retrobulbar hematoma after blepharoplasty. Ophthal Plast Reconstr Surg. 2001; 17(2):126–130

[3] Kloss BT, Patel R. Orbital compartment syndrome from retrobulbar hemorrhage. Int J Emerg Med. 2010; 3(4):521–522

[4] Lee KYC, Tow S, Fong K-S. Visual recovery following emergent orbital decompression in traumatic retrobulbar haemorrhage. Ann Acad Med Singapore. 2006; 35(11):831–832

[5] Lelli GJ, Jr, Lisman RD. Blepharoplasty complications. Plast Reconstr Surg. 2010; 125(3):1007–1017

[6] Mahaffey PJ, Wallace AF. Blindness following cosmetic blepharoplasty–a review. Br J Plast Surg. 1986; 39(2):213–221

[7] Medina FMC, Pierre Filho PdeT, Freitas HB, Rodrigues FK, Caldato R. Blindness after cosmetic blepharoplasty: case report. Arq Bras Oftalmol. 2005; 68(5):697–699

[8] Winterton JV, Patel K, Mizen KD. Review of management options for a retrobulbar hemorrhage. J Oral Maxillofac Surg. 2007; 65(2):296–299

[9] Wolfort FG, Vaughan TE, Wolfort SF, Nevarre DR. Retrobulbar hematoma and blepharoplasty. Plast Reconstr Surg. 1999; 104(7):2154–2162

5 Periocular Infection

Ted H. Wojno

Summary

Periocular bacterial infection is relatively common but, fortunately, quite rare after eyelid surgery. This chapter reviews the causes of such infections and their treatment. The differential diagnoses are discussed.

Keywords: preseptal cellulitis, orbital cellulitis, orbital abscess, subperiosteal abscess, contact dermatitis, inflammatory orbital pseudotumor, thyroid eye disease, dacryocystitis

5.1 Patient History Leading to the Specific Problem

The patient is a 28-year-old woman with a history of progressive, tender swelling of the right upper and lower eyelids for the last 3 days (▶ Fig. 5.1). She has a low-grade fever and feels ill. The week prior to presentation she had an upper respiratory tract infection that cleared with no treatment. She complains of decreased vision in the right eye and double vision.

5.2 Anatomic Description of the Patient's Current Status

Examination reveals firm, warm swelling of the right upper and lower eyelids and moderate proptosis. The visual acuity is 20/60 on the right and 20/20 on the left. The extraocular movements of the right eye are diffusely restricted in all directions. Pupils and dilated retinal examination are normal. A complete blood count (CBC) shows a polymorphonuclear leukocytosis. A computed tomography (CT) scan performed on the day of presentation shows opacification of the right ethmoid sinuses and an abscess along the roof of the right orbit (▶ Fig. 5.2). Examination of the left eye is normal. The diagnosis is right orbital cellulitis and abscess secondary to previous upper respiratory tract infection.

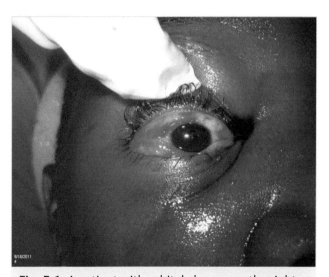

Fig. 5.1 A patient with orbital abscess on the right.

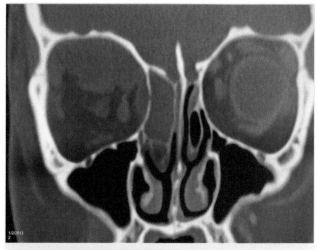

Fig. 5.2 CT scan of the patient showing opacification of the right ethmoid sinus and an abscess along the orbital roof and medial wall on the same side.

5.3 Recommended Solution to the Problem

- Begin broad-spectrum intravenous antibiotics.
- Perform an anterior orbitotomy to drain the orbital abscess and obtain a specimen for culture and sensitivity.
- Otolaryngology performs an ethmoidectomy to drain the affected sinuses.
- Continue oral antibiotics for 10 days to 2 weeks after discharge from the hospital.

5.4 Technique

A variety of incisions are possible for access to the orbit (▶ Fig. 5.3a). Selection depends on the location of the abscess. In this case, we chose an incision located in the inferior edge of the right eyebrow to provide easy access to the soft tissues of the right orbit and moderate amount of pus was

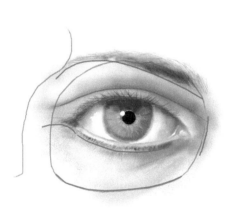

a

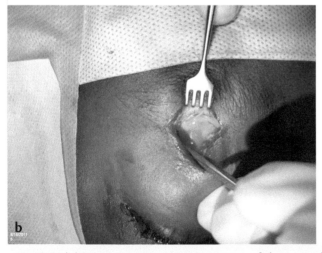

b

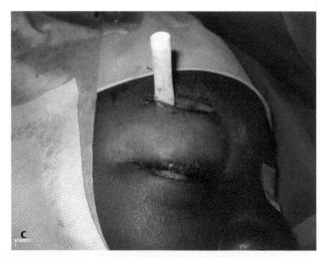

c

Fig. 5.3 **(a)** Diagrammatic representation of the typical incisions to access the orbit. **(b)** An incision is made in the lateral half of the right brow just below the hairline with drainage of pus. **(c)** Penrose drain in the orbit at completion of the procedure.

drained (▶ Fig. 5.3b). After drainage of the abscess and irrigation of the wound, a drain is placed to be removed in 3 days (▶ Fig. 5.3c). Otolaryngology performed an endoscopic ethmoidectomy at the same time.

5.5 Postoperative Photographs and Critical Evaluation of Results

Culture showed mixed aerobic bacterial flora and the patient was discharged on the fourth postoperative day on appropriate oral antibiotic therapy. She did well with complete return of vision and ocular motility. She had a mild ptosis, which was corrected 6 months later (▶ Fig. 5.4).

This report is representative of a typical presentation of bacterial orbital abscess. The vast majority of cases of orbital and preseptal abscess/cellulitis are secondary to bacterial infection of the adjacent sinus cavities. The infection can be confined to the subperiosteal space or invade the intraconal and extraconal orbital soft tissues. If the infection does not respond quickly to intravenous antibiotics or if the vision is threatened, surgical drainage of the abscess and the involved sinuses is indicated. In both adults and children, *Staphylococcus aureus* and *Streptococcus* species are the typical isolates, with gram-negative species playing a somewhat larger role in adults. In both adults and children, methicillin-resistant *S. aureus* (MRSA) is increasing in frequency. MRSA-infected patients characteristically complain of severe pain and often have pustules on the skin of the eyelids (▶ Fig. 5.5a). MRSA-infected patients also can have remarkable swelling and induration of the tissues with seemingly little actual abscess formation. Less common causes of preseptal and orbital cellulitis/abscess are lid trauma, otitis media, sepsis, dacryocystitis, conjunctivitis, and dental infection. Acute dacryocystitis in particular can present with dramatic inflammation, which is always more remarkable over the area of the lacrimal sac (▶ Fig. 5.5b). Given the excellent blood supply to the periocular area, eyelid surgery is only very rarely a culprit in such infections.

There are other causes of periocular inflammation that can mimic infection. The most common problem seen in the postoperative period of eyelid surgery is contact dermatitis and allergic reactions secondary to the use of ointments and eye drops. The swelling in such patients often looks more edematous, is not warm to the touch, and can display a very distinct boundary between the

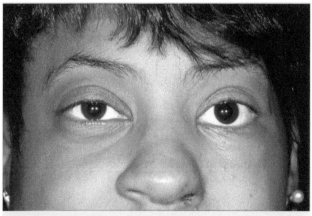

Fig. 5.4 The patient 1 month after surgery showing mild right ptosis.

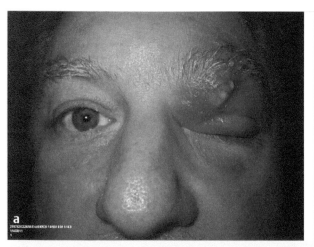 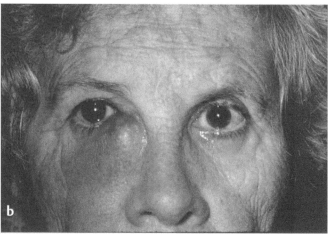

Fig. 5.5 (a) A patient with MRSA preseptal cellulitis on the left eye. **(b)** A patient with acute bacterial dacryocystitis of the right eye.

involved and uninvolved tissues (▶ Fig. 5.6). Discontinuance of the offending agent results in rapid improvement of symptoms.

Idiopathic orbital inflammation (orbital "pseudotumor") is often mistaken for infection. This is a common entity with a rapid onset of painful swelling without antecedent cause or sinus involvement that responds quickly to oral or intravenous corticosteroids (▶ Fig. 5.7a). An acute chalazion of the eyelid can simulate a bacterial cellulitis (▶ Fig. 5.7b). Examination of the tarsal conjunctiva will reveal the characteristic appearance of the swollen meibomian gland (▶ Fig. 5.7c). Thyroid eye disease rarely presents with acute inflammatory signs similar to infection but such patients almost always have a history of recently diagnosed thyroid problems (▶ Fig. 5.7d). Entities such as sarcoidosis and connective tissues disorders of the periocular tissue occasionally cause some diagnostic confusion but the onset is usually much slower than seen in infection.

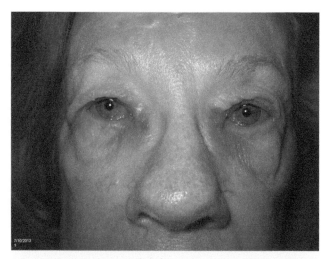

Fig. 5.6 A patient with bilateral contact dermatitis secondary to the use of ophthalmic ointment after eyelid surgery.

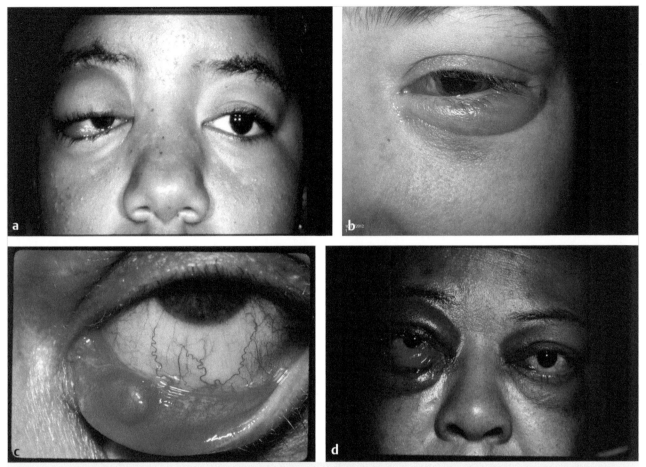

Fig. 5.7 **(a)** A patient with right-sided idiopathic orbital inflammation. **(b)** Acute chalazion affecting the left lower eyelid. **(c)** The conjunctival surface of the left lower eyelid of the patient in ▶ Fig. 5.7b showing the acute chalazion in the medial tarsal plate. **(d)** Severe thyroid eye disease with remarkable lid and conjunctival swelling and erythema.

5.6 Teaching Points

- Periocular bacterial infection is relatively common but almost always associated with adjacent sinusitis.
- Eyelid surgery as a cause of periocular infection is very rare given the excellent blood supply of the eyelids.
- Allergic reactions to topical medications applied to the eyelids in the postoperative period of eyelid surgery are perhaps the most common cause of swelling that can mimic infection.

Suggested Reading

[1] Donahue SP, Schwartz G. Preseptal and orbital cellulitis in childhood. A changing microbiologic spectrum. Ophthalmology. 1998; 105(10):1902–1905, discussion 1905–1906

[2] Garcia GH, Harris GJ. Criteria for nonsurgical management of subperiosteal abscess of the orbit: analysis of outcomes 1988–1998. Ophthalmology. 2000; 107(8):1454–1456, discussion 1457–1458

[3] Harris GJ. Subperiosteal abscess of the orbit: computed tomography and the clinical course. Ophthal Plast Reconstr Surg. 1996; 12(1):1–8

6 Blindness with Blepharoplasty and Injectables

Francesco M. Egro and Foad Nahai

Summary

Blindness is fortunately a rare, yet devastating, complication that may occur following blepharoplasty or filler injections. Knowledge of the etiology and risk factors is key to preoperative preparation and adoption of appropriate measures to minimize risk and ensure patient safety. Avoidance strategies include reduction in risk factors, optimization of the patient's health, surgical technique in the operating room, and close postoperative monitoring. Early recognition and timely management are key for a successful resolution of blindness. A variety of medical and surgical techniques have been described and should be tailored to tackle the initial insult. This chapter explores the incidence, avoidance strategies, and management of blindness following blepharoplasty or filler injections.

Keywords: blindness, complications, blepharoplasty, injections, injectables, filler, incidence, prevention, management

6.1 Incidence

Blindness is fortunately a rare, yet devastating, complication that may occur following blepharoplasty or filler injections. Every physician operating on the eyelids or injecting fillers in the periorbital should be aware of this risk, take precautions to minimize it, and be prepared for emergency treatment.

The first report of blindness following blepharoplasty was published in 1962 by Hartmann et al, and since then, there have been several other publications discussing current strategies for prevention, diagnosis, and management of this complication (▶ Table 6.1). The incidence of blindness following blepharoplasty was first published by DeMere et al in 1974. The authors surveyed 3,000 ophthalmologists and plastic surgeons in the United States, who reported 40 cases of blindness out of the 98,514 eyelid operations, an incidence of approximately 0.04%. Hass et al surveyed 237 members of the American Society of Ophthalmic Plastic and Reconstructive Surgery in 2004. The authors collected reports of 269,433 blepharoplasties, with 48 cases of orbital hemorrhage associated with temporary blindness and 12 cases of orbital hemorrhages associated with permanent blindness. The incidence of temporary blindness was 0.0425%, and that of permanent blindness was 0.0045%. In 2011, we published a large international study where we surveyed a total of 648 members of the American Society for Aesthetic Plastic Surgery (ASAPS) and 72 members of the British Association of Aesthetic Plastic Surgeons (BAAPS). Of the 752,816 blepharoplasties performed by the respondents, blindness was reported in 39 cases: 25 permanent and 14 temporary. The overall incidence of blindness following blepharoplasty was 0.0052% (5 in 100,000, or 1 in 20,000); the incidence of temporary blindness was 0.0019% (2 in 100,000, or 1 in 50,000) and that of permanent blindness was 0.0033% (3 in 100,000, or 1 in 30,000). A summary of the studies reporting the incidence of blindness following blepharoplasty is presented in ▶ Table 6.2.

Blindness is also seen following injection of fillers and adipose tissue. As yet, no incidence rate has been identified. However, a few studies summarized the current strategies for prevention, diagnosis, and management of this

Table 6.1 Published papers on blindness following blepharoplasty

Authors	Symptoms	Time of presentation	Time of LOV	Associated factors	Management	Diagnosis
Hartmann et al (1962)						
(1) P V	Pain, LOV	24 h[a]	36–48 h[a]	Hyperthyroidism, Raynaud's syndrome	Evacuation of hematoma, Novocain, vasodilator (Acecoline-Priscol)	Retinal ischemia caused by arterial spasm or occlusion
(2) P	Hematoma, chemosis	48 h	48 h	Congenital amblyopia	None	Retinal or optic nerve ischemia caused by arterial spasm or occlusion
(3) P V	LOV	24 h	24 h	–	Evacuation of hematoma	Optic nerve ischemia caused by arterial spasm or occlusion
(4) P	Pain, LOV	24 h	24 h	Transitory hyperthyroidism	Isotonic fluid, Novocain, heparin, vasodilators, vasoplegic	Retinal or optic nerve ischemia caused by arterial spasm or occlusion
Morax and Blanck (1969)						
(1) T > P	LOV	0 h	0 h	–	Novocain, Priscol, Nicyl, Hydergine	–
Moser et al (1973)						
(1) P	LOV	5 h	5 h	Hx PUD	Steroids	Retrobulbar optic neuritis
(2) P	Swelling	1 h	5 d	Hx phlebitis	ACTH	Retrobulbar optic neuritis
(3) P	LOV, hematoma, ecchymosis	18 h	18 h	Questionable HTN	Steroids, ACTH	Retrobulbar optic neuritis
(4) P	LOV	4 d	4 d	Arteriosclerosis, preexisting LOV	Diamox, O_2, CO_2	CRAT
(5) P	Hematoma, ecchymosis		7 d	Hx HTN	None	CRVT

Table 6.1 Published papers on blindness following blepharoplasty

Authors	Symptoms	Time of presentation	Time of LOV	Associated factors	Management	Diagnosis
(6) P V	Bleeding, ecchymosis, pain	6–7 h	55–60 h	Hx thrombo-cytopenia	Diamox, steroids, streptokinase, multivitamins, Arlidin	Optic nerve injury
(7) P	Swelling, pain	0–3 h	12–24 h	Cardiospasm, esophagus	–	–
Hartley et al (1973)						
(1) None	Proptosis, edema, pain, reduced extraocular movements	Intra-op	No visual loss	–	Anterior chamber decompression	Retrobulbar hemorrhage
Jafek et al (1973)						
(1) P V	Pain, bleeding, proptosis, ecchymosis, pupil dilation, no light perception	1.5 h	1.5 h		Lateral canthotomy, mannitol, Demerol, antibiotics	Retrobulbar hemorrhage
Putterman (1975)						
(1) T	Pain, proptosis, no light perception, no ocular mobility	2 h	2 h		Incision and drainage	Retrobulbar hemorrhage and retinal artery occlusion
Hueston and Heinze (1974)						
(1) T	Pressure, proptosis, ecchymosis	0–1 h	3 h	–	AC paracentesis, acetazolamide, hydrocortisone, chloramphenicol, atropine	Retrobulbar hemorrhage,[a] central retinal artery occlusion
Hueston and Heinze (1977)						
(1) T	LOV, pain, proptosis, dilated pupils, ecchymosis	3 h	3 h	–	Wound decompression, acetazolamide, mannitol	Retrobulbar hemorrhage,[a] central retinal artery occlusion
Heinze and Hueston (1978)						
(1) T	Pain, proptosis, tension	20–35 min	No visual impairment	–	Wound decompression, acetazolamide, ice packs	Retrobulbar hemorrhage[a]

Table 6.1 Published papers on blindness following blepharoplasty

Authors	Symptoms	Time of presentation	Time of LOV	Associated factors	Management	Diagnosis
(2) P V	Pain, edema	1 h	7 d	–	Incision and drainage	Anterior ischemic optic neuropathy and partial central retinal artery occlusion
Waller (1978)						
(1) P	Pain	0–12 h	12 h		Incision and drainage	Optic nerve injury
Gate et al (1979)						
(1) P	Pain	2 h	12 h	–	Steroids, vasodilators, hyperbaric oxygen	Arterial spasm
Rafaty (1979)						
(1) T	Swelling, pupil dilation, discoloration	Intra-op	Intra-op	Hx ZMC fx	Steroids, incision, and drainage	Reflex vasospasm of retinal vessels[a]
Morgan (1979)						
(1) P	Pain, swelling, "white spots" visual disturbance, proptosis, palsy, anesthesia	2–3 d	7 d	–	Opened wound and IV penicillin	Orbital cellulitis
Anderson and Edwards (1980)						
(1) Right P and left T V	Pain, tension, proptosis, IOP, ecchymosis, hemorrhage	Intra-op	Right < 24 h; left 48 h	Hx HTN and HTN crisis intra-op	Bilateral orbital decompression, drainage	Optic nerve ischemia
Kelly and May (1980)						
(1) T	Pain, swelling	2 h	3 h	–	Lateral canthotomy, incision and drainage, massage, acetazolamide, mannitol	Occlusion of central retinal artery or branches Venous stasis
Lloyd and Leone (1985)						
(1) T	Swelling, ptosis, proptosis, mobility, LOV	7 h	7 h	ASA	Incision and drainage	Retrobulbar hemorrhage

Table 6.1 Published papers on blindness following blepharoplasty

Authors	Symptoms	Time of presentation	Time of LOV	Associated factors	Management	Diagnosis
Goldberg et al (1990)						
(1) P	Swelling	Intra-op	4 h	Bleeding dyscrasia[a]	Incision and drainage, acetazolamide, steroids. Lateral orbitotomy canthotomy, hyperbaric oxygen	Optic nerve injury
(2) P	Pain	6–12 h	48 h	–	Erythromycin, sulfa, steroids	Orbital hematoma
Brancato et al (1991)						
(1) V P/T[a]	Visual acuity	1 d	1 d	–	–	Occlusion of branches of the supero-temporal and infero-temporal retinal arteries and revealed ischemia
Gayton and Ledford (1992)						
(1) TV	Pain, visual acuity, fixed and dilated pupil, swollen lens, anterior chamber shallow, tension	2 d	2 d	–	Acetazolamide, mannitol, timolol, steroids, phacoemulsi-fication, and IOL implant	Angle-closure glaucoma
Good et al (1999)						
(1) P	Swelling, bruising	0–12 h	12–24 h	–	–	Retrobulbar hemorrhage
Cruz et al (2001)						
(1) T V	Pain, proptosis, ecchymosis, extraocular motility, chemosis, conjunctival hemorrhage, visual acuity, IOP	7 d	7 d	–	Mannitol, acetazolamide, Beta-blocker eye drops	Retrobulbar hemorrhage
Oliva et al (2003)						
(1) T V	Decrease vision and visual fields, dilated and fixed pupils, ocular motility	Intra-op	Intra-op	Hx of HTN, dyslipidemia, cerebrovascular accident	–	Hemorrhage, ischemia, anesthetic effect

Table 6.1 Published papers on blindness following blepharoplasty

Authors	Symptoms	Time of presentation	Time of LOV	Associated factors	Management	Diagnosis
Wride and Sanders (2004)						
(1) P	Bleeding, red and painful eye, reduced vision, fixed and dilated pupil, IOP	Intra-op	24 h	Hx of hypermetropia	Acetazolamide, mannitol, pilocarpine, timolol, steroids, augmented trabeculectomy	Angle-closure glaucoma
Yachouh et al (2006)						
(1) P	Edema, bleeding	6 h	11 h	Hx of HTN	Steroids, ice, surgical revision	Vascular spasm involving the retinal or the optic nerve circulation
Teng et al (2006)						
(1) P V	Proptosis, extraocular movements, chemosis, subconjunctival hemorrhage, eyelid ecchymosis	9 d	9 d	–	Wound decompression, lateral canthotomy, cantholysis, cephalexin, Timoptic drops, Bacitracin	Retrobulbar hemorrhage
Chiu et al (2006)						
(1) T	Edema, erythema	4 d	5 d	–	Unasyn, vancomycin, Zosyn, gentamicin, Timoptic, and Alphagan. Orbital decompression.	Orbital apex syndrome (orbital cellulitis)

Abbreviations: AC, anterior chamber; ACTH, adrenocorticotropic hormone; ASA, aspirin or nonsteroidal anti-inflammatory use; CRAT, central retinal artery thrombosis; CRVT, central retinal venous thrombosis; Fx, fracture; HTN, hypertension; Hx, history; IOL, intraocular lens implant; IOP, raised intraocular pressure; IV, intravenous; L, visual loss without hemorrhage; LOV, loss of vision; P, permanent visual loss; PUD, peptic ulcer disease; T, temporary visual loss; V, visual disturbance, including decreased visual acuity or field; ZMC, zygomatic-maxillary complex.
Source: Adapted from Mejia JD, Egro FM, Nahai F. Visual loss after blepharoplasty: incidence, management, and preventive measures. Aesthet Surg J 2011;31(1):21–29. Refer to this article for full referencing of each case report and case series listed in this table.
ªUnclear data presented in the original article.

Table 6.2 Reported incidence of blindness following blepharoplasty

	DeMere et al (1974)	Hass et al (2004)	Mejia et al (2011)
Blepharoplasty cases	98,514	269,433	752,816
Blepharoplasty incidence: overall	0.04%	0.05%	0.0052%
Permanent	–	0.0045%	0.0033%
Temporary	–	0.0425%	0.0019%

complication. Park et al in 2012 reported a consecutive series of 12 patients who suffered ophthalmic, central retinal, and branch retinal vascular occlusions following cosmetic filler injections: 7 patients following adipose tissue injections, 4 following hyaluronic acid, and 1 following collagen. Lazzeri et al published in 2012 a systematic review of 32 cases of blindness following cosmetic filler injections: 15 patients following adipose tissue injections and 17 patients following injections of hyaluronic acid, calcium hydroxyapatite, corticosteroids, silicone oil, paraffin, polymethylmethacrylate, and bovine collagen. Ozturk et al in 2013 published a review of 61 cases of facial vascular occlusion following cosmetic filler injections other than adipose tissue. They reported that 12 patients were complicated by blindness following injections with hyaluronic acid, calcium hydroxylapatite, poly-L-lactic acid, collagen, and dermal matrix. More recently in 2014, Park et al conducted a national survey of the members of the Korean Retina Society who reported a total of 44 cases of blindness following cosmetic filler injections: 22 patients following adipose tissue injections, 13 following hyaluronic acid, 4 following collagen, 2 following poly-L-lactic acid, 1 following calcium hydroxyl apatite, and 2 cases of unknown injections.

6.2 Avoidance

Knowledge of the etiology and risk factors is key to preoperative preparation and adoption of appropriate measures to minimize risk and ensure patient safety. The etiology of blindness after blepharoplasty is varied, as illustrated in ▶ Table 6.1. Retrobulbar hemorrhage remains the most common cause and was reported in 51% of cases. It typically is secondary to continued deep orbital bleeding or superficial bleeding draining through the opened septum into the retrobulbar space. This leads to an increase in intraorbital pressure, which may exceed the central retinal artery pressure (80 mm Hg), compressing the vessel and leading to optic nerve ischemia and permanent neuropathy if untreated. Other causes include central retinal artery occlusion (13%), optic nerve injury (10%), branch retinal artery occlusion (3%), optic neuritis (3%), acute narrow angle glaucoma (3%), and globe perforation. Hypertension has been reported as the most common comorbidity (up to 36% of cases) associated with blindness following blepharoplasty; therefore, it is imperative that hypertension be controlled preoperatively. Aspirin consumption has been associated with 26% of patients with retrobulbar hemorrhage and with 15% of patients who developed blindness, whereas postoperative anticoagulant use was associated with 3% of blindness cases. Therefore, any medication that increases bleeding time (e.g., anticoagulants, aspirin, nonsteroidal anti-inflammatory drugs, or certain supplements) should be suspended 2 weeks preoperatively and should not be restarted for at least 1 week postoperatively. Other steps to reduce the development of retrobulbar hemorrhage include thorough hemostasis, avoidance of excessive traction of the fat pads, and avoidance of rupture of vessels within the posterior orbital fat. Patients who have been injected with epinephrine are at risk of rebound vasodilation and subsequent bleeding; therefore, observation for 2 to 3 hours postoperatively is warranted to ensure no bleeding occurs. Nausea and vomiting has been associated in 16% of retrobulbar hemorrhage and 15% of blindness, whereas coughing has been associated in 5% of retrobulbar hemorrhage and 8% of blindness; therefore, limiting Valsalva maneuvers (such as vomiting and coughing) by administering antiemetics and antitussives may help. Applying occlusive dressings to decrease postoperative edema is not recommended, as it prevents the nursing and surgical staff to promptly identify any acute deterioration. Our study showed that other factors such as glaucoma, increased physical activity, history of vascular disease, trauma, and radiotherapy also predispose patients to blindness.

Blindness following filler injections may cause vascular occlusion due to external pressure on the vessel or more commonly retrograde embolic intravascular occlusion. The latter occurs after injecting a bolus of filler into one of the local arteries, for example, the supraorbital artery if injecting the glabellar region (▶Fig. 6.1). The injection pressure initially forces the filler in retrograde fashion into the ophthalmic artery. Once the pressure is relieved, the normal arterial flow is resumed, carrying the bolus toward one of the smaller branches and leading to occlusion. Park et al conducted a survey among the members of the Korean Retina Society and identified six occlusion sites that can lead to blindness: ophthalmic artery occlusion; generalized posterior ciliary artery occlusion with relative central retinal artery sparing; central retinal artery occlusion; localized posterior ciliary artery occlusion; branch retinal artery occlusion; and posterior ischemic optic neuropathy (▶Fig. 6.2). A variety of facial arteries traverse the areas commonly treated with injectables, including the facial artery, supratrochlear artery, supraorbital artery, angular artery, and lateral nasal artery (▶Fig. 6.1). These are found along the glabellar, nasal, and nasolabial fold areas, and needle aspiration may or may not show any flashback of blood. For this reason, knowledge of their location and caution when injecting near them are essential to minimize the risk of inadvertent injection within the arterial lumen.

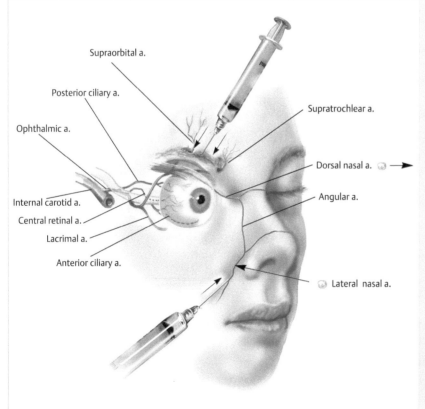

Fig. 6.1 Blood supply of the face and periorbital region in relation to the sites of facial filler injections. The supratrochlear and supraorbital arteries are the possible inlets for retrograde flow in the glabellar region. The anastomosis of the dorsal nasal artery from the ophthalmic artery, angular artery, and lateral nasal artery from the facial artery is the possible inlet for retrograde flow in the nasolabial fold. The arrows indicate the route of retrograde flow of embolic filler.

Supraorbital a.

Posterior ciliary a.

Ophthalmic a.

Internal carotid a.

Central retinal a.

Lacrimal a.

Anterior ciliary a.

Supratrochlear a.

Dorsal nasal a.

Angular a.

Lateral nasal a.

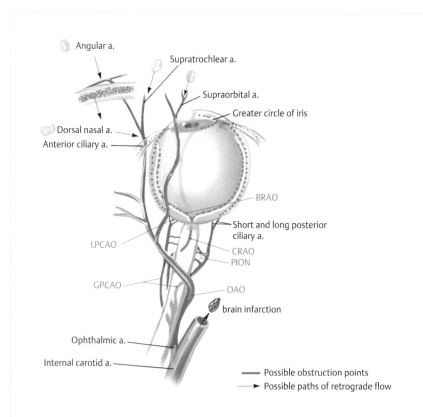

Angular a.

Supratrochlear a.

Supraorbital a.

Greater circle of iris

Dorsal nasal a.

Anterior ciliary a.

BRAO

Short and long posterior
ciliary a.

LPCAO

CRAO

PION

GPCAO

OAO

brain infarction

Ophthalmic a.

Internal carotid a.

Possible obstruction points
Possible paths of retrograde flow

Fig. 6.2 Anatomy of the blood supply to the eye, illustrating the ophthalmic artery, its branches, and possible obstruction points.

Because treatment has usually been proven unsuccessful, prevention is key to avoid blindness, and a variety of strategies have been described in the literature to minimize the risk. Injection of large volumes of filler into any one area can cause a greater degree of arterial obstruction. In fact, the most severe cases of blindness have occurred from the accidental release of more than 0.1 mL of filler. Therefore, complications can be prevented by injecting a maximum of 0.1 mL into any one location and by changing the position of further injections. Attempts to clear a partially blocked needle should be discouraged because this causes an increase in the syringe pressure and a potential accidental discharge of a larger volume of filler. Blood vessels found in healthy fatty tissue usually roll out of the way at the touch of a needle. Deep tissue scarring may fix the vessel in place, making them more vulnerable and easier to be penetrated by small sharp needles. Repeated filler treatments can also be the cause of collagenous tissue scarring, which often presents as "gritty" subcutaneous tissue noticed during repeated injections. Small-gauge needles are more likely to penetrate the arterial lumen. Therefore, larger needles are recommended because not only do they tend to side-cut or roll arteries out of the way rather than penetrating their lumen, but also they facilitate the "back flash" of blood following aspiration, thus alerting the physician about the incorrect position of the needle. The use of blunt cannulas is thought to reduce the risk of accidental intraluminal perforation, especially in cases where scarring is an issue. Nonetheless, there have been reports of accidental intra-arterial injection. Blunt cannulas have the disadvantages of being prone to bending with multiple passes, and the blunt tip may make breaching of planes challenging, resulting in accumulation of the filler. Despite these disadvantages, most injectors believe that blunt cannulas are the best option because of the increased safety, less bruising, and less hematoma. For these reasons, the use of blunt cannulas is strongly recommended when injecting fillers around the orbit. The use of epinephrine injection prior to the filler has been advocated to induce vasoconstriction and reduce the size of vessels, thus reducing the risk of intra-arterial injection. The choice of injectable is also crucial. Size variation of the injected material predisposes the patient to different clinical occlusion patterns, for example, small-sized hyaluronic acid is less likely to completely occlude the ophthalmic artery. Park et al showed that adipose tissue injections are more likely to cause diffuse occlusion (86 vs. 39%), have a higher rate of long-term (≥ 6 months) blindness (100 vs. 43%), and have a higher prevalence of brain lesions on magnetic resonance imaging (MRI; 46 vs. 8%) when compared to hyaluronic acid injections. For these reasons, one might consider a reversible agent such as hyaluronic acid because of the lower complication rates and it can be dissolved by hyaluronidase if blindness occurs.

6.3 Management

Blindness is a true emergency, and appropriate immediate action can avoid permanent loss of vision. The surgeon must be able to recognize early symptoms and signs in order to initiate prompt treatment. The most common symptoms in patients who develop blindness after blepharoplasty are pain and pressure (found in 46 and 36% of cases, respectively); vomiting (13%), nausea (10%), proptosis (5%), diplopia (5%), and blurred vision (5%) are not as common. The majority of affected patients (82%) develop symptoms and/or signs within the first 24 hours, especially within the 1st postoperative hour (26%) or between the 6th to 12th hour (36%). This is why postoperative monitoring is vital as these early symptoms alert the nursing staff and the surgeon that the patient is at risk of developing blindness.

In our study several options to manage blindness following blepharoplasty were mentioned, with orbital decompression being the most common procedure (52%), followed by administration of steroids (21%), canthotomy (10%), mannitol (8%), acetazolamide (5%), and tarsorrhaphy (3%). Twenty-three percent of patients were referred to an ophthalmologist and 8% were merely kept under observation. Irreversible blindness can occur after 90 to 120 minutes of optic ischemia; therefore, it should be immediately treated aggressively as a true surgical emergency. When retrobulbar hemorrhage is suspected, immediate relief of intraorbital pressure is important to reestablish blood flow to the optic nerve. This is achieved by immediate bedside suture removal and lateral canthotomy, followed by surgical exploration in the operating room as soon as possible. Ophthalmology should be involved as early as possible, and the patient should be administered adjuvant medical treatment to lower the intraocular pressure: methylprednisolone (100 mg), 20% mannitol (1.5–2 g/kg; 12.5 g over 3 minutes), acetazolamide (500 mg intravenous [IV]), betaxolol hydrochloride ophthalmic suspension (one drop, then twice daily), and 95% oxygen/5% carbon dioxide. Vision should be monitored by frequent assessment of visual acuity, visual field, light perception, pupillary light reaction, accommodation, fundoscopy, tonometry, and oculomotor function. Once the patient is back in the operating room, the surgical wound should be explored and hematoma should be evacuated and any active bleeding controlled; however, exploration of the retrobulbar space is not advocated. In patients in whom blindness resolves, the wounds can be resutured; however, in patients in whom blindness persists, the surgical wounds and canthotomy should be left open until the swelling resolves, and a delayed closure should be attempted, usually a few days later. If blindness persists despite these medical and surgical measures, an emergent computed tomography (CT) scan without contrast should be carried out to identify the underlying pathology. In the presence of a posteriorly organized hematoma, the patient would benefit from bony orbital decompression to relieve compression of the orbital apex caused by the hematoma. Anterior chamber paracentesis has also been described to emergently lower intraocular pressure; however, its use remains controversial and most surgeons warn against it—the reason being that the majority of blindness is secondary to retrobulbar hemorrhage, which is most effectively treated by decompression of the retrobulbar space. Furthermore, anterior chamber paracentesis carries risks such as intraocular hemorrhage, iris prolapse, and cataract formation. A summary of the management of blindness following blepharoplasty is presented in ▶ Fig. 6.3.

Blindness following filler injections may initially present with ophthalmoplegia, strabismus, ocular pain, anterior segment ischemia, ptosis, neurologic symptoms (e.g., contralateral hemiplegia, dysarthria), and skin lesions (e.g., pallor, blanching, livedo reticularis, erythromelalgia, ulceration, or frank dermal necrosis). Park et al showed that the majority of cases (84%) sought medical attention within 24 hours of symptom onset and were most often managed with observation (30%) or anterior chamber paracentesis (25%). Interestingly, 71% of patients had undergone brain MRI, which showed focal or multifocal brain infarctions in 39% of patients, but only 14% had concomitant neurological symptoms.

Similar to blepharoplasty, blindness following injectables must be treated as an emergency. However, the recommended treatment is different from the description above for blepharoplasty, and unfortunately has rarely been

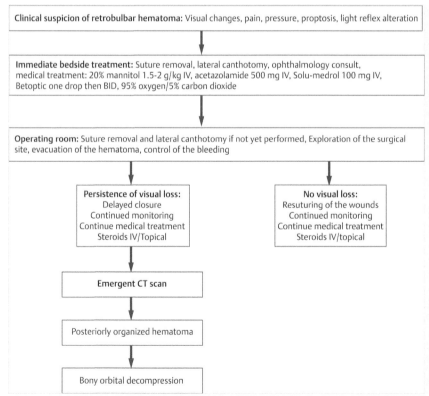

Clinical suspicion of retrobulbar hematoma: Visual changes, pain, pressure, proptosis, light reflex alteration

Immediate bedside treatment: Suture removal, lateral canthotomy, ophthalmology consult, medical treatment: 20% mannitol 1.5-2 g/kg IV, acetazolamide 500 mg IV, Solu-medrol 100 mg IV, Betoptic one drop then BID, 95% oxygen/5% carbon dioxide

Operating room: Suture removal and lateral canthotomy if not yet performed, Exploration of the surgical site, evacuation of the hematoma, control of the bleeding

Persistence of visual loss:
Delayed closure
Continued monitoring
Continue medical treatment
Steroids IV/Topical

No visual loss:
Resuturing of the wounds
Continued monitoring
Continue medical treatment
Steroids IV/topical

Emergent CT scan

Posteriorly organized hematoma

Bony orbital decompression

Fig. 6.3 Treatment algorithm for blindness following blepharoplasty. (Reproduced with permission from Mejia JD, Egro FM, Nahai F. Visual loss after blepharoplasty: incidence, management, and preventive measures. Aesthet Surg J 2011;31(1):21–29.)

successful. Whereas the changes following blepharoplasty are initiated by pressure over the vessels, those resulting from injectables result from embolization. Blindness caused by injection of autologous adipose tissue has been particularly problematic and has always been permanent. Regardless of the type of filler injected, the onset of sudden blindness or prodromal symptoms should prompt the injector to immediately terminate the procedure, and seek urgent consultation with an ophthalmologist or oculoplastic surgeon. In cases where hyaluronic acid was injected, hyaluronidase has been shown to dissolve it both within the vessel and the surrounding tissues. Hyaluronidase can be injected intravenously for systemic action. It can be injected directly into the ophthalmic artery by a neuroradiologist. More commonly, 2 to 4 mL (150–200 units/mL) of hyaluronidase can be injected next to an occluded vessel in the inferolateral orbit because it catabolizes the hyaluronic acid without needing to actually canalize the affected artery. The response to hyaluronidase depends on the type of hyaluronic acid filler, for example, Restylane (Galderma S.A., Lausanne, Switzerland) responds faster than Juvéderm (Allergan, Inc., Irvine, California). Patients might also benefit from administration of 80-mg aspirin as an antiplatelet agent, gentle localized massage to distribute the material throughout the tissues, warm compresses, and topical nitropaste to increase vasodilation. Vital signs should be monitored when using vasodilating agents because of possible decompensation. Other therapies have been attempted to reduce intraocular pressure and move the retinal artery embolus peripherally; these include ocular massage, mannitol, acetazolamide, timolol eye drops, Solu-Medrol 100 mg IV, and anterior chamber fluid evacuation using a needle or Graefe knife. DeLorenzi advocates the use of a "filler crash kit" to include all the drugs mentioned above, making them easily and readily accessible to all injectors. This kit promotes a culture of patient safety and medical staff awareness of this devastating complication, and should be part of every physician's office performing filler injections.

Visual evoked potentials or brain MRI may be helpful in confirming the diagnosis and ruling out brain involvement. The latter is of particular help considering that of 71% of the patients who had undergone brain MRI, 39% were found to have focal or multifocal brain infarctions, but only 14% had concomitant neurological symptoms. A positive MRI should prompt the physician to consult neurology immediately to initiate the appropriate stroke management. A summary of the management of blindness following injectables is presented in ▶ Fig. 6.4.

Blindness following blepharoplasty or injectables is a rare and most feared complication. Knowledge of its etiology, pathology, and presentation can help the surgeon to act promptly and convert a permanent complication into a temporary one. Needless to say, avoidance is preferred over emergency treatment, and for this reason, preventive measures should be adopted and the surgeon should maintain constant vigilance for such a catastrophic event.

6.4 Teaching Points

- Blindness following blepharoplasty or injectables is an extremely rare, yet devastating, complication.
- Avoidance strategies include reduction in risk factors, optimization of the patient's health, surgical technique in the operating room, and close postoperative monitoring.
- Early recognition and timely management are key for a successful resolution of blindness.

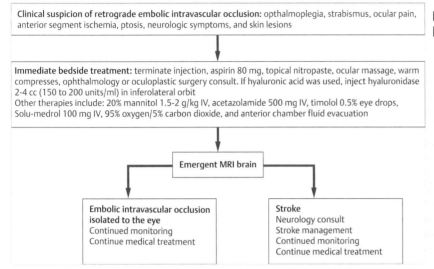

Clinical suspicion of retrograde embolic intravascular occlusion: opthalmoplegia, strabismus, ocular pain, anterior segment ischemia, ptosis, neurologic symptoms, and skin lesions

Immediate bedside treatment: terminate injection, aspirin 80 mg, topical nitropaste, ocular massage, warm compresses, ophthalmology or oculoplastic surgery consult. If hyaluronic acid was used, inject hyaluronidase 2-4 cc (150 to 200 units/ml) in inferolateral orbit
Other therapies include: 20% mannitol 1.5-2 g/kg IV, acetazolamide 500 mg IV, timolol 0.5% eye drops, Solu-medrol 100 mg IV, 95% oxygen/5% carbon dioxide, and anterior chamber fluid evacuation

Emergent MRI brain

Embolic intravascular occlusion isolated to the eye
Continued monitoring
Continue medical treatment

Stroke
Neurology consult
Stroke management
Continued monitoring
Continue medical treatment

Fig. 6.4 Treatment algorithm for blindness following injectables.

- A variety of medical and surgical techniques have been described and should be tailored to tackle the initial insult.
- Injections around the orbit should be performed with blunt needles or cannulas, and physicians should always inject while withdrawing the needle or cannula.

Suggested Reading

[1] Carruthers JD, Fagien S, Rohrich RJ, Weinkle S, Carruthers A. Blindness caused by cosmetic filler injection: a review of cause and therapy. Plast Reconstr Surg. 2014; 134(6):1197–1201
[2] DeLorenzi C. Complications of injectable fillers, part 2: vascular complications. Aesthet Surg J. 2014; 34(4):584–600
[3] DeLorenzi C. Complications of injectable fillers, part I. Aesthet Surg J. 2013; 33(4):561–575
[4] DeMere M, Wood T, Austin W. Eye complications with blepharoplasty or other eyelid surgery. A national survey. Plast Reconstr Surg. 1974; 53(6):634–637
[5] Hartmann E, Morax PV, Vergez A. Grave visual complications of surgery of eyelid pouches [in French] Ann Ocul (Paris). 1962; 195:142–148
[6] Hass AN, Penne RB, Stefanyszyn MA, Flanagan JC. Incidence of postblepharoplasty orbital hemorrhage and associated visual loss. Ophthal Plast Reconstr Surg. 2004; 20(6):426–432
[7] Lazzeri D, Agostini T, Figus M, Nardi M, Pantaloni M, Lazzeri S. Blindness following cosmetic injections of the face. Plast Reconstr Surg. 2012; 129(4):995–1012
[8] Lelli GJ, Jr, Lisman RD. Blepharoplasty complications. Plast Reconstr Surg. 2010; 125(3):1007–1017
[9] Mejia JD, Egro FM, Nahai F. Visual loss after blepharoplasty: incidence, management, and preventive measures. Aesthet Surg J. 2011; 31(1):21–29
[10] Ozturk CN, Li Y, Tung R, Parker L, Piliang MP, Zins JE. Complications following injection of soft-tissue fillers. Aesthet Surg J. 2013; 33(6):862–877
[11] Park SW, Woo SJ, Park KH, Huh JW, Jung C, Kwon OK. Iatrogenic retinal artery occlusion caused by cosmetic facial filler injections. Am J Ophthalmol. 2012; 154(4):653–662.e1
[12] Park KH, Kim YK, Woo SJ, et al; Korean Retina Society. Iatrogenic occlusion of the ophthalmic artery after cosmetic facial filler injections: a national survey by the Korean Retina Society. JAMA Ophthalmol. 2014; 132(6):714–723
[13] Rohrich RJ, Coberly DM, Fagien S, Stuzin JM. Current concepts in aesthetic upper blepharoplasty. Plast Reconstr Surg. 2004; 113(3):32e–42e
[14] Wolfort FG, Vaughan TE, Wolfort SF, Nevarre DR. Retrobulbar hematoma and blepharoplasty. Plast Reconstr Surg. 1999; 104(7):2154–2162

7 Ocular Motility Disorders

Ted H. Wojno

Summary

Diplopia is a bothersome and often disabling condition. Complaints of "double vision" after periocular surgery are very common and, fortunately, are usually of minor consequence. This chapter discusses the common reasons for this complaint and their management.

Keywords: strabismus, ocular motility, cardinal positions of gaze, forced duction test, phoria, tropia

7.1 Patient History Leading to the Specific Problem

The patient is a 64-year-old African American woman who underwent a transconjunctival lower eyelid blepharoplasty performed under general anesthesia 1 month previously; she complains of double vision since the surgery (▶Fig. 7.1). She became aware of this problem in the recovery room. The diplopia has improved slightly since the surgery and is not associated with any loss of vision or discomfort. She is otherwise completely healthy and has no history of ophthalmic problems other than wearing reading glasses.

7.2 Anatomic Description of the Patient's Current Status

By report from the referring surgeon, the procedure was remarkable for significant bleeding in the area of the nasal fat pocket of the right lower eyelid that required vigorous cautery and retraction of the tissues to control (▶Fig. 7.2). Her postoperative course was said to be remarkable for significant swelling and bruising of the right lower eyelid that has now almost completely cleared. Ophthalmologic exam discloses 20/20 vision in both eyes. Pupils, intraocular pressure, and dilated retinal examination are normal. Motility examination shows that the patient has difficulty elevating the right eye especially in the

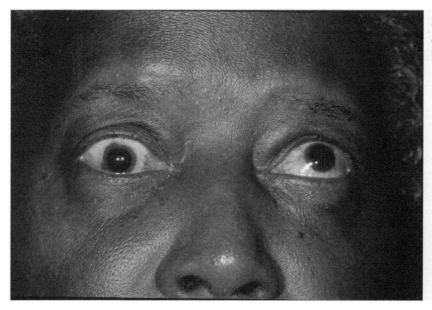

Fig. 7.1 A patient with complaints of double vision after lower eyelid blepharoplasty.

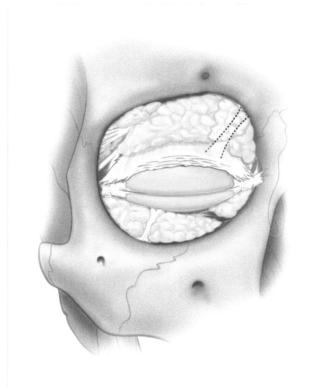

Fig. 7.2 Diagrammatic view of the lower eyelid fat pockets and their proximity to the inferior oblique muscle. (Reproduced with permission from Codner MA, McCord Jr CD. Eyelid & Periorbital Surgery. 2nd ed. New York, NY: Thieme; 2016.)

adducted position (looking to her left). Forced duction testing performed with topical anesthetic was normal. The diagnosis is palsy of the inferior oblique muscle.

7.3 Recommended Solution to the Problem

We will approach this problem as the surgeon encountering it in the recovery room. This assumes that the patient is fully awake and cooperative.
- Perform a basic assessment of the patient's visual acuity.
- Examine the patient's ocular alignment and motility.
- Consider forced duction testing.

7.4 Technique

Check the patient's vision one eye at a time. This is easily accomplished with a pocket vision screener or "near card," which is typically calibrated from 20/20 to 20/800. Allow the patient to hold it at a comfortable reading distance. If the patient wears reading glasses or bifocals for near vision correction (as do most individuals over the age of 40), be certain that these are used. If a near card is not available, use a magazine or newspaper, which is approximately 20/50 vision.

Check the ocular alignment by having the patient look at a penlight held approximately 2 feet away. With normal alignment, the light reflexes will be centered at exactly the same spot on the pupil of each eye (►Fig. 7.3). With a unilateral exotropia, the light reflex will be decentered nasally (►Fig. 7.4) as compared to the normal eye, while in esotropia the reflex will be decentered temporally (►Fig. 7.5). Likewise, with a hypertropia the reflex will be decentered inferiorly on the cornea and in hypotropia it will be seen more superiorly than in the uninvolved eye.

Check the patient's motility in the cardinal positions of gaze (►Fig. 7.6). In medial gaze, the edge of the iris will normally be slightly hidden by the soft tissues of the medial canthus (►Fig. 7.7). In lateral gaze, the temporal limbus will typically just reach the lateral canthus (►Fig. 7.8). In downgaze and upgaze, it is normal for the eyes to move about 45 degrees from the midline (which would put a light reflex just outside of the upper or lower limbus, respectively). Upgaze decreases as patients age and by 94 it is normal to be able to look upward only 16 degrees. Of course, lid and conjunctival edema may obscure these findings, making these observations more difficult.

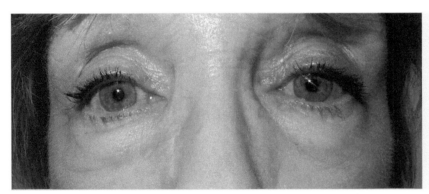

Fig. 7.3 Corneal light reflexes demonstrating normal ocular alignment.

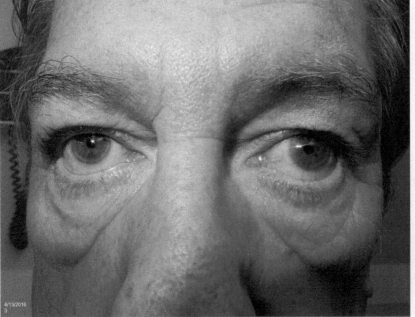

Fig. 7.4 Corneal light reflex demonstrating left exotropia.

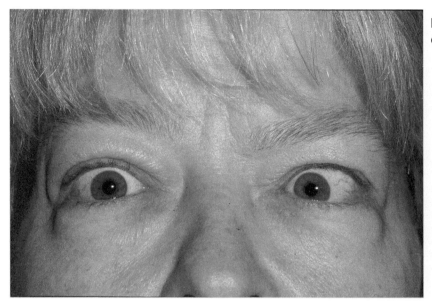

Fig. 7.5 Corneal light reflex demonstrating left esotropia.

The Nine Cardinal Positions of Gaze

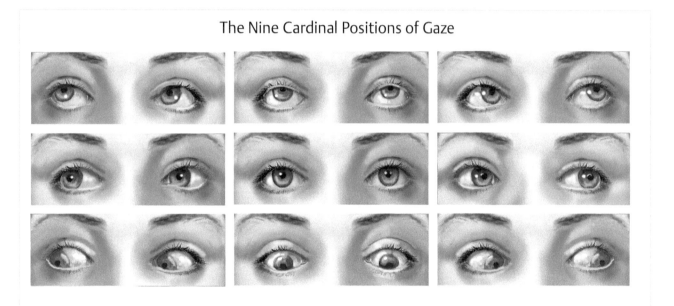

Fig. 7.6 The nine cardinal positions of gaze.

If a motility defect is suspected, the physician may decide to perform forced duction testing. First, apply a drop of a topical ocular anesthetic. Next, apply a cotton-tipped applicator soaked in 2% xylocaine for 30 seconds just outside the corneoscleral limbus 180 degrees opposite to the direction of the suspected underaction (▶ Fig. 7.9a). For instance, if the right globe fails to fully rotate inferiorly, place the applicator near the corneoscleral limbus of the right eye at the 12 o'clock position. Next, grasp the conjunctiva at this position near the limbus with a small toothed forceps and rotate the eye inferiorly (▶ Fig. 7.9b). The eye should easily and fully move to the normal end point of gaze. Difficulty moving the eye suggests a restrictive process such as entrapment in a fracture or orbital edema and hemorrhage. A false-positive result may be found, however, in an anxious patient who may resist the examiner's attempt

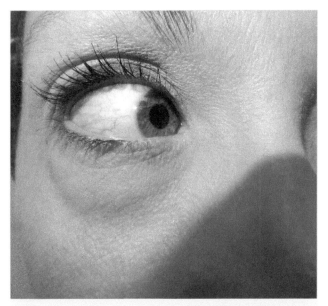

Fig. 7.7 Normal medial gaze (adduction) of the right eye.

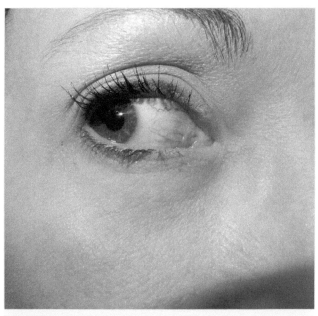

Fig. 7.8 Normal lateral gaze (abduction) of the right eye.

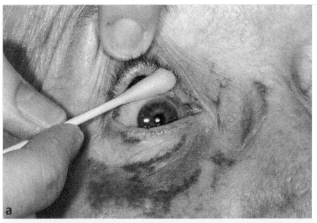

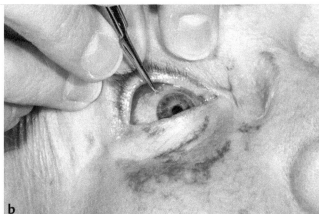

Fig. 7.9 (a, b) A cotton-tipped applicator soaked in xylocaine is placed just outside of the limbus.

to move the eye. If the eye can be moved easily into the field of obvious underaction, a paretic muscle is suspected.

7.5 Postoperative Photographs and Critical Evaluation of Results

Motility disorders can arise in the postoperative period of periocular surgery for many reasons. Direct injury to an extraocular muscle or the motor nerve to the muscle will result in immediate underaction of the involved muscle accompanied by findings of muscle paresis on examination and patient complaints of diplopia. Orbital hemorrhage and edema will also lead to immediate postoperative motility disorders often accompanied by obvious signs of proptosis, eyelid swelling, and/or ecchymosis. In such cases, forced duction testing will usually be positive. Diplopia due to hemorrhage and edema will resolve over several days, while that due to direct injury to the muscle or nerve can sometimes be permanent.

A less frequent cause of diplopia in the postoperative period is the decompensation of a phoria to a tropia. A phoria is a relatively common latent misalignment of the oculomotor system that is normally held in check by the patient's fusional abilities. A phoria can decompensate (become a manifest tropia) due to the effects of sedation, general anesthesia, orbital edema, or even lack of sleep. A decompensated phoria will generally quickly recover in a few days as the patient heals.

Without doubt, the most common cause of complaints of diplopia after periocular surgery is the frequent tendency for patients to label any disturbance in visual function as "double vision." Swelling, ocular ointments, excess tearing, and sedation from pain medicine and anesthetic agents are the usual causes. This can be determined by asking the patient if they frankly see two distinct images of a single object such as the examiner's finger held 2 feet in front of the patient. The patient will often then elaborate by further describing that the disturbance is really more of a blurring that may be cleared by blinking or wiping the eyes (much to the relief of the physician). Such patients can be safely reassured that what they are experiencing is normal and an expected consequence of the surgery that will soon resolve. Obviously, for problems that do not improve quickly or for a clear disturbance of ocular motility, a referral to an ophthalmologist is indicated.

This case was remarkable for excessive bleeding from the area of the nasal fat pocket of the right lower eyelid. This pocket often contains the medial palpebral vessels, which can be very large in some patients and cause vision-threatening hemorrhage if cut (▶ Fig. 7.10). The inferior oblique muscle is typically found just lateral to the medial fat pocket. Surgical manipulation in this area can lead to damage to the inferior oblique muscle or its motor nerve. The motility defect in this patient cleared without treatment over the next 2 months with resolution of diplopia.

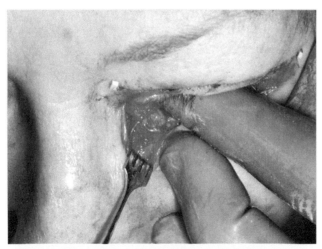

Fig. 7.10 A large medial palpebral artery in the medial fat pocket of the left lower eyelid.

7.6 Teaching Points

- Patients frequently complain of "double vision" after periocular surgery.
- In most cases, complaints of double vision in the postoperative period of periocular surgery are benign and self-limited.
- The surgeon can usually make a determination as to whether there is a pathological change that would warrant a referral to an ophthalmologist.

Suggested Reading

[1] Chamberlain W. Restriction in upward gaze with advancing age. Am J Ophthalmol. 1971; 71(1, Pt 2):341–346

[2] Von Noorden GK. Burian-von Noorden's Binocular Vision and Ocular Motility. 2nd ed. St. Louis, MO: CV Mosby; 1980

Part III

Upper Eyelid

8 Upper Eyelid: Clinical Overview

Ted H. Wojno

The chapters in this section on the upper eyelid address many critical issues. In one way or another, most will have to take the levator muscle into consideration. As the main functional structure in the upper eyelid, the levator muscle must always be considered when doing surgery here. It must be carefully avoided or appropriately treated as the case may be. It is critically important in ptosis repair and in the formation of the upper eyelid crease and fold.

The levator muscle arises from the lesser wing of the sphenoid bone just above the annulus of Zinn. It inserts into the upper tarsal border, the anterior surface of tarsus, the medial canthal tendon, the lateral canthal tendon (after splitting the orbital and palpebral lobe of the lacrimal gland), the pretarsal skin, and orbicularis. It contains Whitnall's ligament (superior transverse ligament) at the level of the equator of the globe at which point it changes direction from posterior-anterior to superior-inferior. The striated portion is 40-mm long and the aponeurosis is 15-mm long, though these measurements vary depending on individual anatomy and ethnicity. The adrenergic Müller's muscle is approximately 10-mm long, arising from the underside of the levator and inserting along the superior tarsal border (▶ Fig. 8.1).

When repairing the ptotic lid, one must differentiate between congenital and acquired ptosis since the surgical parameters are significantly different. Congenital ptosis is most often unilateral and can be considered to be a dystrophic muscle. In general, the more severe the ptosis, the more dystrophic

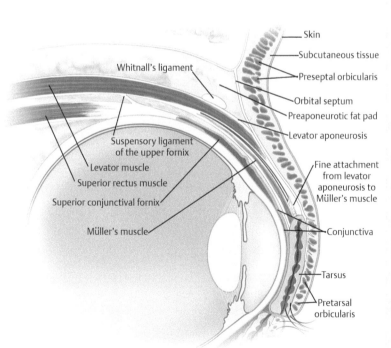

Fig. 8.1 Sagittal view of the structures in the upper eyelid.

Whitnall's ligament

Suspensory ligament of the upper fornix

Levator muscle

Superior rectus muscle

Superior conjunctival fornix

Müller's muscle

Skin

Subcutaneous tissue

Preseptal orbicularis

Orbital septum

Preaponeurotic fat pad

Levator aponeurosis

Fine attachment from levator aponeurosis to Müller's muscle

Conjunctiva

Tarsus

Pretarsal orbicularis

the levator muscle and the more likely to be associated with anisometropia, amblyopia, or strabismus. Congenital ptosis can be accompanied by blepharophimosis syndrome, Marcus-Gunn "jaw-winking," or superior rectus weakness. Surgical repair involves relatively large shortenings of the levator muscle in the range from 12 mm to more than 20 mm and is typically referred to as "levator resection surgery." This resection sometimes includes the Müller muscle at the same time. In severe congenital ptosis, there is not enough functional levator muscle to shorten and will necessitate performance of a frontalis sling procedure utilizing alloplastic materials or autogenous fascia lata. Congenital ptosis repair can be expected to result in lagophthalmos, which, if done before age 10, is well tolerated for the life of the patient.

Sometimes, if the history is unclear, the physician may have to determine if the ptosis is congenital or acquired. Congenital ptosis typically has reduced levator function (2–10 mm) as compared to acquired ptosis (>12 mm). To measure levator function, hold a ruler over the center of the eye with the patient looking down and the brow stabilized so as to negate any contribution from the frontalis muscle (▶ Fig. 8.2a). Then, have the patient look up and measure the excursion of the upper eyelid from downgaze to upgaze to obtain the levator function (▶ Fig. 8.2b).

A helpful clue in unilateral cases is the position of the ptotic lid on downgaze. In unilateral congenital ptosis, the upper eyelid will not descend as far in downgaze as compared to the normal eyelid (▶ Fig. 8.3). This is due to the fact that the muscle in congenital ptosis is partially replaced by fibrous tissue and is, in effect, less elastic and thus tends to hang up a bit in downgaze. In contrast, the eyelid with acquired ptosis behaves as if the muscle/aponeurosis is stretched out and thus descends to a lower level than the normal eyelid on downgaze (▶ Fig. 8.4). This finding will, of course, not be helpful in bilateral ptosis.

The majority of ptosis cases encountered in routine practice will be acquired and age-related. This is typically conceptualized as a thinning and/or stretching of the levator aponeurosis and the repair is often referred to as "aponeurotic surgery." True aponeurotic disinsertion, although frequently discussed, is probably very uncommon since the surgeon can almost always appreciate a continuous, albeit a very diaphanous, aponeurosis. Surgical tightening of the

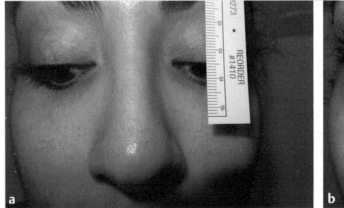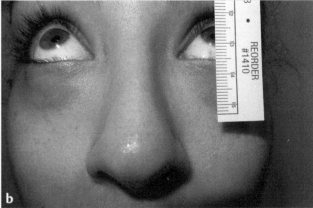

Fig. 8.2 (a) To measure levator function, stabilize the eyebrow, have the patient look down, and place a ruler over the eyelid at the level of the pupil. (b) While holding the brow and ruler still, have the patient look up and measure the excursion in millimeters.

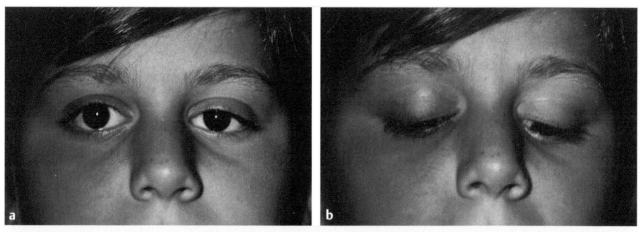

Fig. 8.3 **(a)** A patient with congenital left upper eyelid ptosis. **(b)** The same patient with congenital ptosis looking down. Note that the left upper eyelid does not descend as far as the normal right upper eyelid in downgaze.

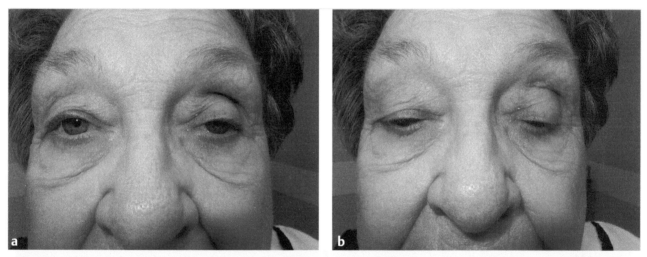

Fig. 8.4 **(a)** A patient with acquired ptosis of the left upper eyelid. **(b)** The same patient with acquired ptosis looking down. Note that the left upper eyelid descends further than the right upper eyelid in downgaze.

levator is relatively smaller than that done in congenital ptosis and is usually in the range of 2 to 10 mm. Postoperative lagophthalmos is uncommon and should generally be avoided given the age of the patients having surgery.

Acquired ptosis can also be treated by shortening of the Müller muscle with or without partial tarsal resection, and this approach has a number of variations. It is often quicker and can be less invasive than levator aponeurosis surgery and is the preferred method for many surgeons.

The eyelid crease is the neglected stepchild in upper eyelid surgery. I believe that it is often overlooked resulting in less-than-optimal results. The upper eyelid margins may be in identical position after ptosis repair, but if the crease and folds are not even, the patient will look asymmetric. From a historical perspective, consideration of the upper eyelid crease and fold traces its origins back over 100 years to Asian "double eyelid" surgery. More contemporary observations were made by Flowers who used the term "anchor blepharoplasty," Sheen who spoke of "supratarsal fixation," and Tenzel who referred to the "high upper eyelid crease." They noted that crease formation in the upper eyelid resulted in a "crisp" invaginated lid fold that tightened and smoothed the pretarsal skin. Although a crease will often spontaneously form at the upper lid incision line, this is not always reliable. The addition of crease formation techniques assures the location and symmetry of a crease and can give pleasing results while minimizing the amount of skin resection needed. The lid crease can be formed in both upper eyelid blepharoplasty and ptosis repair. For a detailed discussion of eyelid crease formation, the reader is referred to the excellent article by doctors Putterman and Urist.

Suggested Reading

[1] Flowers RS. Upper blepharoplasty by eyelid invagination. Anchor blepharoplasty. Clin Plast Surg. 1993; 20(2):193–207

[2] Mikamo M. Plastic operation of the eyelid. J Chugaiijashimpo. 1896; 17:1197

[3] Millard DR, Jr. Oriental peregrinations. Plast Reconstr Surg (1946). 1955; 16(5):319–336

[4] Putterman AM, Urist MJ. Reconstruction of the upper eyelid crease and fold. Arch Ophthalmol. 1976; 94(11):1941–1954

[5] Sayoc BT. Plastic construction of the superior palpebral fold in slit eyes. Bull Phil Ophthalmol Otolaryngol Soc. 1953; 1:2

[6] Sheen JH. Supratarsal fixation in upper blepharoplasty. Plast Reconstr Surg. 1974; 54(4):424–431

[7] Tenzel R. Upper eyelid crease formation. In: Putterman AM, ed. Cosmetic Oculoplastic Surgery. Grune & Stratton, Inc.; 1982:179–186

[8] Uchida K. A surgical method for the double eyelid operation. Jpn J Ophthalmol. 1926; 30:593

9 Scars

Kathleen F. Petro and Brent Hayek

Summary

Some known risk factors for hypertrophic scarring include wound tension, bacterial colonization, younger age, and possibly ethnicity. There are few randomized clinical trials studying nonsurgical hypertrophic scar treatment, and none specific to the periorbital region. Some evidence supports pressure, occlusion, intralesional injections of steroid such as triamcinolone acetonide, fluorouracil, dermabrasion, and certain lasers.

Keywords: hypertrophic scar, silicone, blepharoplasty, triamcinolone acetonide, 5-fluorouracil, nonsurgical scar treatment

9.1 Patient History Leading to the Specific Eyelid Problem

The patient is a 55-year-old Asian woman who gives a history of previous eyelid surgeries, including a bilateral upper eyelid blepharoplasty, medial epicanthoplasty, and lateral canthoplasty (►Fig. 9.1).

Her first surgical intervention was a bilateral medial epicanthoplasty, performed via the Park Z design, and closed with 6–0 nylon interrupted sutures. The bilateral blepharoplasty was done 2 months later, and consisted of skin, orbicularis, and fat removal. She had a concurrent lateral canthoplasty, but the details were not available to us. Hemostasis was achieved with bipolar cautery, and the skin was closed with 6–0 nylon and Steri-Strips.

Postoperatively, she had a wound dehiscence of the lateral right upper eyelid incision. This was allowed to heal by secondary intention. She presented to us 1 month after this surgery, complaining of discomfort and aesthetically unacceptable scars of both upper lids and lateral canthi. She also had asymmetry of her upper eyelid creases, as demonstrated in ►Fig. 9.1.

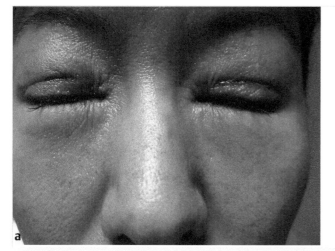
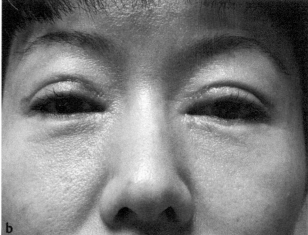

Fig. 9.1 This patient presented with a history of bilateral upper eyelid blepharoplasty, medial epicanthoplasty, and lateral canthoplasty with significant upper eyelid scarring. This was most apparent with **(a)** the eyes closed, but was also visible with **(b)** eyes open.

9.2 Anatomic Description of the Patient's Current Status

The patient had hypertrophic scarring of the incision in the right greater than left upper eyelid and left lateral canthus. The scars were irregular, elevated, indurated, and erythematous (▶Fig. 9.2).

The surgical crease on the right side was 9 mm above the lid margin, being 1 mm higher than that on the left side.

9.2.1 Analysis of the Problem

With proper preoperative planning and closure, upper blepharoplasty incisions are known to heal well with minimal complications. However, there are several potential issues related to wound healing that are demonstrated by this patient, including right upper lid wound dehiscence, hypertrophic scarring, and postoperative asymmetry. Wound dehiscence typically occurs laterally along the thicker skin when the blepharoplasty incision is closed with running suture. This may have been avoided by instructing the patient to avoid eye rubbing, or with additional interrupted sutures and closer spacing of the running suture along the incision at time of closure.

Postoperative asymmetry is a common source of dissatisfaction after double-eyelid "Asian blepharoplasty" surgery, occurring in 13 to 35% patients. Contributing factors may include unrecognized asymmetric eyelids, asymmetric brow, or mild preoperative unilateral ptosis, which may be amplified after resection of eyelid skin. Stretching eyelid skin during operative planning, double checking measurements and markings, and careful fixation of the eyelid may minimize postoperative asymmetry.

Hypertrophic scarring, although not completely understood, is caused by a combination of hypercellularity, augmented neovascularization, inflammatory cytokines, and excessive collagen production. The resultant imbalance between collagen production and collagenases leads to dysfunctional remodeling of granulation tissue and resultant scar hypertrophy. Risk factors for hypertrophic scar formation are young age, bacterial colonization, and skin

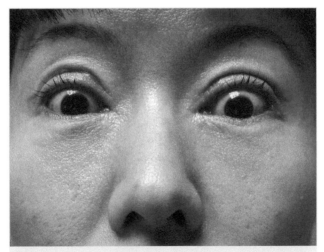

Fig. 9.2 The hypertrophic scars of her eyelids were raised, erythematous, and irregular, leading to asymmetry and increased visibility of the surgical crease discrepancy.

subjected to stretch. Cigarette smoking, chemotherapy, and statins may have a protective effect against hypertrophic scarring.

Although infrequently seen with blepharoplasty, the potential for hypertrophic scar formation exists from trauma to the dermis including surgery. The eyelid dermis of Asians contains a relatively higher concentration of collagen and tends to be thicker compared with that of Caucasians, potentially increasing the risk of hypertrophic scarring. According to studies of breast reduction and sternotomy incisions, approximately 60 to 65% of patients develop hypertrophic scarring within the first postoperative year, typically within the first 3 months. Around 30 to 35% of surgical wounds result in persistent hypertrophic scarring at 1 year, representing a spontaneous regression rate of nearly 50% by postoperative month 12. To our knowledge, no study has been performed evaluating the incidence of scar formation after blepharoplasty and the spontaneous involution rate if hypertrophic scarring occurs. However, it is well known that upper eyelid hypertrophic scar formation is much less frequent than in other areas of skin.

A multitude of treatments have been proposed to reduce the appearance of hypertrophic scars. There is insufficient evidence to support treatment of hypertrophic scars with vitamin E, onion extract, imiquimod cream, and massage therapy. Studies have suggested silicone products, pressure garments, corticosteroids, chemotherapeutics, and Botox to prevent excessive scarring, but many of these treatment options are presented without clinical trials.

A recent review of hypertrophic scar interventions by Kafka et al details the few clinical trials available that provide evidence-based treatment for hypertrophic scars. Silicone gel dressings have been proven effective for treatment and prevention of hypertrophic burn and posttraumatic scars with level 1 evidence. These silicone gel dressings have been shown to reduce scar thickness, increase pliability, alleviate pain and pruritus, and improve pigmentation. The effect was enhanced with concurrent pressure dressings in one controlled clinical trial by Li-Tsang et al. A recent clinical trial of a silicone elastomeric dressing, the "embrace device," demonstrated that an elastic silicone dressing with resulting reduction in wound tension resulted in improved scar appearance. Most silicone gel dressings are available over the counter, or patients may cut the silicone sheets down to an appropriate size and apply them to eyelid scars overnight.

Intralesional triamcinolone acetonide (TAC) is frequently used to suppress aberrant scar formation, and has been shown effective in multiple low-power studies. However, it has been associated with side effect such as injection site pain, hypopigmentation, skin and subcutaneous fat atrophy, and telangiectasias at a rate of approximately 37%.

In three prospective, randomized, blinded, controlled clinical trials with level 1 evidence, treatment with intralesional TAC was compared with a combination of TAC and 5-fluorouracil (5-FU). Combination therapy (TAC + 5-FU) resulted in reduced side effects, decreased scar height, improved pigmentation/erythema, and pliability compared to the TAC-only treatment groups. Asilian et al included an additional treatment group that added irradiation with 585-nm pulsed-dye laser to the TAC + 5-FU treatments. This group demonstrated improved pigmentation/erythema relative to the TAC + 5-FU group. In a large meta-analysis including many smaller studies, Ren et al supported these findings, demonstrating improved scar height, patient satisfaction, and erythema when TAC was combined with 5-FU for the treatment of hypertrophic scars and keloids.

Given the paucity of clinical trials with strong evidence of effectivity, there are no universally accepted guidelines for treatment of hypertrophic scars. Of the options presented above, intralesional injections of TAC + 5-FU appear to be the most effective, evidence-based approach to hypertrophic scar treatment. Unfortunately, these studies were not specifically targeting facial scarring and the results may not be directly applicable to hypertrophic scars due to blepharoplasty.

9.3 Recommended Solution to the Problem

- Steroid ointment (e.g., fluorometholone ophthalmic) with massage with or without occlusive dressings > 8 hours per day (e.g., overnight).
- Intralesional injections of TAC, TAC + 5-FU, or 5-FU alone.
- Consider laser therapies such as pulse dye or other resurfacing.

9.4 Technique

Three months of daily digital massage and twice daily application of fluorometholone ointment to the scars by the patient had no visible effect. Because of this, we injected 0.05 mL of TAC (40 mg/mL) to bilateral blepharoplasty and lateral canthus scars at postoperative months 4 and 7. Care must be taken as this concentration of TAC may lead to visible subdermal deposits. Also, 10 mg/mL is available and less likely to cause deposits.

9.5 Postoperative Photographs and Critical Evaluation of Results

The intralesional TAC injections yielded significant improvement in her blepharoplasty scar quality (▶ Fig. 9.3). The thickness and elevation of the scars improved, and the erythema faded. The patient noted improved symmetry of the eyelids. As seen in the photographs in ▶ Fig. 9.3 taken 2 years later, she still has subtle asymmetry of the eyelid creases that is less noticeable with substantial decrease of her hypertrophic scarring.

9.6 Teaching Points

- Risk factors for hypertrophic scar formation include younger age, bacterial colonization, and skin healing under stretch and possible Asian ethnicity.
- Silicone-based products (gel > sheets) may offer effective nonsurgical management of hypertrophic scars.
- Intralesional triamcinolone is a frequently used and often successful option.
- Combination therapy of intralesional TAC + 5-FU or intralesional 5-FU alone is an evidence-based therapy, which may reduce TAC side effects and enhance resolution of hypertrophic scarring.
- Radiation therapy can be effective in scar reduction but is not recommended in the eyelid.
- Laser treatment may be of value but optimal wavelength and energy level is not well defined.

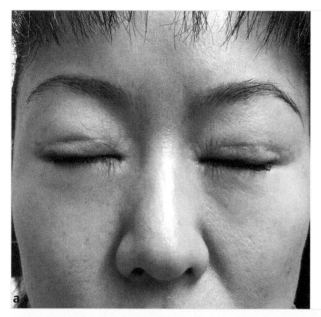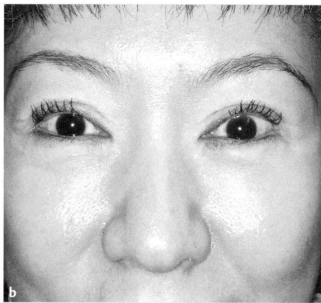

Fig. 9.3 (a,b) The erythema, induration, and elevation of the blepharoplasty scars improved, and the patient noted better symmetry of her eyelids 2 years later.

Suggested Reading

[1] Asilian A, Darougheh A, Shariati F. New combination of triamcinolone, 5-fluorouracil, and pulsed-dye laser for treatment of keloid and hypertrophic scars. Dermatol Surg. 2006; 32(7):907–915

[2] Butzelaar L, Ulrich MM, Mink van der Molen AB, Niessen FB, Beelen RH. Currently known risk factors for hypertrophic skin scarring: a review. J Plast Reconstr Aesthet Surg. 2016; 69(2):163–169

[3] Darougheh A, Asilian A, Shariati F. Intralesional triamcinolone alone or in combination with 5-fluorouracil for the treatment of keloid and hypertrophic scars. Clin Exp Dermatol. 2009; 34(2):219–223

[4] Kafka M, Collins V, Kamolz LP, Rappl T, Branski LK, Wurzer P. Evidence of invasive and noninvasive treatment modalities for hypertrophic scars: a systematic review. Wound Repair Regen. 2017; 25(1):139–144

[5] Khan MA, Bashir MM, Khan FA. Intralesional triamcinolone alone and in combination with 5-fluorouracil for the treatment of keloid and hypertrophic scars. J Pak Med Assoc. 2014; 64(9):1003–1007

[6] Kim DW, Bhatki AM. Upper blepharoplasty in the Asian eyelid. Facial Plast Surg Clin North Am. 2007; 15(3):327–335, vi

[7] Leventhal D, Furr M, Reiter D. Treatment of keloids and hypertrophic scars: a meta-analysis and review of the literature. Arch Facial Plast Surg. 2006; 8(6):362–368

[8] Li-Tsang CW, Zheng YP, Lau JC. A randomized clinical trial to study the effect of silicone gel dressing and pressure therapy on posttraumatic hypertrophic scars. J Burn Care Res. 2010; 31(3):448–457

[9] Longaker MT, Rohrich RJ, Greenberg L, et al. A randomized controlled trial of the embrace advanced scar therapy device to reduce incisional scar formation. Plast Reconstr Surg. 2014; 134(3):536–546

[10] Mahdavian Delavary B, van der Veer WM, Ferreira JA, Niessen FB. Formation of hypertrophic scars: evolution and susceptibility. J Plast Surg Hand Surg. 2012; 46(2):95–101

[11] Momeni M, Hafezi F, Rahbar H, Karimi H. Effects of silicone gel on burn scars. Burns. 2009; 35(1):70–74

[12] Niessen FB, Schalkwijk J, Vos H, Timens W. Hypertrophic scar formation is associated with an increased number of epidermal Langerhans cells. J Pathol. 2004; 202(1):121–129

[13] Rabello FB, Souza CD, Farina Júnior JA. Update on hypertrophic scar treatment. Clinics (Sao Paulo). 2014; 69(8):565–573

[14] Ren Y, Zhou X, Wei Z, Lin W, Fan B, Feng S. Efficacy and safety of triamcinolone acetonide alone and in combination with 5-fluorouracil for treating hypertrophic scars and keloids: a systematic review and meta-analysis. Int Wound J. 2017; 14(3):480–487

[15] van der Wal MB, van Zuijlen PP, van de Ven P, Middelkoop E. Topical silicone gel versus placebo in promoting the maturation of burn scars: a randomized controlled trial. Plast Reconstr Surg. 2010; 126(2):524–531

10 The Eyelid Crease

Ted H. Wojno

Summary

Eyelid crease formation is often ignored in upper eyelid surgery. Techniques presented here that incorporate crease formation can improve aesthetic results and provide more reliable surgical outcomes.

Keywords: crease, fold, supratarsal fixation, anchor blepharoplasty

10.1 Patient History Leading to the Specific Problem

The patient is a 66-year-old white woman who underwent bilateral upper eyelid blepharoplasty 1 year previously. She was unhappy with the cosmetic appearance of the right eye and presented requesting additional skin removal from the right upper eyelid to obtain better symmetry with the left eye (▶ Fig. 10.1).

10.2 Anatomic Description of the Patient's Current Status

This patient demonstrates a common problem after upper eyelid blepharoplasty—asymmetry of the level of the upper eyelid folds. The most common cause of this appearance is removal of unequal amounts of skin, muscle, or fat at the time of the original blepharoplasty. In such a case (all other things being equal), the side with more redundancy will have a lower upper eyelid skin fold postoperatively. This situation is easily remedied by removal of additional tissue from the lid with greater redundancy. This case is different, however, in that although equal amounts of skin were removed from each upper eyelid, the incision was placed at a lower level on the right than on the left. This resulted in a lower crease on the right side. This is obvious in the downgaze photo where one can observe the unequal height of the two lid creases (▶ Fig. 10.2). This gives the appearance of excess skin remaining on the

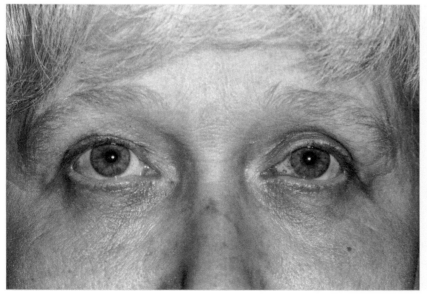

Fig. 10.1 The patient appears to have excess skin on the right upper eyelid.

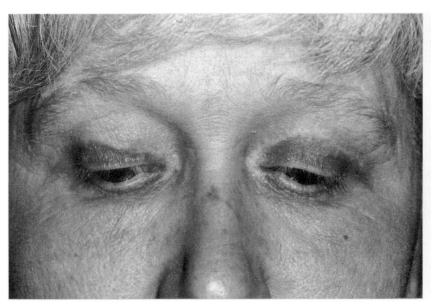

Fig. 10.2 In downgaze, it is apparent that the crease is lower on the right upper eyelid.

right upper lid. Since removing additional skin from the right upper eyelid in this particular patient might lead to lagophthalmos, this solution is not viable.

10.3 Recommended Solution to the Problem

- Elevate the crease in the right upper eyelid.
- Measure the height of the eyelid crease in the left upper eyelid.
- Transpose those measurements to the right upper eyelid and create a new lid crease at this level.

10.4 Technique

Before injecting with local anesthetic, measure from the lash line to the crease in the left upper eyelid centrally, medially, and laterally with the lid in downgaze. Transpose those measurements to the right upper eyelid. ▶ Fig. 10.3

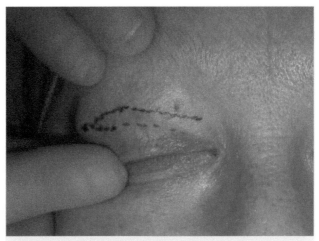

Fig. 10.3 The proposed new, higher crease incision is outlined above the old eyelid crease.

shows the old crease as the lower line and the proposed new crease as the higher line. Anesthetic may be injected at this time. Incise with a blade through skin and orbicularis across the right upper eyelid in the new crease line. Expose the levator aponeurosis in this area by undermining superiorly below the level of the orbicularis muscle across the length of the wound. This may necessitate opening tissue over any preaponeurotic fat that may remain from the prior surgery. If fat remains, dissect the fine attachments between the underside of the fat to the levator muscle to expose the levator. With scissors (I prefer blunt or sharp Westcott scissors), undermine deep to the level of the orbicularis on the anterior surface of the tarsal plate to a point inferior to the old, lower eyelid crease (▶ Fig. 10.4). It is important to do this across the entire old eyelid crease in order to divide all the fibrotic attachments from the tarsus to the underside of skin that form the old crease.

Reform the new, higher eyelid crease using three 6–0 polyester or 6–0 polyglactin buried sutures. Take a bite of the levator aponeurosis at the level of the new crease (▶ Fig. 10.5) and then a bite of the orbicularis at the lower edge of the incision (▶ Fig. 10.6). ▶ Fig. 10.7 shows this in cross-section. Do this centrally, medially, and laterally (▶ Fig. 10.8). Close the skin with a running monofilament suture.

Alternatively, the crease can be formed with three 6–0 silk or 6–0 plain gut sutures placed centrally, medially, and laterally. To do this, first take a bite of the skin on the lower edge of the incision as shown in ▶ Fig. 10.9. Next, take a bite of the levator aponeurosis just deep to the skin edge (▶ Fig. 10.10). Then, take a bite of the upper skin edge (▶ Fig. 10.11). This is shown diagrammatically in cross-section in ▶ Fig. 10.12.

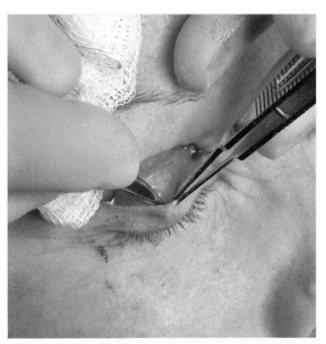

Fig. 10.4 After making the incision in the new crease, skin and orbicularis are undermined on the anterior surface of the tarsal plate deep to the old crease to release the adhesion.

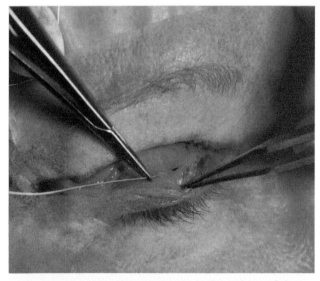

Fig. 10.5 A 6–0 polyester suture takes a bite of the levator aponeurosis at the level of the new crease.

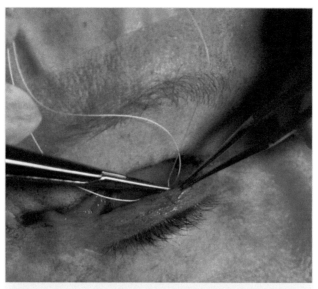

Fig. 10.6 The suture is then passed through the orbicularis at the lower edge of the incision.

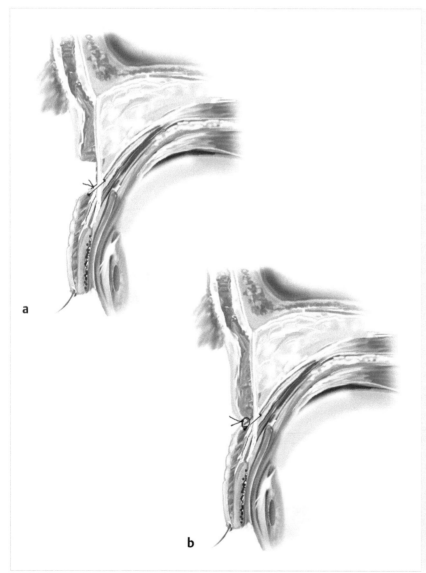

Fig. 10.7 A cross-sectional diagram illustrating passage of the crease suture.

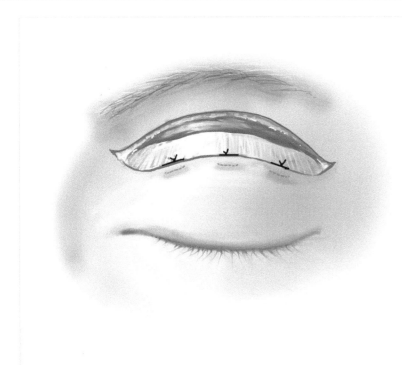

Fig. 10.8 A frontal diagram of the placement of the three crease sutures.

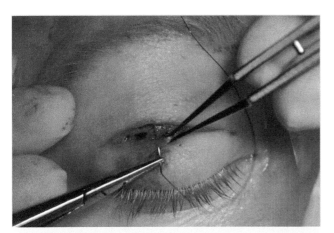

Fig. 10.9 An alternative method of crease formation illustrated in Chapter 6. Here a 6–0 silk suture takes a bite of the lower skin edge.

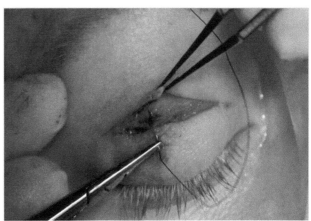

Fig. 10.10 Next the suture is passed through the levator aponeurosis just deep to the lower skin edge.

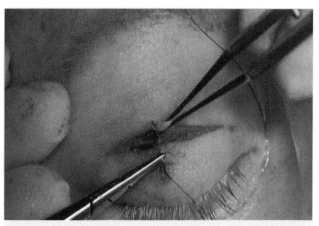

Fig. 10.11 The suture is then passed through the upper skin edge.

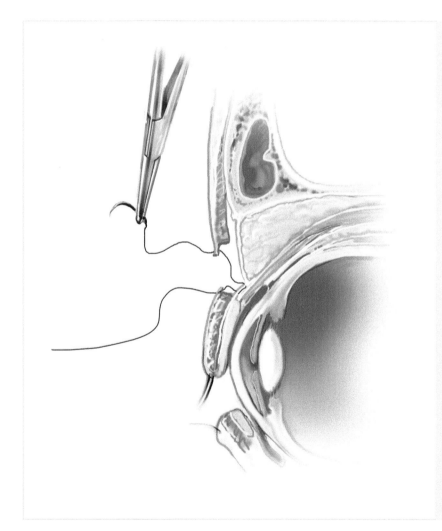

Fig. 10.12 A cross-sectional diagram illustrating passage of the silk suture.

Then, tie the knot (▶Fig. 10.13). A 6–0 silk or 6–0 gut sutures are good for this technique since they are relatively strong and inflammatory and will create a "spot-weld" at each location. This may be easier to perform than the first technique but occasionally results in loss of the crease when the silk sutures are removed the following week or the gut sutures dissolve.

A third and simplest way to reform the crease is to incorporate the levator aponeurosis into the running monofilament suture closure of the skin. This is done by taking a bite of the levator aponeurosis with every second or third passage of the needle through the skin edges (▶Fig. 10.14). This is shown diagrammatically in ▶Fig. 10.15. Like the second technique described in the

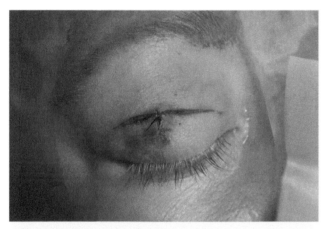

Fig. 10.13 The silk suture is tied.

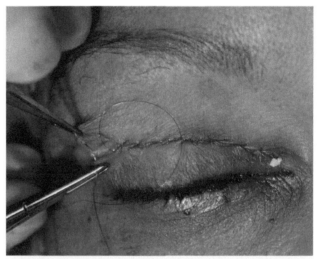

Fig. 10.14 Another alternative for crease formation involves taking multiple bites of the levator aponeurosis with the running monofilament suture used to close the skin.

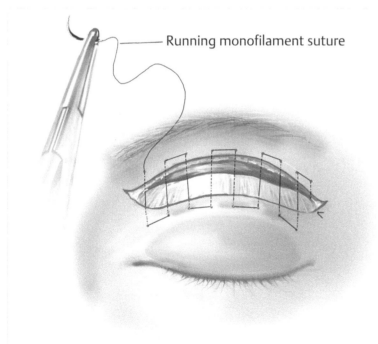

Running monofilament suture

Fig. 10.15 Diagram of the running monofilament suture technique of crease formation.

previous paragraph, the crease is sometimes lost after removal of the running monofilament suture. Additionally, suture removal is somewhat more difficult and uncomfortable because of the deeper bites into the levator.

10.5 Postoperative Photographs and Critical Evaluation of Results

The patient now has good cosmetic symmetry of the folds and creases without having had additional skin removed from the right upper eyelid as seen in ▶Fig. 10.16.

10.6 Teaching Points

- The eyelid crease after upper lid blepharoplasty is due to an adhesion between the levator aponeurosis and the skin.
- The eyelid crease usually, but not always, forms at the level of the upper lid blepharoplasty incision.
- Crease sutures insure the presence of an aesthetically appealing, crisp, and invaginated eyelid crease and lid fold.
- Asymmetry in the level of the upper eyelid crease results in asymmetry of the upper eyelid fold.
- To assure that a secure crease is formed at the incision, utilize one of the fixation methods described here.
- To assure that the creases are formed at the same level, measure carefully from the lid margin up to the proposed incision line centrally, medially, and laterally. Do this identically on each side.
- It is easier and more reliable to raise a low lid crease than it is to lower a high lid crease. Attempting to lower a high crease may result in the formation of two creases in the upper eyelid.
- There are numerous techniques to form a lid crease. Each has advantages and disadvantages.

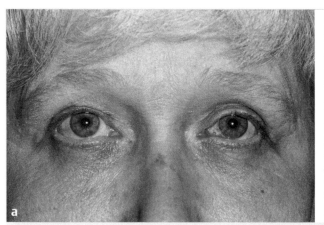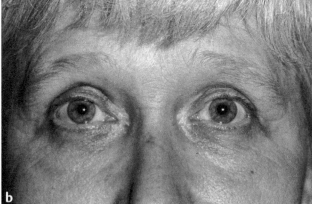

Fig. 10.16 The patient **(a)** before and **(b)** after the crease revision.

Suggested Reading

[1] Boo-Chai K. Plastic construction of the superior palpebral fold. Plast Reconstr Surg. 1963; 31:74–78

[2] Fernandez LR. Double eyelid operation in the Oriental in Hawaii. Plast Reconstr Surg Transplant Bull. 1960; 25:257–264

[3] Flowers RS. Upper blepharoplasty by eyelid invagination. Anchor blepharoplasty. Clin Plast Surg. 1993; 20(2):193–207

[4] Leone CR, Jr, Glover AT. Lipocauterization and thermal fixation in blepharoplasty. Am J Ophthalmol. 1988; 106(5):635–637

[5] Millard DR, Jr. Oriental peregrinations. Plast Reconstr Surg (1946). 1955; 16(5):319–336

[6] Pang HG. Surgical formation of upper lid fold. Arch Ophthalmol. 1961; 65:783–784

[7] Putterman AM, Urist MJ. Reconstruction of the upper eyelid crease and fold. Arch Ophthalmol. 1976; 94(11):1941–1954

[8] Sayoc BT. Plastic construction of the superior palpebral fold. Am J Ophthalmol. 1954; 38(4):556–559

[9] Sheen JH. Supratarsal fixation in upper blepharoplasty. Plast Reconstr Surg. 1974; 54(4):424–431

[10] Thomas CB, Pérez-Guisado J. A new approach: resection and suture of orbicularis oculi muscle to define the upper eyelid fold and correct asymmetries. Aesthetic Plast Surg. 2013; 37(1):46–50

11 Upper Eyelid Crease Malposition

William Pai-Dei Chen

Summary

The use of a superiorly beveled approach in revisional Asian blepharoplasty allows the glide zone to be partially restored and the middle lamellar scar reduced through removal. The preaponeurotic platform can be cleared of any interfering tissues. The combination of techniques described here often allows an abnormally high, static scar line to be repositioned and formatted into a lower, more dynamic crease to the point of being acceptable for the patient. The need for skin grafting may often be avoided.

Keywords: Asian upper blepharoplasty, beveled approach, revision of high crease, glide zone, midlamellar scar, clearance of preaponeurotic platform, reset of anterior and posterior lamellae, dynamic crease

11.1 Introduction

Variation in the position of the upper eyelid crease is a common postoperative finding following upper blepharoplasty. There are myriad factors that can challenge the surgeon's attempt to set the crease at an intended height. The following are some of the factors that come to mind immediately:

- Variable interpretation (definitions) of what an eyelid crease really is.
- Unequal brow position between two sides.
- Variable residual skinfold affecting the apparent crease height.
- Different state of levator function between the two eyes.
- Latent ptosis of one or both eyes.
- Variable ratios of pretarsal versus preseptal segment.

Variation of crease height between two upper lids and higher than expected crease-anchoring are especially distressing to Asian patients as well as surgeons performing this type of aesthetic surgery, commonly called double eyelid surgery in Asia.

11.2 Technique of Resetting a High Crease Height

For the purpose of discussion, this author defines an *upper lid crease* as the area where the upper lid skin invaginates, typically along the level of the superior tarsal border (STB), due to terminal insertions of levator aponeurotic fibers along the STB as well as the upper boundary of the pretarsal segment (skin, orbicularis oculi, upper tarsus). Various authors have identified histological as well as electron microscopic (EM) evidences that showed microfibrils (microtubules) emanating from the distal levator aponeurosis ending in the subcutaneous space along the STB, or fusion with the intermuscular septa and muscle sheath within fibers of the orbicularis oculi. Excluded are skin wrinkle lines as a result of dermatochalasis or depression as a result of supratarsal sulcus, whether they were congenital, acquired from fat excision following blepharoplasty, or involutional. The author ascribes to a dynamic definition for an upper lid crease, one that is a result of levator action through an animated posterior lamella (levator muscle/aponeurosis, Müller's muscle, and tarsal plate) against a passive, gravitating anterior lamella (composed of upper lid fold of skin, orbicularis oculi, and orbital septum; the preaponeurotic fat can be considered as part of the anterior layer while acting as an intermediary "glide zone interface" between the two lamellae' opposing actions). This definition is highly specific, physiologic, and conforms to known anatomy.

The abnormally high crease height we see in consideration for revisional upper blepharoplasty often fails this physiological definition of a crease. There are subcutaneous scar tissues along the vicinity of the STB, which interferes with the normal vectoring of the posterior tarsoaponeurotic segment against a fluidic anterior lamella. The result is a thickened band of skin–fibrous tissue scar attached to levator aponeurotic tissues that extends from the STB upward to a variable height. Physiologically, the levator aponeurosis here is tethered and fails to indent the eyelid crease. The resultant "crease" may appear to be a static crease line or wrinkle, a line that is part of a wrinkled placoid area of immobile lid tissue (glide zone). The most common etiological reasons include high anchoring where the surgeon places sutures to help form the crease on the levator aponeurosis above the STB, placement of buried, nondissolvable sutures toward this attempt, and less-than-meticulous tissue handling and hemorrhage intraoperatively.

11.3 Clinical Findings Seen in Patients Seeking Revisional Surgery

The eyelid may show spreading of the incision scar, high placement of the crease, secondary lagophthalmos on downgaze, and acquired secondary ptosis on straight gaze as well as upgaze. Intraoperatively, one sees thickened middle lamellar scar involving the orbicularis oculi as well as the orbital septum, or the presence of dense scar tissue plaques that may bind the anterior orbicularis oculi as well as the posterior levator aponeurosis (▶Fig. 11.1). Rather than having a physiologically preserved "glide zone" of preaponeurotic fat pad, there is now an apronlike plaque of fibrosis that is preventing the posterior layer from vectoring upward against a passive skin–orbicularis layer. Despite all efforts, there is no observable crease formation. Patients often complain of strain and fatigue, and a feeling of tightness, and may show brow and forehead overaction.

In dealing with revision cases, whether simple or complicated, one of the greatest dilemmas is where to make the incision so that it does not compound the scarring, both from an anterior aesthetic viewpoint as well as middle lamellar scarring and contracture that may cause further functional compromise. To succeed with improved aesthetic results as well as without further functional setbacks is a major triumph for any surgeon familiar with this type of revision surgery. Not only is it difficult, but also often the patient is anxious for a rapid and successful outcome, something that is never easily realized when dealing with scarring and suboptimal outcomes. I am often struck by how devastated these patients are and how grateful when the improvement proves significant. It is important for both patient and surgeon to be realistic in their expectations, as well as projection of the time course of healing following revision.

All these factors funnel into the same conclusion: if there is insufficient skin in reserve, it is unlikely that there is any chance of revisional improvement unless one wishes to supplement the skin with a free full-thickness skin graft. The latter will require precise techniques and experience, with special splinting over the graft in order to end up with an aesthetic improvement. There are, however,

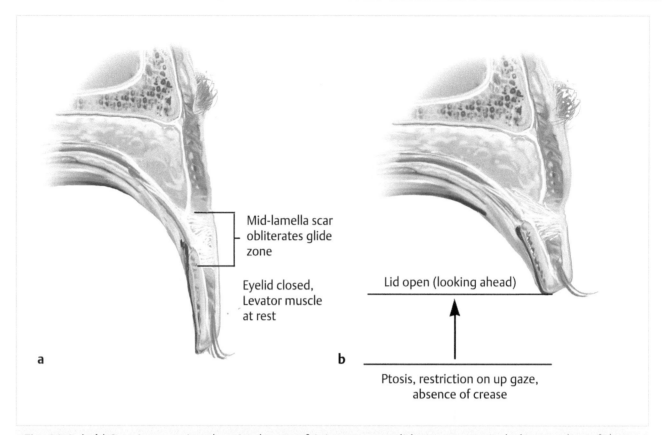

Mid-lamella scar obliterates glide zone

Eyelid closed, Levator muscle at rest

Lid open (looking ahead)

a

b

Ptosis, restriction on up gaze, absence of crease

Fig. 11.1 (a,b) Scarring seen in suboptimal cases of Asian upper eyelid surgery may include spreading of the incision, high placement of the crease, induced lagophthalmos on downgaze, and acquired ptosis on straight gaze as well as upgaze. Intraoperatively, middle lamellar scar involving the orbicularis oculi as well as the orbital septum may be observed; the presence of dense scar plaques may bind the anterior lamella's orbicularis oculi as well as the posterior lamella's levator aponeurosis. Rather than having a physiologically preserved "glide zone" of preaponeurotic fat pad, there is now an apronlike plaque of fibrosis that is preventing the posterior layer from vectoring upward against a passive skin–orbicularis layer. Despite all efforts, there is no observable crease formation. Patients often complain of strain and fatigue, and a feeling of tightness, and may show brow and forehead overaction.

many young adults or middle-aged patients who need revisions and whose problems are severe but are unlikely to have any skin reserves in the near future from aging. Patients with just enough eyelid closure to avoid corneal exposure may develop ocular exposure symptoms if the usual methods of excision of scars and lysis of adhesion of the middle lamella are followed. The amount of skin fragment removed may be only 2 mm, and poor eyelid closure may result.

An ideal solution to this dilemma is to approach the scarred anterior and middle lamellar complex through a superiorly beveled approach without significant removal of viable skin. To do this, the following conditions must be met.

The crease height is evaluated, and if it is high then the degree of planned lowering (in millimeters) will determine the minimum amount of skin redundancy above the existing crease in the preseptal region that needs to be in reserve. For example, if the height of an abnormally high crease is currently at 10.5 mm, which is considered extremely high, and you plan to lower it to 7.5 mm, then the patient will need to have 3 mm of skin in reserve above the crease before this is feasible. If there is only 2 mm, then this needs to be discussed with the patient, as the crease most probably may only be revised down to 8.5 mm in the current situation, or the patient can opt to wait for some skin to become available as a result of natural aging (and then they may proceed to revision at that time). If the patient is desperate for either functional or psychological reasons, then one must discuss the option of a skin graft.

For the majority of revision candidates who can get by without the need for skin grafting, my surgical approach proceeds initially along the same path as in primary cases, the major exception being that the upper and lower incision lines are marked across from each other on either side of the existing scar. Patients in this category for revision are more likely to have had their lid crease incision made in the 8- to 9-mm range, as measured from the central lid margin. The space between the upper and lower incision lines should be no more than 1 mm, and very rarely 2 mm. A no. 15 Bard-Parker blade is used to make a full-thickness incision along the marked upper and lower lines (▶ Fig. 11.2). Now, instead of using cutting cautery to go through the orbicularis to reach the orbital septum, one uses a sharp-tipped Westcott spring scissors to incise across the upper line of incision in a superiorly beveled fashion (▶ Fig. 11.3). At this stage, it is cutting through skin–orbicularis adhesions. Small scissoring motions are then used as the scissor blades transect the middle lamellar scar, opening the whitish, scarred fascial layers between the orbicularis and the underlying levator aponeurosis (▶ Fig. 11.4). This is carried out across the width of the incision along the previous scar. This beveled approach is similar but steeper than in primary Asian blepharoplasty cases (▶ Fig. 11.5). In this scarred middle zone, there will be much less preaponeurotic fat as it will have been previously excised; some residual fat globules, combined with scattered smaller amorphous specks or thin apron of scattered fat droplets, may be seen (▶ Fig. 11.6). After the forehead/eyebrow/preseptal skin layers are carefully reset by loosening the surgical drape over the patient's forehead, the scarred tissues within the space between the dotted superiorly beveled vector and the lower skin incision along the STB may be excised for as long as the remaining skin allows passive eyelid closure. All fat is

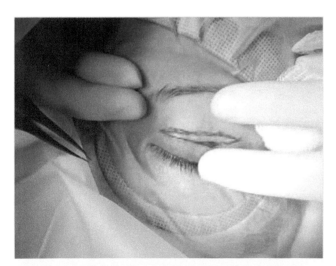

Fig. 11.2 A full-thickness skin incision has been made along the upper as well as the lower lines of the crease marking (left upper lid).

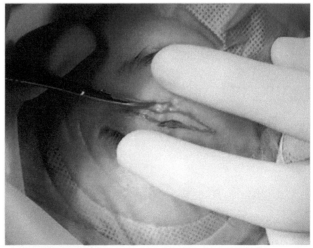

Fig. 11.3 Westcott spring scissors are used to lyse along the upper incisional edge in a beveled fashion. It is cutting through skin–orbicularis adhesions (left upper lid).

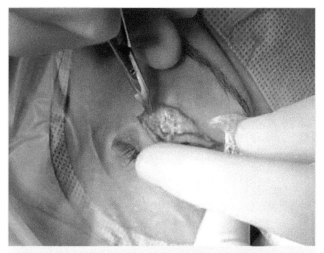

Fig. 11.4 Small scissoring motions are applied as the scissor blades transect the middle lamellar scar, going through whitish, scarred fascial layers between the orbicularis and the underlying levator aponeurosis (left upper lid).

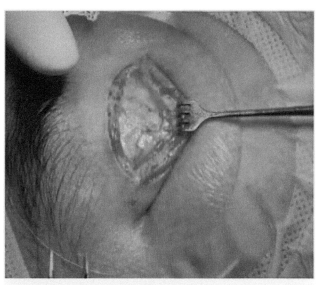

Fig. 11.6 After the preaponeurotic space is reached, within this scarred middle zone one may find some small residual fat globules combined with scattered fat droplets (right upper lid).

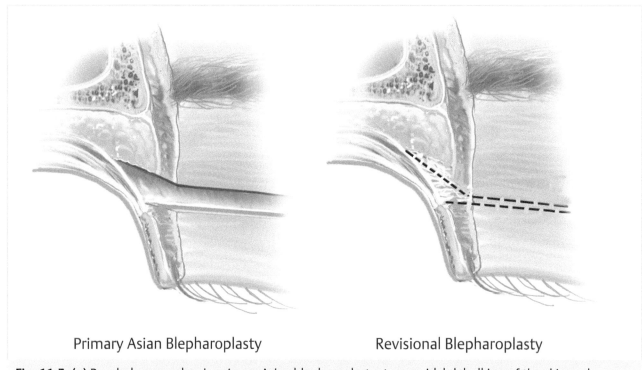

Primary Asian Blepharoplasty   Revisional Blepharoplasty

Fig. 11.5 (a) Beveled approaches in *primary* Asian blepharoplasty: trapezoidal debulking of the skin and preaponeurotic platform. (b) Superiorly beveled approach in *revisional* Asian blepharoplasty. Note the much steeper (oblique) approach taken in revisional attempt; this is necessary in the latter situation to preserve skin and to allow identification of the former preaponeurotic zone. In this scarred middle zone, one frequently finds some residual fat pads combined with scattered smaller amorphous fat globules or a thin apron of scattered fat droplets. After the forehead/eyebrow/preseptal skin layers are carefully reset by loosening the surgical drape over the patient's forehead, the scarred tissues within the space between the dotted superiorly beveled vector and the lower skin incision along the superior tarsal border may be excised, for as long as the remaining skin allows passive eyelid closure. All fat is preserved.

preserved. The levator and levator aponeurosis can be identified when the scar is released, and it is important to check for restriction objectively (by gently pulling the tarsal plate down) as well as subjectively by asking the patient to perform upgaze and downgaze.

The benefits and advantages of this beveled approach for revisional Asian upper blepharoplasty are as follows:

1. By approaching the preaponeurotic space very close to and barely above the scarred crease, one can avoid removal of any skin.
2. By making the upper line of incision close to the scarred crease, one avoids adding an incisional scar.
3. This beveled approach provides a safer passage to the already-explored preaponeurotic space, without injury to underlying levator muscle and Müller's muscle, as well as avoiding any anastomotic vessels of the superior tarsal arcade.
4. In some cases, the beveled maneuver toward the preaponeurotic space frees up the levator excursion significantly, releasing any restriction that may have contributed to lagophthalmos and acquired ptosis. This maneuver in itself may correct the mild ptosis, such that resetting of the previously high crease is then feasible.
5. By approaching the preaponeurotic space in a beveled fashion, it allows one to identify residual preaponeurotic fat that may have spread out and become plastered down on the levator muscle. This residual fat can be peeled off and repositioned to a higher level within the sulcus to help reverse some of the hollow sulcus often seen in patients needing revisional blepharoplasty.
6. The midlamellar scarring that has previously bounded the anterior and posterior lamellae of the upper lid can be safely removed or reduced, allowing partial restoration of the glide zone.

Following revisional Asian blepharoplasty with a superiorly beveled approach, the glide space has been partially restored and the scar carefully removed (▶ Fig. 11.7).

The preaponeurotic platform is cleared of most of the interfering tissues. Although the surgeon is often forced to make a skin incision that is still further from the lid margin than one would for a primary Asian blepharoplasty, upon closure the incision wound (white dot) is free to indent inward when the levator contracts, forming a better crease. The residual fat pads in the middle (glide) zone are preserved and allowed to fill in this glide space where appropriate. Supratarsal skin denoted by the red and blue dots above the incision is now free to gravitate and form the upper lid fold.

The restoration and preservation of the preaponeurotic space is an essential element in the surgical creation of a crease for an Asian with single eyelid, for it is the up-vectoring of the tarsal plate initiated by levator muscle and the presence of preaponeurotic fat in the glide space that facilitates a well-formed crease to form under a lid fold. In primary Asian blepharoplasty, it would be undesirable to excise all preaponeurotic fat, thereby obliterating the glide function of the preaponeurotic space, collapsing the supratarsal midsection of the lid, and creating a hollow sulcus on an Asian upper lid.

These reasonings are applied to revisional blepharoplasty as well, especially when it comes to resetting a high crease. This beveled approach allows the surgeon to reach the preaponeurotic space safely, to reposition any remaining preaponeurotic fat superiorly to fill in the hollow sulcus, and to approach the

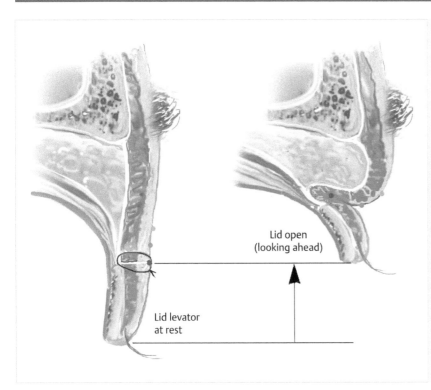

Fig. 11.7 Following revisional Asian blepharoplasty using a superiorly beveled approach, the glide space has been partially restored and the scar removed. The preaponeurotic platform is cleared of any interfering tissues. Although the surgeon is often forced to make a skin incision that is still further (higher in crease height) from the eyelid margin than one would for a primary Asian blepharoplasty, upon closure the incision wound (white dot) is free to indent inward when the levator contracts, forming a better crease. The residual fat pads in the middle (glide) zone are preserved and allowed to fill in this glide space where appropriate. Supratarsal skin denoted by the red and blue dots above the incision is now free to gravitate and form the upper lid fold.

preaponeurotic space without having to excise precious millimeters of skin along the upper skin incision line (▶ Fig. 11.8; ▶ Fig. 11.9).

In the author's practice, a series of 26 patients and 48 eyelids underwent revisional blepharoplasty over a four-year period for the specific purpose of revising a postsurgical high crease to a lower position. Excluded from this series were all primary Asian blepharoplasty candidates including any patients with preexistent high crease, touch-up surgery for the purpose of enhancing (deepening) an existing or surgically created crease that was in

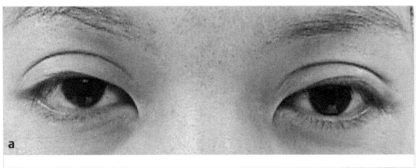

Fig. 11.8 (a) Preoperative appearance of a patient with high crease prior to revision. **(b)** Postoperative appearance at only 2 weeks following revision showing reduction of abnormal crease height.

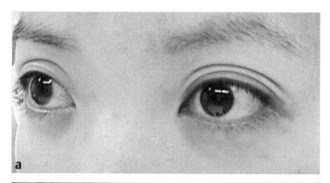
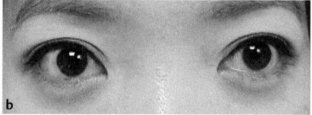

Fig. 11.9 (a) Preoperative appearance of a patient who presented with a high crease with some fat loss and an additional false crease in the pretarsal segment. **(b)** Postoperative view shows that the true crease has been revised downward, with improvement to her sulcus by fat repositioning. The double presence of a high crease with a false crease in the midpretarsal segment has been eliminated.

the correct position, correction of incomplete crease or crease shape alone, and simultaneous correction of acquired or involutional ptosis in conjunction with primary Asian blepharoplasty. There were 5 males and 21 females, and with the exception of 4 patients who requested unilateral crease revisions, all others were bilateral. The data were arranged in two separate sets of columns (►Table 11.1).

OD stands for the right upper lid and OS for the left upper lid. The third column of each of these two clusters of data reflects the difference between the preoperative and postoperative measurements. There were 24 eyelids in each category, for a total of 48 eyelids. The data were pooled together to arrive at the overall statistical mean. The prerevisional crease height was measured in the office using a millimeter scale and varied between 8 and 14 mm, with the overall mean being 9.9 mm. The crease height designed during revision (in 0.5-mm increments) varied between 6.0 and 8.5 mm based on the circumstances, with the mean being 7.15 mm; and 7 mm was the most often applied measurement during surgery under local anesthetic.

The effective lowering of the crease height ranges from 1 to 6 mm when reassessed during their 2-month postrevisional visits. The mean lowering of crease height is 2.75 mm in this series based on 2-month follow-up. Therefore, a 10-mm crease height on average can be reduced and reset to a height of 7.0 to 7.5 mm, which is a very acceptable position. The typical course is such that the crease height will continue to settle down with egress of swelling and wound healing, such that the effective lowering of the crease will likely increase had it been possible for all these patients to return for a longer follow-up period.

Table 11.1 Revisional data in a series of 48 eyelids showing age, gender, and degree of lowering of crease height in millimeters

	Age and Gender	Pre-op OD	Post-op OD	Change	Pre-op OS	Post-op OS	Change
1	42F	12	7.5	4.5	11	7.5	3.5
2	38F	11	7.5	3.5	10	7.5	2.5
3	46F	11	7	4	10	7	3
4	60F	10	6	4	10	6	4
5	54F	9.5	7.5	2	9.5	7.5	2
6	32F	9	7	2	9	7	2
7	32F				8.5	6.5	2
8	22F	8.5	7	1.5	8.5	7	1.5
9	23M	8	7	1	8	7	1
10	63F	9	7	2	9	7	2
11	36F	12	8	4	14	8	6
12	58F	12	7	5	12	7	5
13	65F	11	7	4	11	7	4
14	29F	9	7	2	9	7	2
15	22F	9	8	1	9	8	1
16	55F	10	7.5	2.5	10	7.5	2.5
17	66F	9	6	3	8.5	6	2.5
18	30F	11	8.5	2.5	10	8	2
19	34F	9.5	8	1.5			
20	25F	8.5	7	1.5	8.5	7	1.5
21	39F	9	7	2	9	7	2
22	47F	11	8	3	11	8	3
23	28F				8	6.5	1.5
24	63F	10	7	3			
25	26F	9.5	6.5	3	9.5	6.5	3
26	28F	12	6	6	12	8	4
Subtotal		240.5	172	68.5	235	171.5	63.5
Statis. mean		10.02	7.17	2.85	9.79	7.15	2.65
Total (OD + OS)		475.5	343.5	132			
Overall mean		9.9	7.15	2.75			

Note: OD stands for the right upper lid and OS for the left upper lid. The third column of each of these two clusters of data reflects the difference between the preoperative and postoperative measurements. There were 24 eyelids in each category, for a total of 48 eyelids. The data were pooled together to arrive at the overall statistical mean. The prerevisional crease height was measured in the office using a millimeter scale and ranges between 8 and 14 mm, with the overall mean being 9.9 mm. The crease height designed during revision (in 0.5-mm increments) varied between 6.0 and 8.5 mm based on the circumstances, with the mean being 7.15 mm; and 7 mm was the most often applied measurement during surgery under local anesthetic. The effective lowering of the crease height ranges from 1 to 6 mm when reassessed during their 2 months' postrevisional visits. The mean lowering of crease height is 2.75 mm in this series based on 2-month follow-up.

The use of a superiorly beveled approach in revisional Asian blepharoplasty allows the glide zone to be partially restored and the middle lamellar scar reduced through removal. The preaponeurotic platform can be cleared of any interfering tissues. This combination of techniques described here often allows an abnormally high, static scar line to be repositioned and formatted into a lower, more dynamic crease to the point of being acceptable for the patient. The need for skin grafting may often be avoided.

Suggested Reading

[1] Chen WPD. Asian blepharoplasty. Update on anatomy and techniques. Ophthal Plast Reconstr Surg. 1987; 3(3):135–140

[2] Chen WPD. Concept of triangular, trapezoidal, and rectangular debulking of eyelid tissues: application in Asian blepharoplasty. Plast Reconstr Surg. 1996; 97(1):212–218

[3] Chen WPD. The concept of a glide zone as it relates to upper lid crease, lid fold, and application in upper blepharoplasty. Plast Reconstr Surg. 2007; 119(1):379–386

[4] Chen WPD. Beveled approach for revisional surgery in Asian blepharoplasty. Plast Reconstr Surg. 2007; 120(2):545–552, discussion 553–555

[5] Chen WPD. Asian Blepharoplasty and the Eyelid Crease. 3rd ed. New York, NY: Elsevier; 2015

[6] Cheng J, Xu FZ. Anatomic microstructure of the upper eyelid in the Oriental double eyelid. Plast Reconstr Surg. 2001; 107(7):1665–1668

[7] Collin JR, Beard C, Wood I. Experimental and clinical data on the insertion of the levator palpebrae superioris muscle. Am J Ophthalmol. 1978; 85(6):792–801

[8] Maheshwari R, Maheshwari S. Muller's muscle resection for ptosis and relationship with levator and Muller's muscle function. Orbit. 2011; 30(3):150–153

[9] Morikawa K, Yamamoto H, Uchinuma E, Yamashina S. Scanning electron microscopic study on double and single eyelids in Orientals. Aesthetic Plast Surg. 2001; 25(1):20–24

[10] Morris CL, Morris WR, Fleming JC. A histological analysis of the Müllerectomy: redefining its mechanism in ptosis repair. Plast Reconstr Surg. 2011; 127(6):2333–2341

[11] Press UP, Schayan-Araghi K, Juranek R, Hübner H. Resection of the Müller muscle. Indications, technique and results [in German] Ophthalmologe. 1994; 91(4):533–535

[12] Ranno S, Sacchi M, Gonzalez MO, Ravula MT, Nucci P. Evaluation of levator function for efficacy of minimally invasive and standard techniques for involutional ptosis. Am J Ophthalmol. 2014; 157(1):209–213.e1

12 Postblepharoplasty Ptosis

Andrew Anzeljc and Brent Hayek

Summary

Postblepharoplasty ptosis involves an abnormally low upper lid margin after blepharoplasty. The most common etiologies are unidentified preexisting blepharoptosis and damage to the levator palpebrae superioris muscle during blepharoplasty. Postblepharoplasty ptosis may be repaired using both external and internal approaches in appropriate candidates.

Keywords: blepharoplasty, ptosis, blepharoptosis, postoperative ptosis, levator palpebrae superioris, levator advancement, müllerectomy, ptosis repair

12.1 Patient History Leading to the Specific Problem

A 65-year-old woman had one previous blepharoplasty 3 years prior to presentation (▶ Fig. 12.1). The patient noted progressive painless ptosis of her right upper lid after the procedure, obstructing her visual axis and causing cosmetic deformity. The patient desired ptosis repair to improve the appearance of her eyelids as well as her visual function. She was a breast cancer survivor status post mastectomy, but otherwise healthy without significant medical issues.

12.2 Anatomic Description of the Patient's Current Status

This patient demonstrates a common problem with postseptal dissection and fat excision during blepharoplasty. Accidental injury to the levator palpebrae superioris during blepharoplasty will lead to postoperative ptosis.

12.3 Analysis of the Problem

Careful preoperative patient evaluation is critical to the surgical success and prevention of postoperative complications in blepharoplasty. The most common cause of permanent postblepharoplasty blepharoptosis is inadequate preoperative patient evaluation and identification of ptosis. Preoperative measurement of the palpebral fissures in primary gaze, margin-reflex distance, and levator function may reveal blepharoptosis and guide appropriate surgical intervention.

The levator palpebrae superioris merges with the preseptal orbicularis oculi muscle near the inferior half of the skin muscle excision during blepharoplasty. Aggressive upper eyelid dissection may damage supratarsal lid crease fibers from the levator aponeurosis to the skin (▶ Fig. 12.2). Posterior dissection during postseptal fat removal may lead to levator damage as well. The septum may be sutured to levator during closure. If injury is noted at the time of surgery, it is corrected immediately.

Transient postoperative ptosis is typically due to mechanical restriction of levator action caused by eyelid edema. Postoperative hematomas, however, may lead to restricted levator function and subsequent fibrosis, leading to permanent levator function deficits. Therefore, if ptosis first presents 2 weeks postoperatively, it is monitored over 3 months for spontaneous resolution.

Management of postoperative ptosis requires evaluation of the type and degree of ptosis present, which will guide surgical intervention.

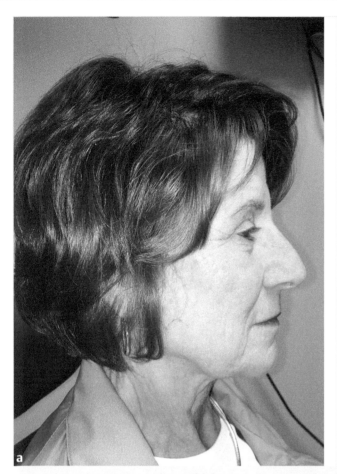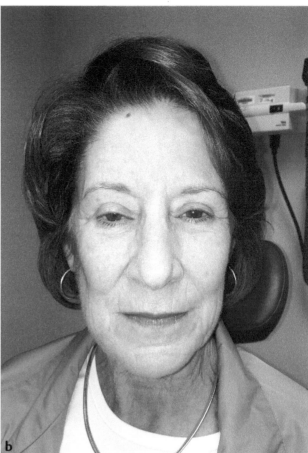

Fig. 12.1 **(a)** Right lateral and **(b)** frontal views reveal right upper lid ptosis. Note the asymmetric margin-reflex distance.

Pertinent history includes age and timing of onset, prior eyelid or periocular trauma or surgery, swelling, contact lens use, and presence of other ocular, systemic, neurologic, or muscular symptoms. Examination of eyelid function involves measurement of palpebral fissures in primary gaze, margin-reflex distance, and levator function. Levator advancement is the procedure of choice in most cases with moderate to severe ptosis, abnormal or poorly formed eyelid creases, or minimal improvement with Neo-Synephrine testing. As an alternative, a posterior approach such as a Müller muscle resection is ideal in cases with ptosis with positive neosynephrine test and normal eyelid creases.

12.4 Recommended Solution to the Problem

Ptosis repair via external or internal approach:
- Levator advancement or resection.
- Müllerectomy.

12.5 Technique

12.5.1 External Ptosis Repair: Levator Advancement

We injected 2 mL of 2% lidocaine with 1:100,000 epinephrine, 0.75% Marcaine, and Wydase at the eyelid crease. The eyelid incision is made through the prior

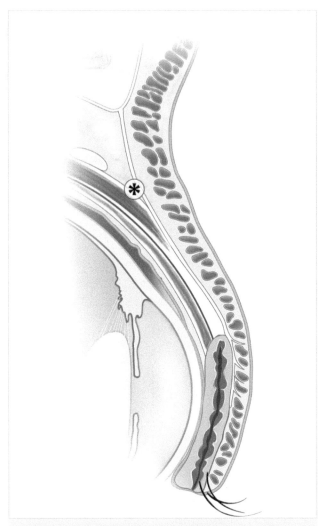

Fig. 12.2 Illustration of upper eyelid anatomy. Asterisk (*) denotes the location of the levator palpebrae superioris muscle posterior to the orbital septum and preaponeurotic fat. (Reproduced with permission from Codner MA, McCord Jr CD. Eyelid & Periorbital Surgery. 2nd ed. New York, NY: Thieme; 2016.)

blepharoplasty scar through skin and orbicularis muscle (▶Fig. 12.3a–c). The orbital septum is opened along the length of the incision (▶Fig. 12.3d). The levator is identified posterior to orbital fat (▶Fig. 12.3e).

Dissection is carried down along the central tarsal plate to free the levator aponeurosis attachments. Levator aponeurosis is freed from the underlying Müller muscle (▶Fig. 12.3f–i).

The levator aponeurosis is then reattached to the superior border of the tarsus using 6–0 Mersilene sutures adjusted for optimal lid height and contour, ensuring the tarsal sutures are not placed full thickness (▶Fig. 12.3j–l).

The patient is placed upright and the eyelids are checked for symmetry, height, and contour. The skin is closed with 6–0 Prolene sutures in a simple running technique (▶Fig. 12.3m).

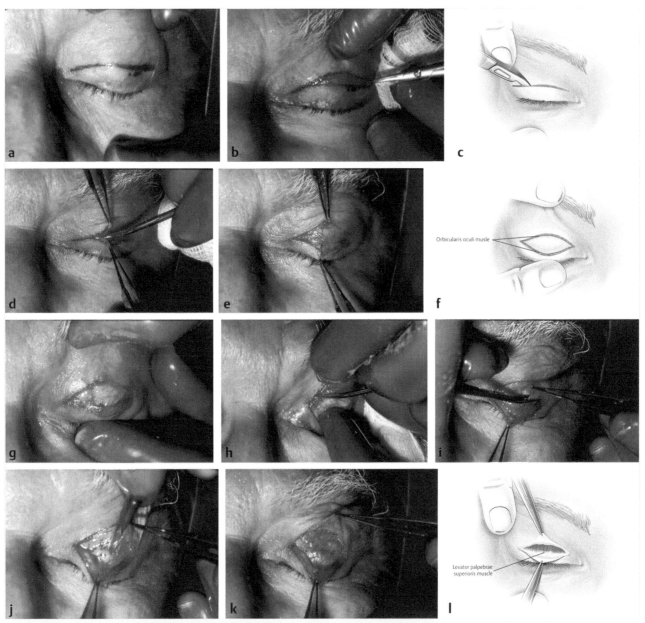

Fig. 12.3 External ptosis repair: levator advancement. (a) The upper eyelid crease incision is marked with a surgical marking pen. (b,c) The skin of the upper eyelid crease is incised at the marked site with a no. 15 blade. (d) The orbicularis muscle is opened with Westcott scissors. (e,f) The incision edges are spread to display the orbital septum. (g) Pressure on the globe allows for preaponeurotic fat to protrude forward behind the orbital septum. (h) The orbital septum is incised exposing preaponeurotic fat. (i) The orbital septum incision is extended medially and laterally. (j) Further septal fibers are dissected free from the levator. (k,l) The levator palpebrae superioris is exposed posterior to the preaponeurotic fat.

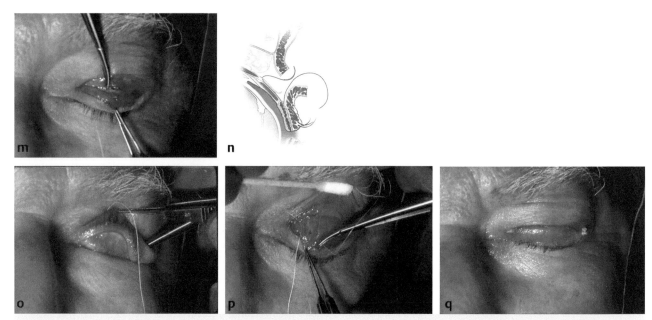

Fig. 12.3 (*Continued*) (m,n) A double armed 5–0 polyester suture is placed partial-thickness through the tarsus. (o) The upper eyelid is everted to ensure the suture was not placed full-thickness through the tarsus. (p) Both arms of the suture are passed through the levator muscle at the appropriate height. (q) The skin of the lid crease incision is closed with a running suture.

12.5.2 Internal Ptosis Repair: Müllerectomy

Local anesthetic consisting of a 50:50 mixture of 2% lidocaine with 1:100,000 epinephrine, 0.75% bupivacaine, and hyaluronidase is injected through the conjunctiva superior to the tarsus. The lid is everted over a Desmarres retractor and a caliper is used to mark 4 mm or more from the superior tarsal border medial, central, and lateral using Bovie cautery with microdissection needle (▶Fig. 12.4a,b).

Next, a 6–0 silk suture is passed through the markings incorporating conjunctiva and Müller's tissue (▶Fig. 12.4c). The tissue is then tented up and clamped with a Putterman clamp (▶Fig. 12.4d).

A 6–0 Prolene suture is passed percutaneously medially through the eyelid skin exiting in the superior fornix and then passed underneath the clamp in a running back-and-forth fashion (▶Fig. 12.4e). The 6–0 Prolene is then passed through the lateral superior fornix exiting onto the skin and drawn tight (▶Fig. 12.4f).

A no. 15 blade is used to excise the clamped tissue (▶Fig. 12.4g,h).

The 6–0 Prolene suture is then tied over the skin (▶Fig. 12.4i).

12.6 Postoperative Photographs and Critical Evaluation of Results

Bilateral upper eyelid levator advancement was performed using an external approach through the patient's prior blepharoplasty lid crease incision.

At 3 months postoperatively, the margin-reflex distance and palpebral fissure

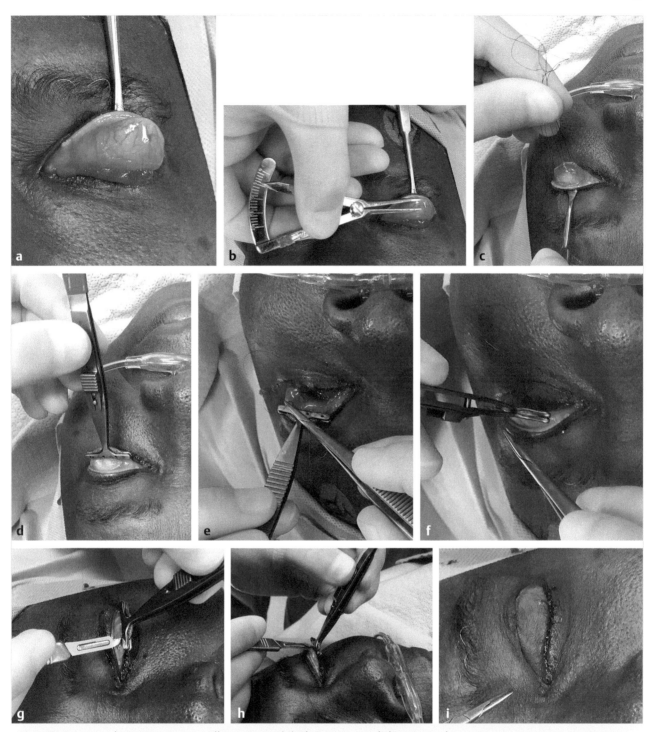

Fig. 12.4 Internal ptosis repair: müllerectomy. **(a)** The upper eyelid is everted on a Desmarres retractor.
(b) A caliper is used to mark 4 mm or more from the superior tarsal border medially, centrally, and laterally.
(c) A 6–0 silk suture is passed through the markings incorporating conjunctiva and Müller's muscle.
(d) A Putterman clamp is used to secure the tissue. **(e)** A 6–0 Prolene suture is passed percutaneously through the medial eyelid skin exiting the superior fornix and then passed beneath the clamp in a running fashion.
(f) The suture is then passed through the lateral superior fornix exiting onto the skin and drawn tight.
(g) A no. 15 blade is placed directly beneath the Putterman clamp. **(h)** The no. 15 blade is used to excise the tissue within the clamp. **(i)** The 6–0 Prolene suture is tied over the skin.

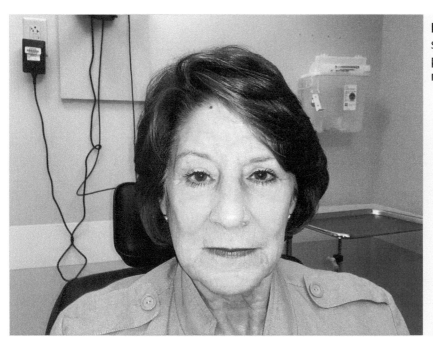

Fig. 12.5 Postoperative results show a symmetric eyelid contour, palpebral fissure height, and margin-reflex distance bilaterally.

height are symmetric bilaterally. The right upper eyelid height has been elevated to match the left upper eyelid. The patient was pleased with the height and contour of both of her upper eyelids (▶ Fig. 12.5).

12.7 Teaching Points

- Careful preoperative eyelid evaluation may identify coexisting ptosis and dermatochalasis.
- Careful dissection and identification of the levator during blepharoplasty is necessary to avoid inadvertent levator injury.
- Postblepharoplasty ptosis may be repaired using both external and internal approaches in appropriate candidates.

12.8 Suggested Reading

[1] Baylis HI, Sutcliffe T, Fett DR. Levator injury during blepharoplasty. Arch Ophthalmol. 1984; 102(4):570–571
[2] Lisman RD, Hyde K, Smith B. Complications of blepharoplasty. Clin Plast Surg. 1988; 15(2):309–335
[3] Lowry JC, Bartley GB. Complications of blepharoplasty. Surv Ophthalmol. 1994; 38(4):327–350
[4] Patrocinio TG, Loredo BA, Arevalo CE, Patrocinio LG, Patrocinio JA. Complications in blepharoplasty: how to avoid and manage them. Rev Bras Otorrinolaringol (Engl Ed). 2011; 77(3):322–327
[5] Pacella SJ, Codner MA. Minor complications after blepharoplasty: dry eyes, chemosis, granulomas, ptosis, and scleral show. Plast Reconstr Surg. 2010; 125(2):709–718

13 Full-Thickness Eyelid Resection in the Treatment of Secondary Ptosis

Allen M. Putterman

Summary
The chapter describes a vertical full-thickness eyelid resection for the treatment of ptosis as related to overcorrection after recession for eyelid retraction from Graves' disease or undercorrected external levator advancement ptosis procedures.

Keywords: blepharoptosis, thyroid, overcorrection, undercorrection, full thickness, retraction

13.1 Patient History Leading to Upper Eyelid Ptosis

This is a 53-year-old woman with a history of thyroid ophthalmopathy associated with exophthalmos and upper and lower eyelid retraction (▶ Fig. 13.1). She was treated with a bilateral four-wall orbital decompression, excision of the upper eyelid Müller muscle and levator recessions, bilateral lateral canthoplasties, and excision of herniated orbital fat. Postoperatively, she had a left upper eyelid ptosis with secondary loss of superior peripheral vision and difficulty reading due to closure of her left eyelids in the down-position of gaze.

Hertel exophthalmometry readings were 20.5/105 on the right and 20/105 on the left.

13.2 Anatomical Description of the Patient's Current Status

The left upper eyelid ptosis was due to the excision of the Müller muscle and recession of levator aponeurosis. It was done to lower her retracted left upper eyelid. The orbital decompression to treat her exophthalmos also contributed to the ptosis by the sinking inward and downward of the eye (▶ Fig. 13.1).

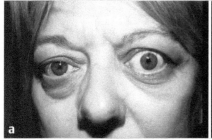 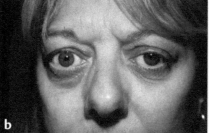

Fig. 13.1 (a) Patient with thyroid ophthalmopathy with upper eyelid retraction following orbital decompressions. (b) Post-op left Müller's muscle excision and levator recession with secondary left upper eyelid ptosis.

This chapter is supported by the Unrestricted Grant from Research to Prevent Blindness.

13.2.1 Analysis of the Problem

The usual method to treat acquired upper eyelid ptosis is by procedures such as a Müller muscle–conjunctival resection or levator aponeurosis advancement or resection. However, in this case, Müller's muscle has already been excised and the levator aponeurosis has already been recessed; also, there is scarring of the upper eyelid tissues from her previous procedures. All this makes the usual procedures more difficult and complicated. Although a full-thickness resection ptosis procedure is not advocated for primary upper eyelid ptosis, it is ideal for secondary ptosis. This is because the upper eyelid tissues are scarred together from the first procedure.

13.3 Recommended Solution to the Problem

- A vertical resection of full-thickness eyelid from the crease incision site.
- The amount of resection is based on the amount of ptosis, with a resection of a millimeter of full-thickness tissue for each millimeter of ptosis.
- Thus, if there are 3 mm of ptosis, 3 mm of full-thickness eyelid is resected.
- The amount of resection is varied nasally, centrally, and temporally, depending on the amounts of the ptosis at each of these segments to create a more normal upper eyelid arch.
- The resection of full-thickness tissue is done below or above the present crease, depending on if there is an abnormally high or low crease and fold.
- Therefore, if the distance from the present eyelid crease is large, there is a resection of full-thickness tissue below the crease-incision site.

13.4 Technique

A sterile surgical marking pen is used to delineate the predetermined eyelid crease on the upper eyelid and local anesthetic is injected subcutaneously (▶Fig. 13.2a).

The upper eyelid is everted over a Desmarres retractor and local anesthetic is infiltrated subconjunctivally at the superior tarsal border (▶Fig. 13.2b).

After placing a 4–0 silk traction suture in the upper eyelid margin, a #15 Bard-Parker blade and Colorado needle are used to create an eyelid incision. Hemostasis is performed with a disposable cautery (▶Fig. 13.2c).

A full-thickness incision is made across the entire upper eyelid (▶Fig. 13.2d).

When the margin distance on the ptotic eyelid is elevated in comparison to the contralateral eyelid, a full-thickness resection of tissue is removed inferior to the crease incision site (▶Fig. 13.2e).

A 6–0 double-arm Vicryl suture is then passed through the central lower eyelid portion of the wound with care given to avoid suture contact with the globe. Often, the sutures pass through tarsus; both arms of the suture then pass securely through the upper portion of the wound (▶Fig. 13.2f). Care is taken to imbricate the levator muscle but not to pierce the conjunctiva.

The suture is then tied with two throws of a surgeon's knot, over a knot-releasing piece of 4–0 silk suture (▶Fig. 13.2g).

The contact lenses are removed from the patient's eyes and the patient is sat upright. If the lid level is too high or low, the 4–0 suture is pulled to release the knot and the sutures are replaced lower or higher, respectively.

The remaining wound is first closed with the open arms of the 6–0 Vicryl suture used to imbricate the underlying levator muscle (▶Fig. 13.2h).

The wound is finally closed with a running 6–0 silk suture (▶Fig. 13.2i).

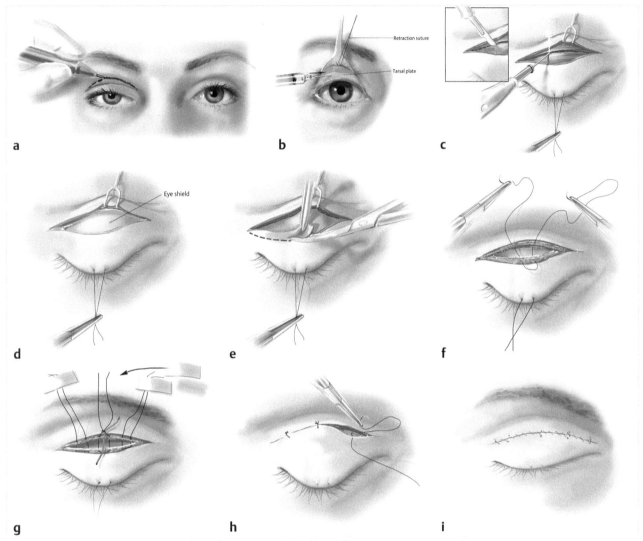

Fig. 13.2 (a) A sterile surgical marking pen is used to delineate the predetermined eyelid crease on the upper eyelid. (b) The upper eyelid is everted over a Desmarres retractor and local anesthetic is again sparingly infiltrated subconjunctivally at the superior tarsal border. (c) After placing a 4–0 silk traction suture in the upper eyelid margin, a #15 blade and Colorado needle are used to create a full-thickness eyelid incision. Hemostasis is performed with disposable cautery. (d) A full-thickness incision across the entire upper eyelid. (e) When the margin-crease distance (MCD) on the ptotic eye is elevated in comparison to the contralateral eyelid, full-thickness tissue is removed inferior to the crease incision. (f) A 6–0 double-armed Vicryl suture is then passed through the central lower portion of the wound with care given to avoid future suture contact with the globe. Often, this suture is passed through the upper portion of the tarsus. Care is taken to imbricate the levator muscle, but not to pierce the conjunctiva. (g) The suture is then tied down with two throws of a surgeon's knot over a knot-releasing piece of 4–0 silk suture. The contact lenses are removed from the patient's eyes, and the patient is sat upright. (h) The remaining wound is first closed with the open arms of the 6–0 Vicryl sutures used to imbricate the underlying levator muscle. (i) The wound is finally closed with a running 6–0 silk suture.

13.5 Postoperative Photographs and Critical Evaluation of Results

The postoperative photograph is 3 months after the full-thickness resection ptosis procedure. The left upper eyelid ptosis has been corrected and the patient has improvement in her superior peripheral vision as well as her reading vision. There is also improvement in the upper eyelid level as well as the left upper eyelid arch, crease, and fold (▶Fig. 13.3).

13.5.1 Additional Patients

Two patients with residual upper eyelid ptosis following previous ptosis procedures who were successfully corrected with the full-thickness ptosis procedure are shown in ▶Fig. 13.4 and ▶Fig. 13.5.

13.6 Teaching Points

- The treatment of secondary upper eyelid ptosis is more complicated due to scarring of tissues from the primary surgery.
- This leads to more difficulty in identifying the eyelid structures, such as the Müller muscle and the levator aponeurosis.
- Advancing and resecting the Müller muscle and the levator aponeurosis is more uncertain with secondary ptosis due to scarring from the primary procedure.

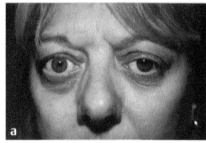
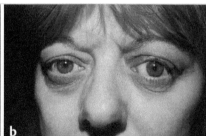

Fig. 13.3 **(a)** Patient in ▶Fig. 13.1 with upper eyelid ptosis following Müller's muscle excision and levator recession. **(b)** Post-op following full-thickness resection ptosis procedure.

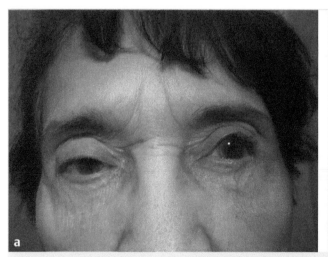
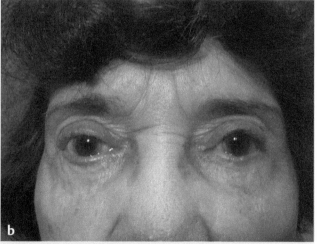

Fig. 13.4 **(a)** Pre-op of patient with right upper lid ptosis after previously having a bilateral Müller muscle resection. **(b)** Post-op after right upper lid full-thickness resection ptosis procedure.

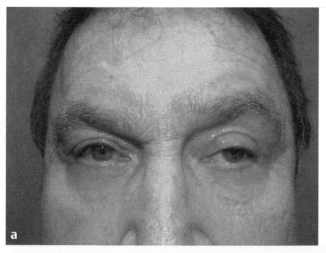 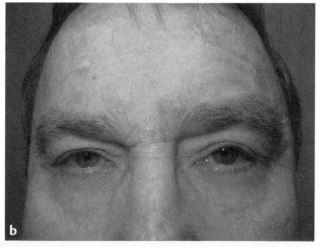

Fig. 13.5 **(a)** Pre-op of patient with left upper lid ptosis after previous bilateral upper eyelid levator resections. **(b)** Post-op after left upper eyelid full-thickness resection ptosis procedure.

- The full-thickness resection ptosis procedure is ideal for secondary upper eyelid ptosis, since the eyelid tissues are scarred together.
- The procedure not only corrects the ptotic lid but also can create a more normal arch to the upper lid.
- The procedure can also create more symmetric upper lid creases and folds by decreasing the distance between the upper eyelid margin and the lid crease through resection of full-thickness tissues beneath a high upper lid crease and fold.

Suggested Reading

[1] Bassin RE, Putterman AM. Full-thickness eyelid resection in the treatment of secondary ptosis. Ophthal Plast Reconstr Surg. 2009; 25(2):85–89

[2] Baylis HI. Full-Thickness eyelid resection for the treatment of uncorrected blepharoptosis and eyelid contour defects. ADV Ophthal Plas Reconstr Surg. 1982; 1:205–212

[3] Gladstone GJ, Putterman AM. Internal vertical shortening for the correction of diffuse or segmental postoperative blepharoptosis. Am J Ophthalmol. 1985; 99(4):429–436

[4] Putterman AM, Fett DR. Müller's muscle in the treatment of upper eyelid retraction: a 12-year study. Ophthalmic Surg. 1986; 17(6):361–367

[5] Putterman AM. Surgical treatment of thyroid-related upper eyelid retraction. Graded Müller's muscle excision and levator recession. Ophthalmology. 1981; 88(6):507–512

[6] Putterman AM. Internal vertical eyelid shortening to treat surgically induced segmental blepharotosis. Am J Ophthalmol. 1976; 82(1):122–128

[7] Putterman AM, Urist M. Surgical treatment of upper eyelid retraction. Arch Ophthalmol. 1972; 87(4):401–405

14 The Missed Ptosis in Upper Eyelid Blepharoplasty

Richard L. Scawn, Sri Gore, and Naresh Joshi

Summary

This chapter highlights the importance of detecting and correcting eyelid and eyebrow ptosis in patients being evaluated for upper lid blepharoplasty surgery. The authors' technique for upper eyelid blepharoplasty surgery is presented with a discussion of managing postblepharoplasty eyelid and eyebrow ptosis.

Keywords: ptosis, blepharoplasty, aesthetic, brow lift, microptosis, botulinum toxin, skin crease

14.1 Introduction

The recognition of ptosis in the postoperative period after cosmetic blepharoplasty may present an unwelcome finding for patients and surgeons.

Incidence data are lacking but qualitatively the phenomenon has been described as common; thus, a preemptive avoidance strategy, alongside a repertoire of corrective techniques, is likely to be worthwhile. A previously unrecognized ptosis should still prompt careful ophthalmic examination, including pupil and motility, to exclude a new-onset neurogenic cause for a ptosis such as a Horner's syndrome.

Upper lid dermatochalasis warranting blepharoplasty rarely manifests in absolute isolation to other periocular involutional changes. The aesthetic continuums of the eyebrow and eyelid both influence the lid margin position and degree of dermatochalasis, so each must be evaluated prior to blepharoplasty. The detection of a small concurrent brow or eyelid ptosis prior to blepharoplasty, even if not considered clinically significant to initially require surgery, warrants discussion with the patient at the outset.

Should ptosis be subsequently recognized postoperatively, the contribution of eyebrow, eyelid, and involutional skin changes must be reassessed in order to correctly target a surgical solution.

14.2 Prevention

"An ounce of prevention is worth a pound of cure" offers an applicable adage to focus our initial attention on preventable causes.

Prevention involves both the preoperative assessment, to exclude brow or eyelid pathology that would benefit from concurrent correction alongside upper lid blepharoplasty surgery, and surgical techniques, to avoid exacerbating or introducing an iatrogenic ptosis.

14.2.1 Preoperative Prevention

At initial assessment, the surgeon should be aware of previous procedures and concurrent aesthetic interventions, such as recent botulinum toxin, especially where designed to elevate the brow position, thus masking an underlying ptotic brow.

In our experience, at least two preoperative assessment visits are preferred, both for the patient's preparation and to give the surgeon more than one opportunity to detect subtle pathology, analyze photographs from the previous clinical visit, and discuss patient expectations.

Preoperative photographs allow static preoperative clinical scrutiny and provide a medical record (▶ Fig. 14.1). A standardized photographic system described by Coombes et al, and utilized in our practice, improves objectivity and also opposes frontalis overaction, helping assess the contribution of the brow to upper lid dermatochalasis.

14.2.2 Intraoperative Prevention

Swelling and bruising after blepharoplasty will frequently generate a transient ptosis. Patients should be forewarned and reassured that signs will typically resolve over forthcoming days to weeks. However, fastidious surgical techniques and postoperative care may mitigate ecchymosis and edema such that these entities need not be considered an inevitable blepharoplasty consequence.

Local anesthetic with adrenaline and dexamethasone is administered, using a previously described "pinch and roll" to avoid puncturing the vascular

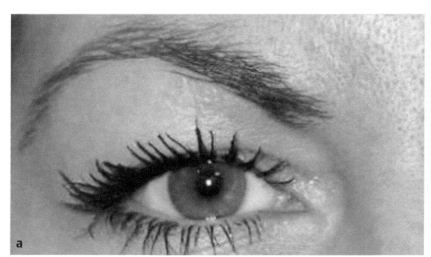
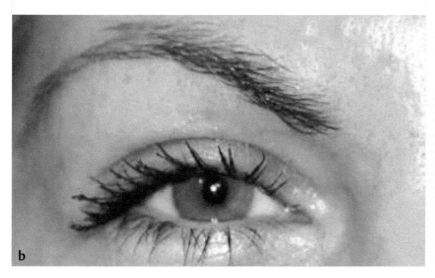

Fig. 14.1 **(a)** Preoperative upper lid blepharoplasty. **(b)** Day 5 postoperative blepharoplasty.

orbicularis that lies beneath the skin and inducing a subcutaneous hematoma. A Colorado microdissector needle is preferred to allow simultaneous cutting and cautery to reduce hemorrhage. Patients should continue their antihypertensive medication, and a risk versus benefit decision regarding suspending concurrent anticoagulation should be made in conjunction with the prescribing internal medicine physician and the patient.

Impaired levator aponeurosis function may occur secondary to hematoma during upper lid blepharoplasty, suturing of the orbital septum to the levator, inadvertent levator disinsertion when opening the orbital septum, or during orbicularis excision. The surgeon performing upper lid blepharoplasty must be confident of the eyelid anatomy, to differentiate orbital septum from levator particularly when fatty degeneration of the levator muscle is present. Racial variations exist in upper lid anatomy, particularly the fusion point of the septum upon the levator, and surgeons should be cognizant of such. When removing orbital fat, opening of the septum "high up" at the point of the fusion with levator has been recommended for less experienced surgeons to avoid unintended levator injury close to point of septal–levator fusion.

14.3 Brow Stability

Involutional brow descent, especially laterally, is a classically cited aging characteristic. The temporal fusion line of the forehead marks an attenuation of the frontalis muscle, the primary brow elevator. The lateral orbicularis oculi coupled with involutional tissue descent can thus act to depress the brow with limited opposition lateral to the temporal fusion line.

Although some authors have shown limited or no postblepharoplasty brow descent, a series from Prado et al, including 45 patients, used quantitative pre- and postoperative digital analysis to demonstrate consistent lateral brow descent after upper lid blepharoplasty. Our preference to promote lateral brow stability is to excise a strip of orbicularis that is much broader laterally, described by Widgerow as an "orbicularis wedge" (▶ Fig. 14.2). This deliberately weakens the lateral brow depressive forces, promoting a neutral or potentially elevated postoperative lateral brow.

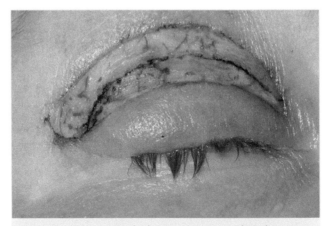

Fig. 14.2 Photograph demonstrating orbicularis excision that is wider laterally to promote lateral brow stability.

14.4 Management of Ptosis after Blepharoplasty

Initial management, as previously discussed, is typically conservative because the majority are transient. A decision to reoperate is usually postponed, pending static clinical findings on at least two clinic visits, and revision surgery preferably deferred 3 to 6 months after initial blepharoplasty.

14.4.1 Brow Ptosis

A small ptosis secondary to brow descent may be managed using surgical and nonsurgical methods.

Botulinum toxin injections offer a less invasive, albeit temporary, correction of brow ptosis and may be most effective in younger patients. Injections can be directed into the glabellar region to weaken the medial brow depressors, while lateral orbicularis injections can elevate the lateral brow.

Surgical techniques to correct a small residual brow ptosis include a temporal pretrichial lift or a direct crenated brow lift (▶Fig. 14.3).

In the pretrichial temporal brow lift, an approximately 1-cm wide, 3 to 4 cm in length skin ellipse is excised just in front of the temporal hair line. Blunt dissection exposes the deep temporal fascia and fashions a subdermal plane beneath the leading (inferior) arc of the ellipse. A 4–0 polypropylene suture is placed in deep tissues of the inferior ellipse and then anchored in the deep temporal fascia, thereby elevating the temporal brow. Skin is closed with 5–0 polypropylene and the incision site usually heals with a barely visible scar. The degree of elevation will attenuate with increasing distance between the lateral brow and the skin excision, so the procedure is most powerful in those with a low hairline (▶Fig. 14.3).

The direct brow offers potentially a more powerful correction of an unexpected ptotic brow after blepharoplasty. It is suited to those in whom a pretrichial brow lift will be insufficient and those with prominent brow cilia,

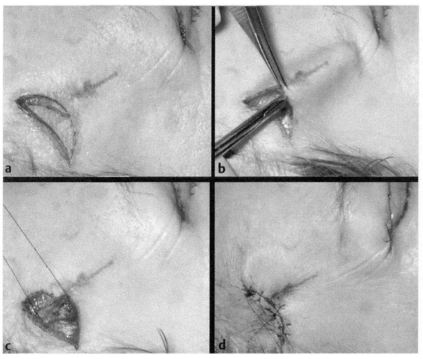

Fig. 14.3 Temporal pretrichial operative series demonstrating **(a)** excision of a pretrichial skin ellipse, **(b)** blunt dissection in subdermal plane, **(c)** placement of 4–0 polypropylene suture from inferior subdermal tissue to deep temporal fascia at superior incision border, and **(d)** incision closure.

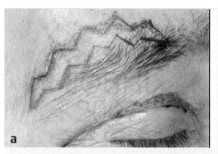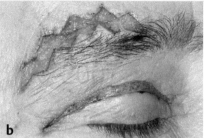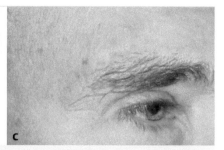

Fig. 14.4 (a) Incision shape. (b) Incision depth. (c) Postoperative cosmetically very acceptable incision healing.

which help to camouflage the incision. Use of a crenated shape further reduces the visible scar, although patients, especially important in those undergoing revision surgery after blepharoplasty, do need to be counseled regarding a postoperative scar (▶ Fig. 14.4). The excision depth extends into the brow fat, as in a traditional direct brow lift, and is closed in two layers: interrupted 5–0 absorbable sutures deep to the epidermis and skin closure with a 5–0 polypropylene suture.

14.5 Case Example

A female patient requested treatment for persistent lateral lid "hooding." Examination demonstrated predominantly lateral dermatochalasis with obscuration of the eyelid crease and a pseudoeyelid ptosis primarily secondary to lateral brow descent. Clinical examination showed that the involutional changes were predominantly in the brow, and with gentle manual lateral brow support, the excess "hooding," that the patient was aware of, resolved. The eyelid margin was normal.

A temporal brow lift with restoration of the natural lateral arch brow was recommended (▶ Fig. 14.5). The broad options for achieving brow support include: browpexy, crenated (direct) brow lift, temporal pretrichial approach, or an endoscopic brow lift. In our experience, browpexy techniques with this degree of brow ptosis may not deliver sufficient elevation and longevity.

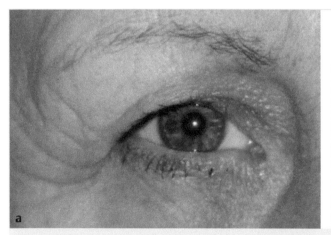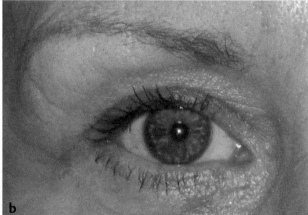

Fig. 14.5 (a) Preoperative. (b) Postoperative after temporal pretrichial brow lift.

While the endoscopic approach has a well-established role in brow rejuvenation, in this situation excellent outcomes with skin excision and minimal scarring may be achieved using the crenated brow lift or the temporal pretrichial lift. In this female patient, the pretrichial lift was favored because the lateral brow cilia were relatively sparse and the distance from the lateral brow to the pretrichial skin was short, which potentiated the potency of a pretrichial brow lift.

14.5.1 Eyelid Ptosis and Skin Crease Symmetry

Before embarking on corrective ptosis surgery, it is important to differentiate asymmetric lid margin position from an asymmetric tarsal platform show or lid crease asymmetry. Patients may perceive an eyelid as ptotic, when in fact the asymmetry results from a difference in the tarsal platform or "lid show" on that side, and surgery should be directed accordingly to raise or lower an eyelid crease.

A moderate (≥ 2 mm) residual bilateral eyelid ptosis with normal levator function can be corrected in a standard fashion, via the surgeon's choice of levator advancement or conjunctival müllerectomy. Although very rare, early postoperative presentation with ptosis, lagophthalmos, lid hang-up in downgaze, and diminished levator function raises a suspicion that the orbital septum may have been sutured to the levator or tarsus; these patients warrant early exploration via an anterior approach and restoration of the normal anatomy.

Correction of a small (≤1.0 mm) but aesthetically unsatisfactory eyelid ptosis may be technically more taxing (▶ Fig. 14.6). A posterior approach with conjunctival müllerectomy offers a predictable method of correcting a small ptosis with preservation of eyelid contour. Published nomograms would advocate approximately 4-mm tissue resection for 1 mm of ptosis correction and preoperative topical phenylephrine testing forms part of many such nomograms. Although there may be a trend among some to perform

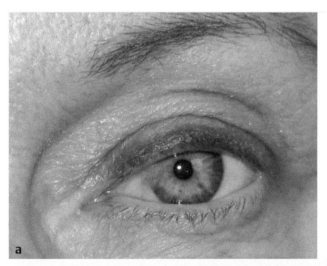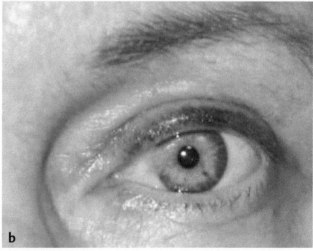

Fig. 14.6 Left small (micro) ptosis and secondary tarsal platform and brow asymmetry corrected with anterior approach small incision. (a) Preoperative photograph revealing small (micro) ptosis. (b) Postoperative photograph after left microptosis correction showing improved symmetry of the lid crease, tarsal platform, and brow asymmetry.

conjunctival müllerectomy for smaller ptosis correction, an anterior approach may offer more options in skin crease shaping. Small anterior incision minimal dissection ptosis repair and standard aponeurosis repair have both proved to be effective methods. A comparison between anterior approach and conjunctival müllerectomy has also shown similarly good outcomes. There will be advocates for each approach, so the ideal procedure for managing a small ptosis probably lies with the technique the individual surgeon is most experienced performing. In our hands, a small incision (10 mm) anterior approach is preferred for correcting a small degree of ptosis. A single 6–0 Prolene suture is used to advance the levator onto the tarsus in the midpupillary. The skin is closed with Prolene, incorporating anterior levator fibers to form a crease.

14.6 Conclusion

Ptosis following blepharoplasty may occur secondary to both eyelid and brow pathology. The management strategy will need to be tailored to the underlying etiology. Surgeons performing blepharoplasty should have a surgical repertoire for ptosis correction. Careful preoperative scrutiny and patient counseling remain paramount and, in our opinion, may reduce the need for subsequent revision surgery after blepharoplasty.

Suggested Reading

[1] Baylis HI, Sutcliffe T, Fett DR. Levator injury during blepharoplasty. Arch Ophthalmol. 1984; 102(4):570–571

[2] Ben Simon GJ, Lee S, Schwarcz RM, McCann JD, Goldberg RA. External levator advancement vs Müller's muscle-conjunctival resection for correction of upper eyelid involutional ptosis. Am J Ophthalmol. 2005; 140(3):426–432

[3] Coombes AG, Sethi CS, Kirkpatrick WN, Waterhouse N, Kelly MH, Joshi N. A standardized digital photography system with computerized eyelid measurement analysis. Plast Reconstr Surg. 2007; 120(3):647–656

[4] Huang W, Rogachefsky AS, Foster JA. Browlift with botulinum toxin. Dermatol Surg. 2000; 26(1):55–60

[5] Mauriello JA. Unfavorable Results of Eyelid and Lacrimal Surgery—Prevention and Management. Boston, MA: Butterworth-Heinemann; 2000

[6] Klapper SR, Patrinely JR. Management of cosmetic eyelid surgery complications. Semin Plast Surg. 2007; 21(1):80–93

[7] Knize DM. An anatomically based study of the mechanism of eyebrow ptosis. Plast Reconstr Surg. 1996; 97(7):1321–1333

[8] Lam VB, Czyz CN, Wulc AE. The brow-eyelid continuum: an anatomic perspective. Clin Plast Surg. 2013; 40(1):1–19

[9] Love LP, Farrior EH. Periocular anatomy and aging. Facial Plast Surg Clin North Am. 2010; 18(3):411–417

[10] O'Doherty M, Joshi N. The "bespoke" upper eyelid blepharoplasty and brow rejuvenation. Facial Plast Surg. 2013; 29(4):264–272

[11] Prado RB, Silva-Junior DE, Padovani CR, Schellini SA. Assessment of eyebrow position before and after upper eyelid blepharoplasty. Orbit. 2012; 31(4):222–226

[12] Scawn R, Joshi N, Kim YD. Upper lid blepharoplasty in Asian eyes. Facial Plast Surg. 2010; 26(2):86–92

[13] Widgerow AD. Upper blepharoplasty with lateral segmental orbicularis excision. Ann Plast Surg. 2003; 50(5):471–474

[14] Yeatts RP. Current concepts in brow lift surgery. Curr Opin Ophthalmol. 1997; 8(5):46–50

15 Postblepharoplasty Lagophthalmos

H. Joon Kim

Summary

This chapter discusses the various causes and symptoms associated with lagophthalmos, with emphasis on postblepharoplasty lagophthalmos. It also summarizes the different nonsurgical and surgical treatment options for alleviating signs and symptoms associated with lagophthalmos.

Keywords: long-standing, cicatricial, blepharoplasty, trauma, facial nerve palsy, dry eyes, exposure keratopathy, full-thickness skin grafts, steroid injections, lubrication

15.1 Patient History Leading to the Specific Problem

The patient is a 67-year-old woman who underwent a bilateral upper eyelid blepharoplasty 10 years ago. She developed lagophthalmos with dry eye symptoms on the left side since the surgery (▶ Fig. 15.1). She tried conservative measures with massage and scar creams, but she had persistent symptoms of foreign body sensation, pain, itching, and redness in her left eye that only temporarily improved with artificial tears and ointments. These symptoms progressively worsened and she presented desiring correction of her lagophthalmos.

15.2 Anatomic Description of the Patient's Current Status

Lagophthalmos, or inability to fully close the eyelids, can develop from a number of causes. Paralytic lagophthalmos can result from any etiology affecting

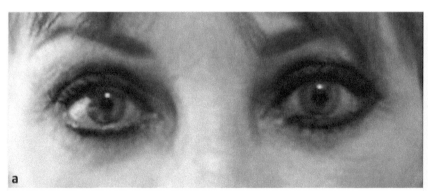
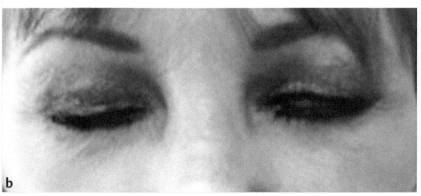

Fig. 15.1 (a) The external photograph shows that the patient has a mild left upper lid retraction, where the upper lid is higher than the ideal position. (b) The photograph shows approximately 3 mm of lagophthalmos of the left side with attempted eyelid closure.

the facial nerve, such as trauma, iatrogenic injuries to the facial nerve, cerebrovascular accidents, tumor resection, infections, or Bell's palsy. Proptosis or retraction of the eyelids can also often lead to lagophthalmos, most notably in patients with thyroid eye disease.

Cicatricial lagophthalmos often stems from trauma or surgery. In cases of postblepharoplasty lagophthalmos, aggressive skin excision is the most common cause for both upper and lower lid blepharoplasty. Although lagophthalmos appears to occur more commonly following a lower lid blepharoplasty, patients are usually more symptomatic after an upper lid blepharoplasty, likely due to more corneal exposure with upper lid involvement. Lower lid retraction and associated lagophthalmos can also result if a horizontal tightening procedure was not performed (canthopexy or canthoplasty) or if physiologic or pathologic exophthalmos was not addressed.

Cicatricial lagophthalmos from anterior lamellar insufficiency can typically be avoided by a thorough examination and careful planning. It is necessary to take into consideration the degree of forward displacement of the eyes when planning for a lower lid blepharoplasty. Exophthalmometer measurement greater than 15 mm generally necessitates an eyelid spacer graft to the lower lids in order to avoid retraction and associated lagophthalmos. Commonly used eyelid spacer grafts include porcine acellular dermal matrix (Enduragen), decellularized porcine derived membrane (TarSys), or an ear cartilage graft. When evaluating for an upper lid blepharoplasty, it is crucial to distinguish true blepharoptosis from dermatochalasis and also to take note of brow ptosis that is contributing to the dermatochalasis. Intraoperatively, excessive skin excision can be avoided by generally leaving at least 20 mm of skin on the upper lid from the brow–lid junction to the eyelid margin, when performing an upper lid blepharoplasty. This can be combined with the "pinch" technique, where the redundant skin can be gently grabbed with a forceps to estimate the amount of skin that needs to be excised (e.g., Green fixation forceps) until slight eversion of the eyelashes is noted.

Although the skin shortage often goes unnoticed when the eyelids are open, it becomes obvious with eyelid closure due to the presence of lagophthalmos. Lagophthalmos often leads to exposure keratopathy, where the surface of the eye becomes dry due to poor corneal coverage and rapid evaporation of the tears. If this progresses, it can cause infections, permanent scarring, or even perforation of the globe and blindness. The degree of lagophthalmos often correlates to the severity of the exposure keratopathy.

15.3 Recommended Solution to the Problem

- Lubrication of the eyes with artificial tears and/or ointment can always be utilized in patients with lagophthalmos with dry eye symptoms. If artificial tears need to be used on a very frequent basis (e.g., more than four times a day), it is best to use preservative-free artificial tears.
- For more severe dry eyes, moisture chamber goggles can be used at night since the eyes are most susceptible to desiccation from nocturnal lagophthalmos.
- For extremely severe cases where the globe is threatened, a tarsorrhaphy could be needed. However, this is not a sound long-term solution as this can severely limit the vision and is aesthetically unappealing.

- Steroid ointments, steroid injections, or 5-flurouracil injections coupled with massage of the lid can be tried in mild cases to relax the cicatrix. These options are most effective in the immediate postoperative phase.
- For lagophthalmos that stems from a lower lid retraction after a lower lid blepharoplasty, placing an eyelid spacer graft coupled with a canthoplasty can improve the retraction and associated lagophthalmos. This is only successful if the patient does not have a severe anterior lamellar insufficiency. Otherwise, it could result in an ectropion, or an anterior rotation, of the lower lid margin that could still necessitate a full-thickness skin graft.
- For patients with long-standing lagophthalmos that has not improved with conservative therapy, a full-thickness skin grafting procedure to the lids is the best option.

15.4 Technique

Mark the natural lid crease and infiltrate the eyelid with a local anesthetic (▶ Fig. 15.2). A blade can be used to incise the skin and the orbicularis at the marked site. Dissect posteriorly to open up the septum. It is critical to open the septum across the entire length of the eyelid to ensure that anterior lamellar scar has been lysed and the full extent of the defect can be appreciated. Otherwise, the graft can be undersized with incomplete resolution of the lagophthalmos. Measure the anterior lamellar defect at this time (▶ Fig. 15.3). Attention is then turned to the retroauricular harvest site. This is an ideal donor site due to similarities in color and thickness to the eyelids. It is usually smooth without hair, readily available, and in a hidden location. Other possible donor sites include the contralateral eyelid, but typically the supply is limited and can result in asymmetry. The supraclavicular region is also another potential site that is a good match, but the scar is more visible. Mark the size of the graft that is needed and infiltrate with a local anesthetic. About 30% of the graft can contract during the healing process, so it is ideal to oversize the graft. A full-thickness skin graft is harvested and the harvest site is closed with a running subcuticular 4–0 Vicryl suture (▶ Fig. 15.4). The skin graft is then sutured into the defect with a 6–0 fast-absorbing gut suture (▶ Fig. 15.5). A Telfa bolster is then sutured over the skin graft with a 4–0 silk suture. The bolster is removed 5 days postoperatively.

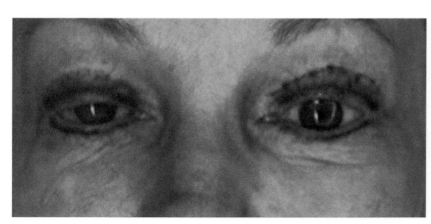

Fig. 15.2 The intraoperative photograph demonstrates the incision site on the left upper lid crease.

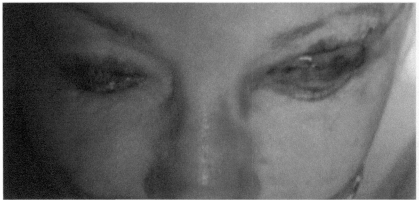

Fig. 15.3 The dissection has been performed through the skin, orbicularis oculi, and septum with scar lysis revealing the size of the anterior lamellar defect measuring approximately 10 mm vertically and 25 mm horizontally.

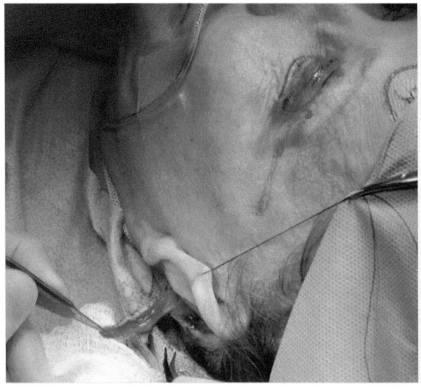

Fig. 15.4 A retroauricular full-thickness skin graft is being harvested followed by closure of the harvest site with a running subcuticular 4–0 Vicryl (not pictured).

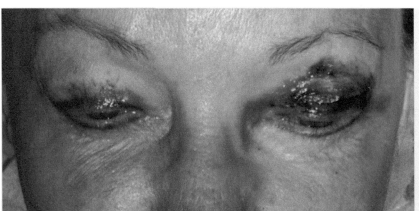

Fig. 15.5 A full-thickness skin graft has been shaped and sized accordingly to fit the defect and sutured into place with a running 6–0 fast-absorbing gut. A Telfa bolster is sutured onto the skin graft for viability (not pictured).

15.5 Postoperative Photographs and Critical Evaluation of Results

The photographs demonstrate the skin graft 3 weeks postoperatively with complete resolution of the lagophthalmos and dry eye symptoms. The lid height is also more symmetric to the contralateral side as the left upper lid is no longer retracted superiorly. As expected, there is residual swelling of the eyelid (as this will take about 2–3 months to resolve) and the graft still looks thickened. The skin graft on average can take about 3 to 6 months to heal, if not longer, in some patients. Massage and use of steroid cream (or other scar creams) can facilitate a more rapid recovery (▶ Fig. 15.6).

15.6 Teaching Points

- Lagophthalmos, or inability to fully close the eyelids, can result from excessive skin removal during an upper or lower lid blepharoplasty or failing to address exophthalmos when performing a lower lid blepharoplasty.
- Lagophthalmos can result in exposure keratopathy and significant discomfort to the patient and, in severe cases, can lead to infections and blindness.

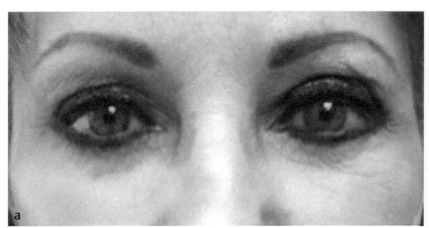

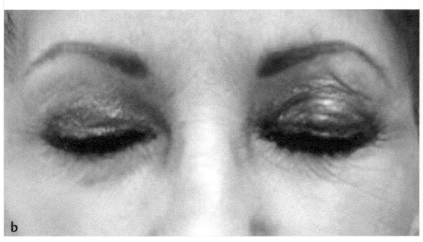

Fig. 15.6 (a) Clinical photograph shows the patient 3 weeks after the full-thickness skin graft to the left upper lid. As anticipated, she still has some edema to the left upper and lower lids but the upper lid is no longer retracted. **(b)** She is also able to close her left eye fully without any lagophthalmos, as shown. The graft is slightly thickened but the appearance will improve over the next 3 to 6 months.

- Lagophthalmos from skin shortage can be avoided by leaving behind at least 20 mm of skin on the upper lid from the brow–lid junction to the lid margin.
- Mild cases of lagophthalmos can be treated with massage, steroid creams or injections, or 5-fluorouracil injections.
- In severe or long-standing cases of lagophthalmos, a full-thickness skin graft is needed to replace the skin shortage and resolve the lagophthalmos.
- Anterior lamellar scar lysis needs to be performed at the level of the septum and the skin graft slightly oversized in order to fully resolve the lagophthalmos.

Suggested Reading

[1] Shorr N, Goldberg RA, McCann JD, Hoenig JA, Li TG. Upper eyelid skin grafting: an effective treatment for lagophthalmos following blepharoplasty. Plast Reconstr Surg. 2003; 112(5):1444–1448

[2] Wilson MC, Groth MJ, Baylis HI. Complications of upper blepharoplasty. In: Putterman AM, ed. Cosmetic Oculoplastic Surgery. 3rd ed. Philadelphia, PA: Saunders; 1993:349

16 Correction of Upper Blepharoplasty Overresection

Oren Tepper, Sergei Kalsow, Elizabeth B. Jelks, and Glenn W. Jelks

Summary

Revision surgery due to overresection of skin and/or fat continues to be a relatively common indication for secondary blepharoplasty. Overresection of skin and/or fat in the upper eyelid leads to a hollowed appearance, which creates not only an overoperated look, but also one of aging. Similar issues of hollowness can occur with overresection of lower eyelid fat, whereas overresection of lower eyelid skin can lead to the dreaded complication of lower eyelid malposition. This chapter discusses correction of common problems associated with overresection in blepharoplasty, and reviews surgical techniques for correction of this secondary deformity.

Keywords: overresection, secondary blepharoplasty, upper eyelid hollowing, lower eyelid hollowing, augmentation blepharoplasty

16.1 Patient History Leading to the Specific Problem

The patient is a 53-year-old woman who presented following an upper lid blepharoplasty elsewhere 2 years prior to presentation. She expressed concerns for an "unnatural" appearance. She felt that she looked "overoperated" and was seeking correction of the appearance of her upper eyelids.

16.2 Anatomic Description of the Patient's Current Status

The patient's upper orbits have a hollowed-out appearance. The hollowing is most apparent medially, producing an A-frame deformity. The skeletonized nature of her deformity accentuates the visibility and prominence of her superior orbital rim. This results in an overall aged and deflated appearance despite her initial goals of looking younger from a blepharoplasty (▶Fig. 16.1).

16.3 Analysis of the Problem

Overresection is a relatively common problem after traditional blepharoplasty due to traditional concepts that emphasize resection of excess skin, muscle, and fat. Laxity and gravitational descent will cause excessive hanging and bulging of tissues in most patients who present for blepharoplasty, but deflation is also a major component of periorbital aging. These bulging tissues often mask the loss of volume, and thus during resection of the apparent "excess" tissue, the surgery contributes to an even greater loss of volume. This only exacerbates the continued deflation that occurs with further aging and increases the risk of skeletonization of the orbit and development of a hollowed-out cadaveric appearance.

The following elements lead to formation of the undesired deep excavation of supraorbital area:
- Overresection of medial and central fat pads will create a central hollow.
- Overresection of preseptal orbicularis muscle will expose superior orbital rim.

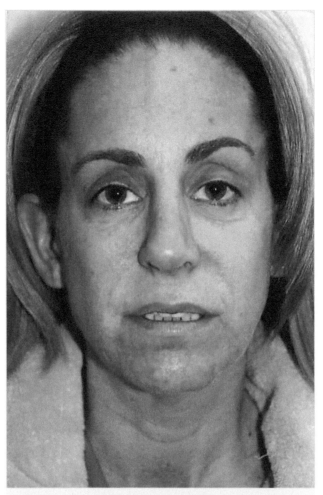

Fig. 16.1 The patient's upper eyelids demonstrate a skeletonized appearance due to overresection of skin and fat from a prior blepharoplasty.

- Overresection of lower fat pads will reduce total amount of fat in the orbit, allow eyeball to sink down, and translate to upper hollowness indirectly.

Avoidance of overresection of volume, which often corresponds to fat, should be a priority in any operation. The surgeon's goal should be to address the apparent excess of tissues while remembering deflation is a central characteristic of the aging eye. If the surgeon pursues a *fat resection* approach, one technique that may be helpful to avoid overresection is to press on the globe during the operation to allow preaponeurotic fat to bulge. The end point of fat resection should not extend beyond the point of resecting preaponeurotic fat back into the orbit. The surgeon should distinguish excess fat that delivers itself from fat that needs to be surgically manipulated and pulled, and focus on excising the former.

Fat preservation approaches have also been described to avoid overresection. One method uses bipolar coagulation (BICO) to reduce the pseudoherniation of bulging fat. The technique simply makes a small incision through skin and preseptal orbicularis muscle to expose the orbital septum and underlying fat. BICO is then applied to the septum to cause shrinkage and disappearance of bulging subseptal fat analogous to "hernia repair." Of note, the authors do not strictly rely on bipolar instruments for this technique, but do feel that coagulation in general can be a valuable means of camouflaging such bulges without traditional resection of fat.

16.4 Recommended Solution to the Problem

The surgical solution to overresection following upper blepharoplasty is volume replacement. This can be accomplished through
- Autologous free fat grafting.
- Hyaluronic acid fillers.
- Orbital fat transposition flap.
- Dermofat graft.

Each option offers unique advantages that should be discussed with the patient and matched to the specific deformity. Regardless of treatment method, all will be affected by previous surgical scarring and iatrogenically altered anatomy.

Autologous fat grafting has long been the mainstay for volume augmentation in our practice, as it is a natural filler that avoids rejection, sensitivity reactions, sterile abscesses, or nodules and has minimal donor-site morbidity. Hyaluronic acid fillers offer an alternative to free fat grafts to provide volume to the overresected postblepharoplasty scenario. These fillers are injected into the subcutaneous or suborbicularis fat, and varying compositions for this have been described, such as Restylane, which may provide greater projection compared to more liquid formulations such as Juvederm, but require more molding. The typical volume required per brow is 0.5 to 1 mL, and in general, too much volume looks worse than does too little. Injections are made parallel to the brow and stop at the inferior border of the supraorbital rim. Visible and palpable irregularities are a concern, and can be addressed with massage, blending injections, or, ultimately, hyaluronidase. Duration of benefit varies among patients, but has been reported to exceed up to 2 years with approximately 10% of patients requiring additional small-volume injections during that time (►Fig. 16.2).

Orbital fat transposition flaps and dermofat grafts have also been described for surgical management of the overresected postblepharoplasty patients. Orbital fat transposition involves rotating the lateral end of the central fat pad 180 degrees to fill volume in the medial region. This procedure may provide only limited benefit for minor volume deficiencies as most overresected eyes have little remaining preaponeurotic fat pads. A dermofat graft may be a better option when the volume deficiency is more severe and involves a visible bony orbital rim. These can be harvested as a full-thickness piece of dermis with a thin layer of subcutaneous fat from the intergluteal crease, de-epithelialized, and placed between the orbital fat sac and orbicularis oculi muscle below the supraorbital rim. The resorption rate is estimated to be only approximately 10 to 20%. Overcorrection with excessive graft weight may impair eye opening and create a ptotic appearance. This usually resolves naturally in 10 to 14 days with full resolution by 2 to 3 months.

As mentioned earlier, the authors feel autologous fat grafting should be the gold standard of treatment for correction of this deformity. When considering factors such as reliability, risk, invasiveness, and longevity, we feel that autologous fat grafting provides the most superior treatment method.

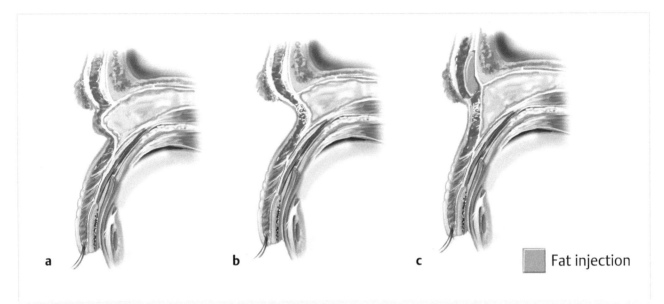

Fat injection

Fig. 16.2 **(a)** The cross-sectional illustration of a typical preoperative contour of the upper eyelid and superior orbit is shown. Note the volume in the superior orbit is provided by pretarsal orbicularis muscle, anterior positioned orbital septum, and preaponeurotic fat. **(b)** Cross-sectional illustration of a typical postoperative situation with overresection of the upper eyelid preaponeurotic fat, scar tissue within the pretarsal orbicularis oculi muscle, and associated contraction producing the upper eyelid orbital-palpebral sulcus deformity. **(c)** Cross-sectional illustration of fat injection to the correct superior orbital palpebral sulcus deformity. The injected fat is placed with a small caliber (20 gauge), blunt tip, side port cannula above the superior orbital rim periosteum and behind the orbital and pretarsal orbicularis oculi muscles. The orbital septum is not disrupted, and the fat is not placed within the orbit.

16.5 Technique

Correction involves replacement of volume. The goal is a smooth contour of the upper lid, correction of the sunken eyelid appearance, and elimination of the visible superior orbit. The harvested fat is deposited between the skin and the periorbital septum. It is not placed retroseptally, where the original fat was overresected, but anterior to the septum. One has to be careful not to overcorrect, so serial fat grafting is often recommended.

Fat grafting can be unpredictable. Even if one distributes the fat evenly, one cannot say that the fat will survive evenly. Thus, fat grafting can lead to irregularity. Alternatively, filler material such as Restylane or Belotero can be used.

16.6 Postoperative Photographs and Critical Evaluation of Results

Postoperative result illustrates a smoother and more natural upper lid contour. The fullness is restored, and the superior orbital rim is no longer as visible. As a result, the deformity is corrected, and the patient's eyes look more youthful, lighter, and softer (▶ Fig. 16.3).

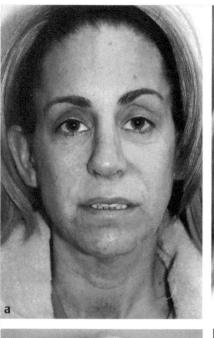
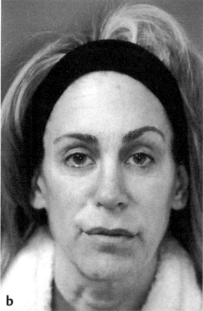
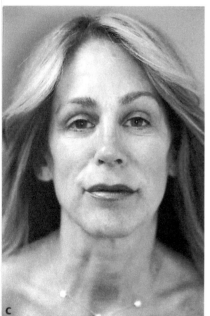
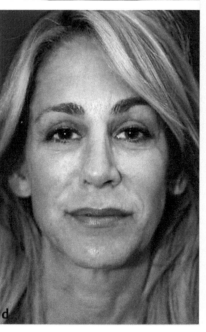

Fig. 16.3 (a–d) Photographs show the progression of the patient's condition after three sessions of lipostructure volume replacement to the upper eyelid. Sessions 1, 2, and 3 took place over the course of 32 months, with session 1 initially, session 2 at 25 months, and session 3 at 32 months. Also of note, the patient had lipostructural compartmental fat grafting for facial volume deficiency. This has created improvement in facial volume, which complements the superior orbital palpebral sulcus deformity treatment.

16.7 Teaching Points

- Aging of periorbital area involves not only gravitational descent but also deflation.
- Be aware of an already deficient tissue volume around the eyes while performing blepharoplasty.
- End point of fat resection is mild protrusion of fat while the globe is pressed.
- Consider fat-preserving techniques, such as skin and muscle excision with simple coagulation around mild areas of bulging septum.

- Treatment of hollowed-out appearance involves replacement of volume in specific locations in correct amounts.
- Volume can be replaced with autologous fat grafting, hyaluronic acid filler materials (Restylane, Juvederm, Belotero), orbital fat transpositioning, or dermofat.
- Safe injection techniques should be practiced that minimize risk of intravascular injection.

Suggested Reading

[1] Hardy TG, Joshi N, Kelly MH. Orbital volume augmentation with autologous micro-fat grafts. Ophthal Plast Reconstr Surg. 2007; 23(6):445–449

[2] Jeon MS, Jung GY, Lee DL, Shin HK. Correction of sunken upper eyelids by anchoring the central fat pad to the medial fat pad during upper blepharoplasty. Arch Plast Surg. 2015; 42(4):469–474

[3] Lambros V. Observations on periorbital and midface aging. Plast Reconstr Surg. 2007; 120(5):1367–1376, discussion 1377

[4] Lambros V. Volumizing the brow with hyaluronic acid fillers. Aesthet Surg J. 2009; 29(3):174–179

[5] Lee W, Kwon SB, Oh SK, Yang EJ. Correction of sunken upper eyelid with orbital fat transposition flap and dermofat graft. J Plast Reconstr Aesthet Surg. 2017; 70(12):1768–1775

[6] Morley AMS, Taban M, Malhotra R, Goldberg RA. Use of hyaluronic acid gel for upper eyelid filling and contouring. Ophthal Plast Reconstr Surg. 2009; 25(6):440–444

[7] Ramil MR. Fat grafting the hollow upper eyelids and volumetric upper blepharoplasty. Plast Reconstr Surg. 2017;140:889-897

[8] Rohrich RJ, Coberly DM, Fagien S, Stuzin JM. Current concepts in aesthetic upper blepharoplasty. Plast Reconstr Surg. 2004; 113(3):32e–42e

[9] Romeo F. Upper eyelid filling with or without surgical treatment. Aesthetic Plast Surg. 2016; 40(2):223–235

[10] Rose JG, Jr, Lucarelli MJ, Lemke BN, et al. Histologic comparison of autologous fat processing methods. Ophthal Plast Reconstr Surg. 2006; 22(3):195–200

[11] Tonnard PL, Verpaele AM, Zeltzer AA. Augmentation blepharoplasty: a review of 500 consecutive patients. Aesthet Surg J. 2013; 33(3):341–352

[12] van der Lei B, Timmerman ISK, Cromheecke M, Hofer SOP. Bipolar coagulation-assisted orbital (BICO) septoblepharoplasty: a retrospective analysis of a new fat-saving upper-eyelid blepharoplasty technique. Ann Plast Surg. 2007; 59(3):263–267

17 Upper Blepharoplasty Overresection

Hisham Seify

Summary

Upper eyelid overresection could often be seen in consultation, and patients frequently request for removal of additional skin. The essential step is the proper diagnosis and the remedy is to reconstruct the missing tissues by adding fat or other fillers.

Keywords: A-frame deformity, upper blepharoplasty, fat grafting, upper lid fat overresection

17.1 Patient History Leading to the Specific Problem

The patient is a 60-year-old white woman who underwent bilateral upper eyelid blepharoplasty 2 years ago (▶ Fig. 17.1). She presented requesting more skin removal for a "tighter" upper eyelid.

17.2 Anatomical Analysis of the Patient's Current Condition

The patient demonstrates asymmetric hollowness of the upper eyelid (A-frame deformity). The most common cause is overresection of the central fat pad and orbicularis muscle during her initial blepharoplasty. The patient's request was initially to remove more skin to obtain a tighter upper eye lid. In this case, removal of more tissues will lead to worsening of the deformity. The condition could be remedied with addition of tissues to the upper lid. Options for reconstruction include injectable fillers, dermis fat graft, or fat graft. Fat grafting was recommended to her as the best option. The volume of fat needed will vary per side due to the existing asymmetry.

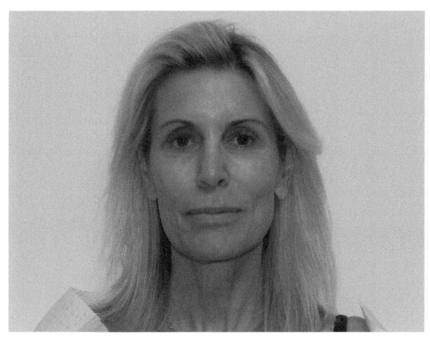

Fig. 17.1 This patient is a 60-year-old white woman who underwent bilateral upper eyelid blepharoplasty 2 years ago. She is presenting with A-frame deformity.

17.3 Recommended Solution to the Problem

- Asymmetric fat injection to the upper lid (right more than left).

17.4 Technique

The procedure could be done under local or general anesthesia. In this case, the patient was undergoing additional procedures, so it was performed under general anesthesia.

Local anesthesia is injected along the superior orbital margins, 1 to 1.5 mL on each side. Preoperative pictures are used as a guide during the injection. The operative plan is to inject 2 mL on the right and 1.5 mL on the left side. In the preoperative consult, saline with lidocaine could be used to demonstrate the effect of the injection to the patient.

The fat is harvested from the abdominal area after infiltration of tumescent fluid (500 mL of saline, 50 mL of lidocaine, 0.5 mL of epinephrine 1:1,000). Only 250 mL were infiltrated in the abdominal area. The fluid was allowed to settle for 20 minutes before harvesting. The harvesting was done using the Tulip system (2-mm cannula) (▶Fig. 17.2). The fat was allowed to settle for separation of the fluid component; this portion is discarded before the injection. Transfer the fat between two syringes to allow a homogeneous filler to be obtained and to avoid lumps (microfat grafting). Centrifuge, PureGraft, or any other method could be used as a way to prepare the fat for injection depending on the surgeon's practice.

A 0.9-mm blunt Tulip fat grafting cannula is used for periorbital injection. The skin puncture is done using an 18-G needle to avoid any incisions. The injection is done along the superior orbital margin (▶Fig. 17.3). It is aimed above the septum to minimize complications. It is done using the right hand in a retrograde manner to avoid injection into a blood vessel. The left hand is used to blend the fat along the undersurface of the bony orbit. A slight overcorrection is aimed for without creating any irregularities, which could be

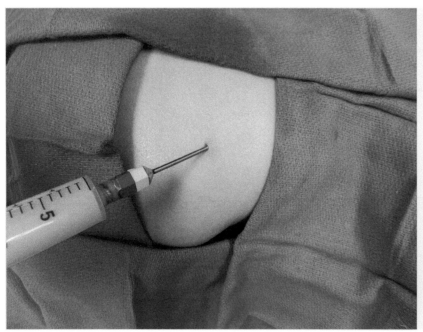

Fig. 17.2 Harvesting of the fat using a 2-mm cannula.

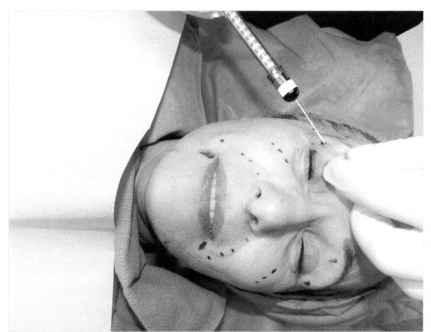

Fig. 17.3 Injection into the superior orbital sulcus using a 0.9-mm cannula.

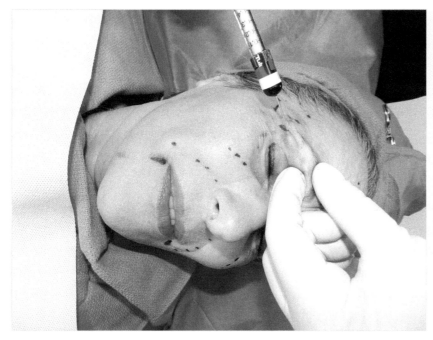

Fig. 17.4 The injection is done in a retrograde manner; the left hand is used to guide the injection and avoid any irregularities.

difficult to correct. Injection directly into the eyelid skin should be avoided and will lead to postinjection bumps (▶ Fig. 17.4).

17.5 Postoperative Photographs and Critical Evaluation of Results

The patient now has a more cosmetic appearance of her upper eyelid without skin removal (▶ Fig. 17.5). We also offered her to add more, especially on the right side, but she was pleased with this result.

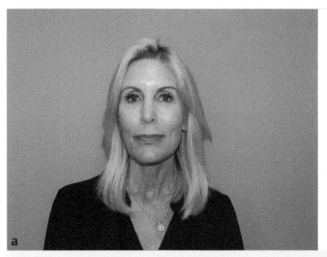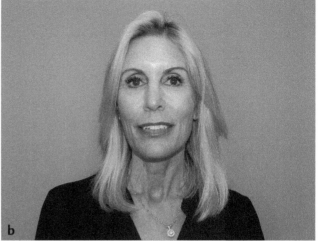

Fig. 17.5 (a,b) The patient's post-op pictures following correction with 2 mL on the right and 1.5 mL on the left.

17.6 Teaching Points

- A-frame deformity is more commonly caused by excessive removal of fat and muscle during upper blepharoplasty.
- In some cases, the condition could present as if there is excess skin and request for additional removal of skin should not be entertained without proper evaluation of the condition.
- From a technical standpoint, fat or hyaluronic acid filler could be used. Using a blunt needle with the retrograde injection technique is preferred in order to avoid inadvertent vascular injection.
- Slight overcorrection should be the goal while avoiding any bumps or irregularities.
- In the case of overcorrection, early massage of the filler should be done. If the patient presents later with bumps, the condition should be evaluated for injection with 5 FU or dilute steroids. In extreme cases, surgical removal could be done.
- Fat grafting is not an exact science. It is very difficult to access the amount of fat that will eventually survive. The aim for overcorrection should be carefully balanced with a conservative approach to avoid complications. The patient should be counseled that additional injections could be needed.

Suggested Reading

[1] Goldwyn R, Cohen M. The Unfavorable Result in Plastic Surgery: Avoidance and Treatment. 3rd ed. Philadelphia, PA: Lippincott; 2001
[2] Persichetti P, Di Lella F, Delfino S, Scuderi N. Adipose compartments of the upper eyelid: anatomy applied to blepharoplasty. Plast Reconstr Surg. 2004; 113(1):373–378, discussion 379–380
[3] Kane MAC. Nonsurgical periorbital and brow rejuvenation. Plast Reconstr Surg. 2015; 135(1):63–71
[4] Pacella SJ, Nahai FR, Nahai F. Transconjunctival blepharoplasty for upper and lower eyelids. Plast Reconstr Surg. 2010; 125(1):384–392
[5] Lindenblatt N, van Hulle A, Verpaele AM, Tonnard PL. The role of microfat grafting in facial contouring. Aesthet Surg J. 2015; 35(7):763–771
[6] Seify H, Roderick, Hester T. The use of microfat grafting in periorbital rejuvenation: review of 100 consecutive facelifts: 24. Plast Reconstr Surg. 2005; 116(3, Suppl):31–32

18 Underresection of Skin and Fat in Blepharoplasty

Oren Tepper, Brian Mikolasko, Elizabeth B. Jelks, and Glenn W. Jelks

Summary

Underresection of skin and/or fat following blepharoplasty is a relatively common complaint necessitating secondary surgery. The incidence of patients with underresection may be exacerbated by recent trends favoring more conservative approaches to blepharoplasty. This chapter discusses relevant periorbital surgical anatomy and presents approaches to address residual excess skin and fat.

Keywords: underresection, secondary blepharoplasty, transconjunctival, lateral fat, medial fat, eyelid fullness

18.1 Patient History Leading to the Specific Periorbital Problem

A patient, who underwent prior upper and lower eyelid blepharoplasty, was unhappy with her postoperative results, and was bothered by the persistent "fullness" in both the upper and lower eyelids (▶ Fig. 18.1).

18.2 Anatomic Description of the Patient's Current Status

The patient's conditions at the time of presentation can be best characterized by the following:
- Residual upper eyelid fullness due to excess skin and residual medial fat.
- Persistent lower lateral fat.

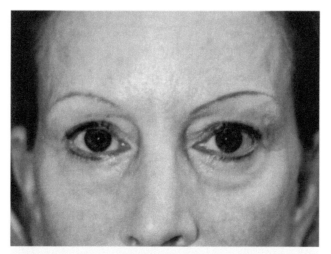

Fig. 18.1 The patient had a previous upper and lower primary blepharoplasty. She was bothered by excess fullness medially on the upper lids, a feeling of persistent heaviness laterally, and irregular contour at the eyelid–cheek junction owing to persistent lower lateral compartment fat.

18.2.1 Analysis

Unsatisfactory results from blepharoplasty can generally be divided into one of two conditions: (1) overresection or (2) underresection. This chapter describes problem scenarios that result from underresection following upper and lower blepharoplasty. The true incidence of secondary blepharoplasty is not entirely known, but in one series of nearly 1,000 blepharoplasties over a 20-year period, the rate of secondary blepharoplasty was found to be 10%. Reasons for secondary blepharoplasty include dermatochalasis, blepharoptosis, and general dissatisfaction from primary blepharoplasty.

The issues highlighted by the above patient represent relatively common complaints/deformities in patients who have undergone previous upper blepharoplasty. For the upper eyelid, it is not uncommon to see redundant skin laterally and inadequate resection of nasal fat. In the lower eyelids, fat persists most often in the lower lateral fat compartments.

Persistent Upper Eyelid Skin

Persistent fullness in the upper eyelid can be a common complaint following primary upper blepharoplasty and is most commonly seen laterally. Anatomically, fullness develops with age due to a tendency of central upper eyelid fat to shift laterally and lateral excess skin's absence of fixation to the tarsal plate. This can be further exacerbated by decreasing frontalis support of the temporal brow and, infrequently, lacrimal gland prolapse. These anatomical changes need to be considered when evaluating patients for both primary and secondary blepharoplasty. In addition, it is also essential that the surgeon be aware of eyebrow position and function, particularly the potential role of compensatory brow elevation. Dermatochalasis and significant temporal hooding are often compensated for by elevating the forehead in an attempt to maintain maximal vision.

Excess upper eyelid skin following blepharoplasty may be due to a number of factors, including difficulty in judging the extent of skin resection as well as limiting the most lateral extent of the incision. Furthermore, brow ptosis may be the culprit in some cases, and may be the result of preexisting or new-onset brow ptosis, such as can occur following Botox therapy. For this reason, it is important to inquire about the Botox status/history of such patients. Of note, underresection can typically be differentiated from brown ptosis by a true excess of skin folds.

Persistent Upper Eyelid Fat

Upper eyelid preaponeurotic fat lives in one of two compartments, central or medial. The central fat pad tends to atrophy with age, while the denser and more stem cell–rich medial fat pad is an extension from deeper orbital fat and tends to become more prominent with age, even after primary blepharoplasty.

Underresection of upper eyelid fat may be seen following primary blepharoplasty, and is most commonly associated with the medial fat compartment. From a technical perspective, this makes sense, as medial fat is typically more difficult to visualize and dissect during upper blepharoplasty. Although nasal fat can often be distinguished by its unique pale "whitish" color, it is important that surgeons identify and remove any excess fat in this distinct compartment during blepharoplasty.

Interestingly, the recent emphasis on fat preservation techniques in upper blepharoplasty may also be increasing the likelihood of "underresected" fat in upper blepharoplasty procedures. As surgeons grow increasingly concerned with avoiding hollowness and skeletonization, overly conservative results are a possible outcome.

Persistent Lower Eyelid Fat

Persistent lateral compartment fat is among the most common findings requiring secondary lower blepharoplasty. One interesting phenomenon with age is the development of pseudoherniation of lower eyelid fat pads, predominately in the lateral aspect, which may result from globe descent inferiorly and laterally in the orbit. In older patients, specifically, atrophic soft tissue coverage further exacerbates contour irregularities to create a fullness that interrupts what ideally should be a single mildly convex line in the sagittal view that defines the youthful eyelid–cheek complex.

The lower lateral fat pocket is prone to underresection during primary blepharoplasty for reasons similar to those noted earlier, including recent trends in conservative blepharoplasty as well as an anatomical location that is relatively challenging to access and identify, particularly so in the transconjunctival approach. Furthermore, recent approaches favoring fat preservation or transposition may also contribute to the risk of persistent lateral fat. For example, some surgeons now favor medial and central fat repositioning techniques, whereby these compartments are mobilized along with redundant septum and transpositioned into a subperiosteal pocket. Notably, this cannot be accomplished with the lateral fat compartment as it is located just above the Lockwood ligament and lacks adequate mobility to be repositioned.

18.3 Recommended Solution to the Problem

- Like all secondary procedures, surgeons must consider unique challenges that result from incisional scars, internal scarring affecting lamellae, and iatrogenically altered anatomy.
- If the problem involves a component of brow ptosis, this should be further discussed with the patient regarding surgical and nonsurgical lift options.
- Residual upper eyelid excess fat and skin should be addressed through a prior upper blepharoplasty incision.
- Residual lower eyelid lateral fat can be removed through the same upper blepharoplasty incision approach.
- Excess skin can removed via a skin pinch procedure with relative ease and safety.

18.3.1 Upper Eyelid Skin

When correcting excess lateral upper eyelid skin, the surgeon should not simply rely on a standard crescent-shaped incision used in primary blepharoplasty since it tends to be the widest at the center and may not adequately address excess fullness from lateral. In this type of scenario, the surgeon should consider an incision that is more "scalpel-shaped," with the widest portion occurring laterally and tapering medially. This tends to take on the shape of a 20-scalpel blade and runs along the supratarsal crease inferiorly, extends laterally in a natural crease just below and slightly past the lateral extent of the eyebrow, and ends medially approximately 1 cm above and lateral to the canthus. Older patients may see an improvement in crow's feet related to position of the lateral suture line, but in younger patients without such natural creases this will leave a visible suture line (▶Fig. 18.2).

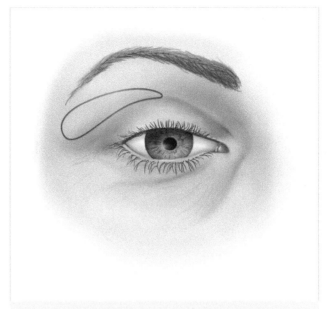

Fig. 18.2 A modified upper eyelid skin excision. Note that the incision is tailored to the patient's specific deformity so that the lateral portion of excess is incorporated.

18.3.2 Upper Eyelid Fat

Upper eyelid fat can be resected through the same initial upper eyelid incision. Once excess skin is removed using needle tip electrocautery, an additional strip of orbicularis oculi may be excised if needed. In cases in which no further skin excision is necessary, but excess fat must be removed, a minor stab incision can be made through skin, muscle, and septum to access underresected fat.

Alternately, an isolated nasal fat pocket may be addressed through the transconjunctival approach. This technique avoids visible scarring and dissection through scarred tissues while preserving the orbital septum. It is performed through a medial incision 3 to 4 mm above the tarsal margin and continued through the conjunctiva until excess fat is visualized. Determining adequate resection can be slightly more difficult, but this approach offers a safe and effective method to address isolated upper medial fullness in the previously operated patient.

Regardless of the approach, excessive fat removal from either compartment will exacerbate the aged appearance of the eye. Thus, the medial fat pad should only be minimally sculpted with an understanding that overresection will leave a hollowed-out, skeletonlike appearance. To avoid overresection, the end point of resection should be mild protrusion of fat when the globe is gently pressed (▶ Fig. 18.3).

18.3.3 Lower Eyelid Fat

The anatomy of the lower eyelid makes it a particularly challenging area to operate, necessitating both aesthetic and functional considerations prior to any approach. In our practice, we favor excision of lower eyelid lateral fat through the upper blepharoplasty incision. A blunt scissor and fine point

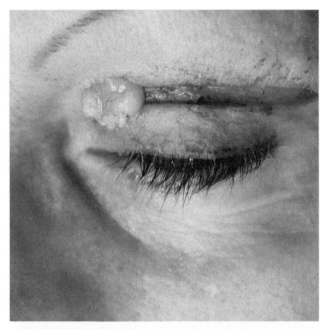

Fig. 18.3 Excision of upper eyelid medial compartment fat was removed from this patient via the prior upper blepharoplasty incision.

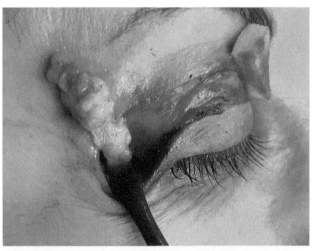

Fig. 18.4 Demonstration of technique of upper eyelid access to the lower lateral fat compartment. If a previous upper eyelid incision exists, or the patient is having a concomitant upper eyelid procedure, this lower eyelid fat compartment can easily be accessed and visualized through an upper eyelid approach. Of note, this approach can also be used to perform canthal tightening procedures.

electrosurgical dissection are used to elevate a 1- to 2-cm submuscular, supraperiosteal skin and muscle flap around the lateral canthus and lower eyelid. The flap begins from the inferior border of the lateral edge of the upper eyelid incision and is elevated using an insulated Desmarres retractor until the lateral retinaculum is visualized. The lower lateral fat compartment is covered by septum just below the lateral retinaculum and excess fat will bulge when gentle pressure is applied to the globe. Resection should again be conservative, as excessive fat removal will leave a hollowed appearance. Removal of as small as 0.5 mL of fat can result in visible changes, and some believe this is due to the globe shifting up and posteriorly. Ultimately, the goal is to gently remove fat with forceps and electrocautery while creating an appropriate contour (▶ Fig. 18.4).

18.4 Postoperative Photographs

(▶ Fig. 18.5)

18.5 Teaching Points

- Underresection of skin in the upper eyelid is most commonly a problem laterally.
- Underresection of fat in the upper eyelid is most commonly a problem medially.
- Underresection of fat in the lower eyelid is most commonly a problem laterally.
- Evaluation of persistent upper eyelid fullness following blepharoplasty should distinguish between dermatochalasis and brow ptosis.
- Excess lateral upper eyelid skin can be resected by extending both the incision and its widest point laterally.

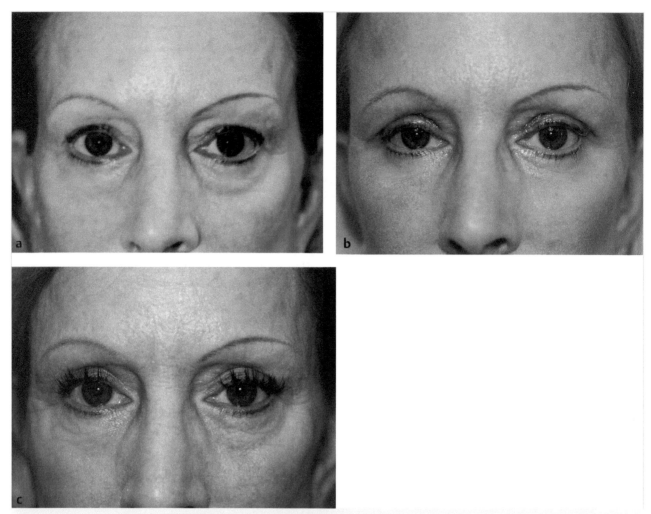

Fig. 18.5 Our patient is shown at **(a)** initial presentation and **(b)** 1 week and **(c)** 1 year following secondary blepharoplasty. Note the improvement in the upper eyelid crease with additional resection of lateral skin. The lower lateral fat compartments also show decreased fullness following resection of excess fat with a softer, more youthful transition at the eyelid–cheek junction.

- Isolated upper eyelid nasal fat can be addressed in secondary blepharoplasty through a transconjunctival approach.
- While the lower eyelid transconjunctival approach in primary blepharoplasty is an effective approach with decreased risk of eyelid malposition, it may increase rates of residual fat in the lateral compartment owing to issues with visualization and access.
- Excess lower eyelid lateral fat lacks the mobility to be repositioned, in contrast to the medial and central fat pads, and, as a result, should be resected.
- Lower lateral eyelid fat can be resected through the upper blepharoplasty incision with relative ease.

Suggested Reading

[1] Baker S, LaFerriere K, Larrabee WF, Jr. Lower lid blepharoplasty: panel discussion, controversies, and techniques. Facial Plast Surg Clin North Am. 2014; 22(1):97–118

[2] Hahn S, Holds JB, Couch SM. Upper lid blepharoplasty. Facial Plast Surg Clin North Am. 2016; 24(2):119–127

[3] Har-Shai Y, Hirshowitz B. Extended upper blepharoplasty for lateral hooding of the upper eyelid using a scalpel-shaped excision: a 13-year experience. Plast Reconstr Surg. 2004; 113(3):1028–1035, discussion 1036

[4] Honrado CP, Pastorek NJ. Long-term results of lower-lid suspension blepharoplasty: a 30-year experience. Arch Facial Plast Surg. 2004; 6(3):150–154

[5] Januszkiewicz JS, Nahai F. Transconjunctival upper blepharoplasty. Plast Reconstr Surg. 1999; 103(3):1015–1018, discussion 1019

[6] Jelks GW, Glat PM, Jelks EB, Longaker MT. The inferior retinacular lateral canthoplasty: a new technique. Plast Reconstr Surg. 1997; 100(5):1262–1270, discussion 1271–1275

[7] Korn BS, Kikkawa DO, Hicok KC. Identification and characterization of adult stem cells from human orbital adipose tissue. Ophthal Plast Reconstr Surg. 2009; 25(1):27–32

[8] Mendelson BC, Luo D. Secondary upper lid blepharoplasty: a clinical series using the tarsal fixation technique. Plast Reconstr Surg. 2015; 135(3):508e–516e

[9] Mullins JB, Holds JB, Branham GH, Thomas JR. Complications of the transconjunctival approach. A review of 400 cases. Arch Otolaryngol Head Neck Surg. 1997; 123(4):385–388

[10] Murri M, Hamill EB, Hauck MJ, Marx DP. An update on lower lid blepharoplasty. Semin Plast Surg. 2017; 31(1):46–50

[11] Rohrich RJ, Coberly DM, Fagien S, Stuzin JM. Current concepts in aesthetic upper blepharoplasty. Plast Reconstr Surg. 2004; 113(3):32e–42e

[12] Stanciu NA, Nakra T. Revision blepharoplasty. Clin Plast Surg. 2013; 40(1):179–189

[13] Whipple KM, Lim LH, Korn BS, Kikkawa DO. Blepharoplasty complications: prevention and management. Clin Plast Surg. 2013; 40(1):213–224

[14] Wong CH, Mendelson B. Extended transconjunctival lower eyelid blepharoplasty with release of the tear trough ligament and fat redistribution. Plast Reconstr Surg. 2017; 140(2):273–282

19 Coronal Foreheadplasty Improves Periorbital Appearance and Rejuvenation Not Achieved by Facial and Eyelidplasties Alone

Jack A. Friedland

Summary

A foreheadplasty should be considered to correct deformities and signs of aging of the forehead and periorbital region, which cannot be adequately treated by facial and eyelidplasties alone.

Keywords: foreheadplasty, periorbital rejuvenation, eyelidplasty, facialplasty, transverse furrows of the forehead, glabellar frown lines, brow ptosis

19.1 Patient History Leading to the Specific Problem

This 64-year-old woman desired aesthetic facial surgical rejuvenation (▶ Fig. 19.1). She was overweight and said that she had tried but could not lose any weight. She accepted her status and wished to proceed with surgery. Though she was advised to undergo forehead surgery as well as eyelid and facialplasties, she opted to only have the latter, which included bilateral lateral canthoplasties and a perioral dermabrasion.

19.2 Anatomic Description and the Patient's Current Status

The patient was initially pleased with the results of surgery, but within a month she became unhappy due to the continued presence of drooping brows, transverse furrows of her forehead, vertical glabellar frown lines, and transverse creases across the radix of her nose and the glabellar region of her forehead (▶ Fig. 19.2).

19.2.1 Analysis of the Problem

An open coronal foreheadplasty was recommended to correct the residual deformities, in spite of the fact that the patient had a high frontal hairline. Alternative procedures were discussed. Since the patient had already undergone upper eyelidplasties, work on the procerus and corrugator muscles through an upper eyelidplasty approach was not recommended. An endoscopic browlift would be an acceptable approach, but the surgeon preferred an open approach because of the long-lasting good results and minimal complications which had been consistently obtained with that procedure.

19.3 Recommended Solutions to the Problem

- When evaluating a patient for rejuvenation of the forehead and eyelids, it is necessary to place the eyebrows at a normal level (1 cm above the superior orbital rim in a woman, at the rim in a man) and then to measure and mark the upper eyelid skin for excision with the patient in an upright position.

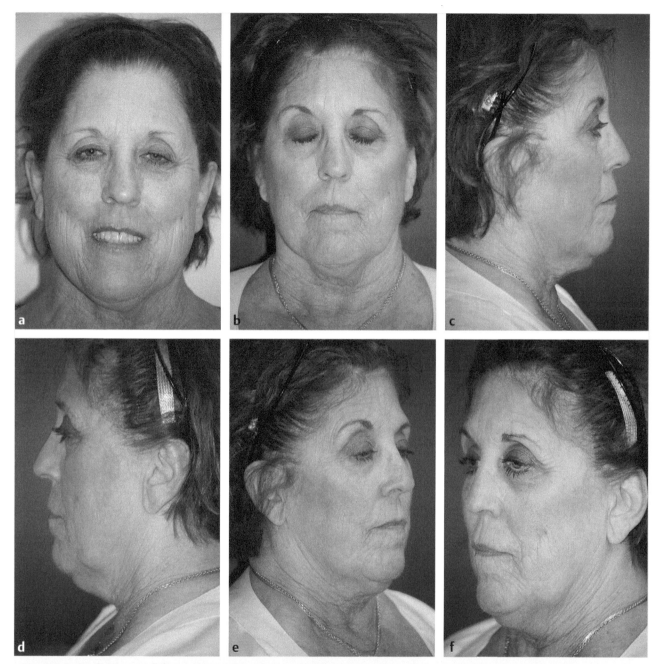

Fig. 19.1 (a–f) Views of the patient prior to any surgery.

- Transverse furrows of the forehead are best obliterated by direct modification of the frontalis muscle through an open approach.
- Resection of a good portion of the corrugator and procerus muscles can easily be done and excellent hemostasis can be achieved, thus eliminating the necessity to insert drains under the forehead flap.
- Though only 1 cm of scalp is usually excised, asymmetrical levels of the brows can be corrected by excising a bit more scalp on the side where the brow needs to be elevated.
- It is not necessary to insert brow suspension sutures, or to fix the scalp flap to the skull with sutures placed through a cortical tunnel or to impale the flap on a fixed absorbable device to hold it in an elevated position.

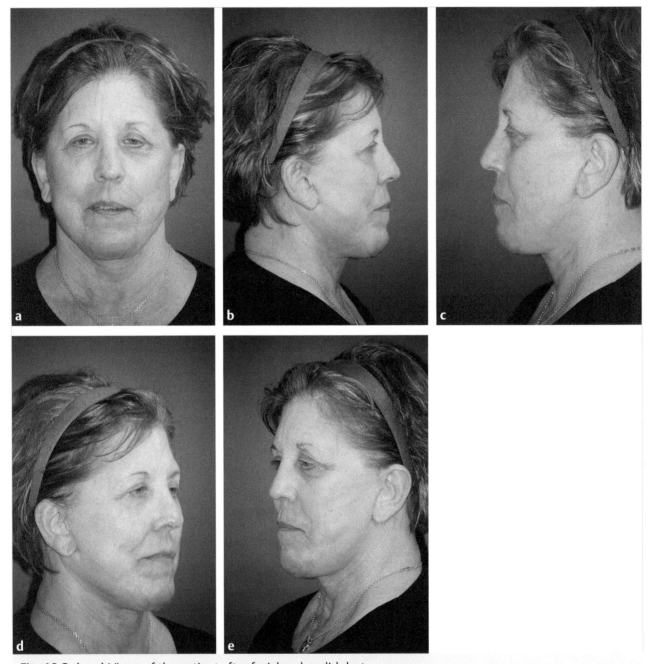

Fig. 19.2 (a–e) Views of the patient after facial and eyelidplasty.

- When performed at the same time, after the scalp incision has been closed, and the foreheadplasty has been completed, the markings for upper eyelid skin excision are re-evaluated and modified if it is felt that less skin needs to be removed.
- It is easier to take less skin from the lids than trying to modify the scalp excision, and it is for that reason that the foreheadplasty is performed before the eyelid surgery.
- In this case, where the lid surgery had already been performed, the decision to remove any scalp at all was determined by observation and determination to make sure that the patient would be able to completely close her eyelids without tension.

19.4 Technique

After the hair is prepared, only a small swath of hair is cut (not shaved) for the incision; 1% xylocaine with 1:100,000 epinephrine added for hemostasis is injected across the entire supraorbital region, extending to the ears and up to include the coronal incision. The coronal flap is elevated at a level above the pericranium, but at about 1 cm above the superior orbital rim, the dissection is converted to a subperiosteal level. Markings are made to identify the area for modification of the frontalis muscles, and then the procerus and corrugator muscles are partially excised, removing about 75%. After hemostasis is assured in the operative field for a final time, the frontal forehead flap is redraped, a small amount of flap is excised, and the incision margins are reapproximated. The galea is reapproximated with 3–0 Monocryl sutures (absorbing the tension for the closure) and simple running 3–0 Nylon sutures are meticulously placed to approximate the scalp skin margins (not interlocking so as to minimize trauma to the hair follicles, preventing hair loss). Suture clips are not used. Attention is turned to performing the eyelidplasties and subsequently to the facialplasty. A light dressing is applied over the face and entire head after completion of all of the procedures.

19.5 Postoperative Photographs and Critical Evaluation of Results

The patient's appearance has been improved and all of the significant signs of aging, transverse furrows, glabellar frown lines, drooping brows, lateral canthal rhytids, and residual excess eyelid skin have disappeared. The patient can still elevate her brows, and the distance between her brows and her frontal hairline has remained the same as it was preoperatively (▸ Fig. 19.3).

19.6 Teaching Points

- The muscles of facial expression in the forehead and periorbital region are antagonistic. When the frontalis muscles are on (contracting), procerus and corrugators are off, and vice versa.
- The object of surgical modification of the muscles is to improve the patient's appearance in repose, yet retaining the ability to raise the eyebrows. The surgical technique recommended and performed achieved that goal.
- There is no reason not to approach rejuvenation of the forehead at the same time the eyelid and lower facial surgery is being performed.
- Knowledge of the anatomy and function of the muscles of facial expression is essential to achieving good and long-lasting results.

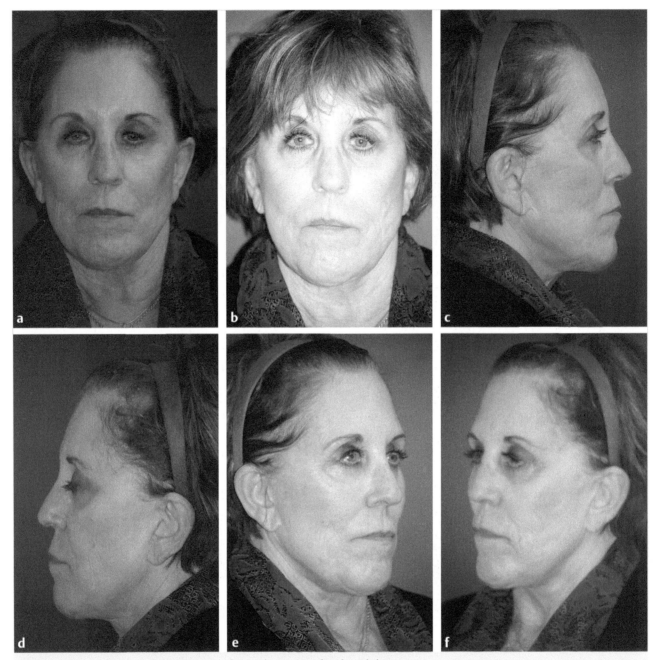

Fig. 19.3 (a–f) Views of the patient after subsequent foreheadplasty.

Suggested Reading

[1] Friedland JA, Jacobsen WM, TerKonda S. Safety and efficacy of combined upper blepharoplasties and open coronal browlift: a consecutive series of 600 patients. Aesthetic Plast Surg. 1996; 20(6):453–462

[2] Friedland JA, Lalonde DH, Rohrich RJ. An evidence-based approach to blepharoplasty. Plast Reconstr Surg. 2010; 126(6):2222–2229

[3] Maffi TR, Chang S, Friedland JA. Traditional lower blepharoplasty: is additional support necessary? A 30-year review. Plast Reconstr Surg. 2011; 128(1):265–273

[4] Elkwood A, Matarasso A, Rankin M, Elkowitz M, Godek CP. National plastic surgery survey: brow lifting techniques and complications. Plast Reconstr Surg. 2001; 108(7):2143–2150, discussion 2151–2152

Part IV

Chemosis

IV

20 Chemosis: Clinical Overview

Foad Nahai

20.1 Introduction

Chemosis or edema of the conjunctiva is one of the more common and relatively benign complications following blepharoplasty. It is most often associated with lower lid procedures, especially those involving the lateral canthal area.

The fluid collects in the natural plane between Tenon's capsule and the conjunctiva (▶ Fig. 20.1).

The typical appearance seen in ▶ Fig. 20.2, where the collection is sharply demarcated at the cornea, results from the firm adherence of Tenon's capsule and conjunctiva to the underlying sclera at the corneoscleral limbus.

Chemosis results from the reaction of the conjunctiva to inflammation following surgery, allergies, trauma, infection, and even Graves' disease. Chemosis following blepharoplasty is most likely the result of inflammation. Its association with canthal procedures also raises the possibility of lymphatic disruption as a contributing factor. Predisposing conditions for chemosis include patients with compromised eyelid closure, lid laxity, ocular surface pathology, and conjunctivochalasis.

Once the initial inflammation has led to accumulation of chemosis fluid, a cycle may begin, prolonging the process (▶ Fig. 20.3). As the conjunctiva becomes desiccated, more inflammation ensues, displacing the eyelid from the cornea and limiting lid closure. This leads to further corneal drying and the cycle continues till interrupted by treatment. Lubrication and patching will temporarily interrupt the cycle till permanent resolution is achieved.

20.2 Management of Chemosis

Chemosis may even be seen intraoperatively. Postoperatively, it may be seen early (the first week) or late (2–3 weeks). Management includes conservative and invasive options (▶ Fig. 20.4; ▶ Fig. 20.5).

20.2.1 Intraoperative

On occasions, we see chemosis during the operation and it should be resolved immediately. Placement of sutures (▶ Fig. 20.6) and opening the conjunctiva and Tenon's ligament (▶ Fig. 20.7) are appropriate options. We routinely place a temporary tarsorrhaphy suture (▶ Fig. 20.8) in all patients we feel may be at risk of postoperative chemosis. We have found that the suture reduces that risk.

20.2.2 Postoperative

Early and mild chemosis within the first week is initially treated conservatively (▶ Fig. 20.5) with dexamethasone, phenylephrine, and lubricants. Moderate chemosis may benefit from eye patching.

Severe chemosis, which prevents eyelid closure, is best treated invasively through a conjunctivectomy (snipping) and drainage. We perform this under local anesthesia in the office exam room. Following the instillation of tetracaine drops, we inject a drop or two of xylocaine 1% with epinephrine 1 in

100,000 into the swelling or 2.5% phenylephrine for vasoconstriction. Then, under loupe magnification, the snip is performed assuring that not only the conjunctiva but also anterior Tenon's capsule is opened. The chemosis is immediately relieved; ointment and occasionally a patch may be applied.

Prolong, over a month, or recurrent chemosis may require evaluation and treatment of eyelid closure problems.

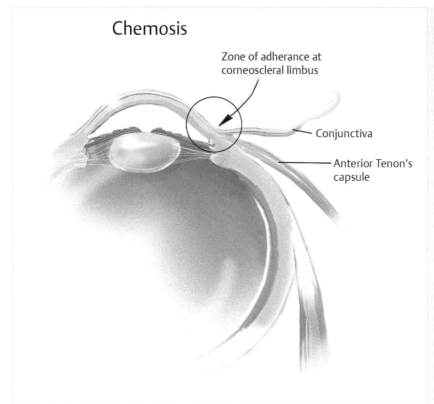

Fig. 20.1 Tenon's capsule, conjunctiva, and chemosis fluid. Note the firm adherence of conjunctiva to underlying sclera at the corneoscleral limbus.

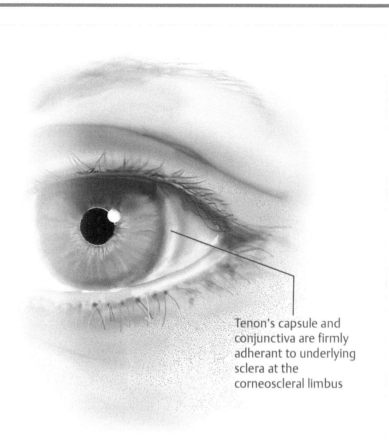

Fig. 20.2 Tenon's capsule and conjunctiva are firmly adherent to underlying sclera at the corneoscleral limbus.

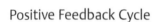

Tenon's capsule and conjunctiva are firmly adherant to underlying sclera at the corneoscleral limbus

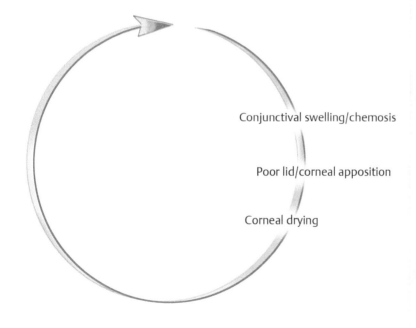

Fig. 20.3 The sequence of events producing a positive "feedback" cycle of chemosis and dellen formation.

Positive Feedback Cycle

Conjunctival swelling/chemosis

Poor lid/corneal apposition

Corneal drying

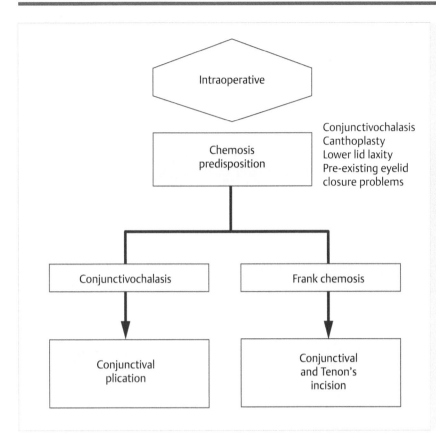

Fig. 20.4 A comprehensive algorithm for chemosis management.

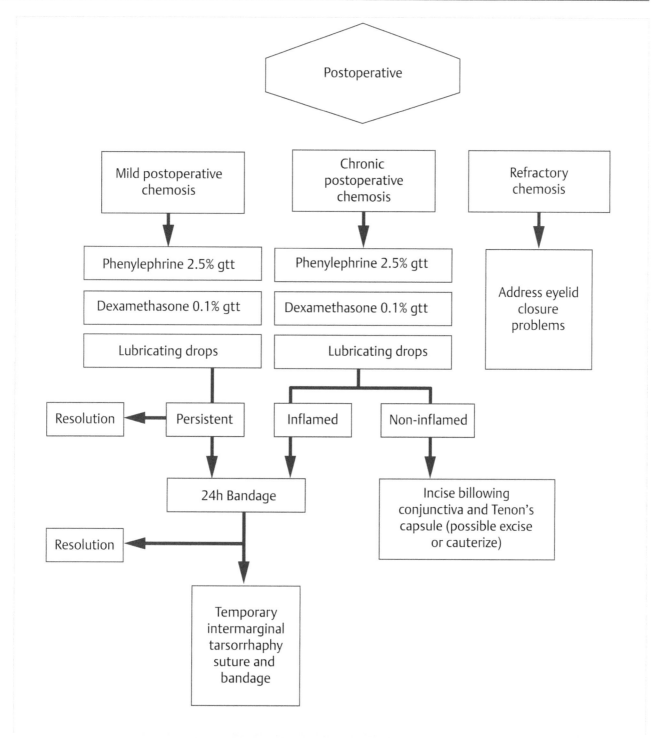

Fig. 20.5 A comprehensive algorithm for chemosis management.

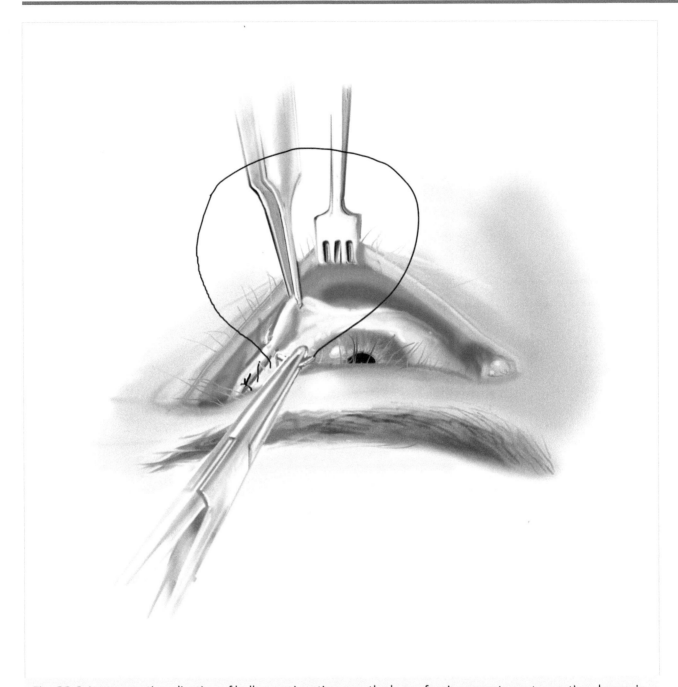

Fig. 20.6 Intraoperative plication of bulbar conjunctiva near the lower fornix prevents postoperative chemosis. A fast-absorbing suture is used and is placed away from the cornea.

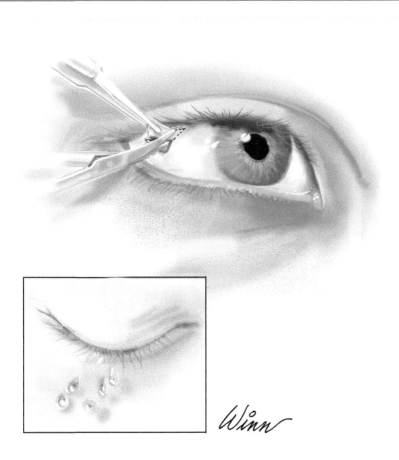

Fig. 20.7 One-snip conjunctivectomy to release chemotic fluid. The underlying Tenon's capsule is spread with scissors to allow fluid egress. The relationship between conjunctiva, Tenon's capsule, and chemotic fluid is shown. Penetration through Tenon's capsule is needed for maximum fluid release.

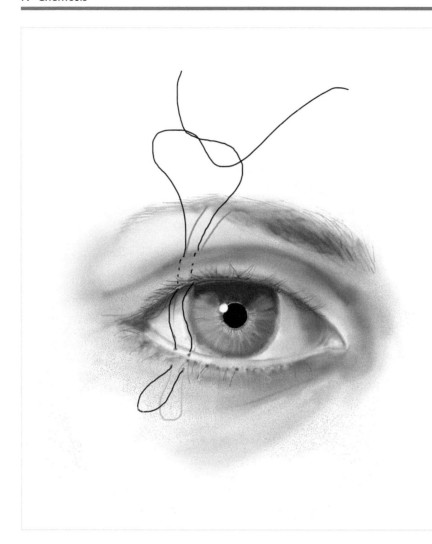

Fig. 20.8 Intraoperative intermarginal suture placement or tarsorrhaphy prevents postoperative chemosis. This maneuver is usually performed with 6–0 nylon. Sutures enter and exit the eyelids at midthickness and are placed to avoid potential contact with the ocular surface.

Suggested Reading

[1] Enzer YR, Shorr N. Medical and surgical management of chemosis after blepharoplasty. Ophthal Plast Reconstr Surg. 1994; 10(1):57–63

[2] Gausas RE, Gonnering RS, Lemke BN, Dortzbach RK, Sherman DD. Identification of human orbital lymphatics. Ophthal Plast Reconstr Surg. 1999; 15(4):252–259

[3] McCord CD, Kreymerman P, Nahai F, Walrath JD. Management of postblepharoplasty chemosis. Aesthet Surg J. 2013; 33(5):654–661

[4] McGetrick JJ, Wilson DG, Dortzbach RK, Kaufman PL, Lemke BN. A search for lymphatic drainage of the monkey orbit. Arch Ophthalmol. 1989; 107(2):255–260

[5] Nijhawan N, Marriott C, Harvey JT. Lymphatic drainage patterns of the human eyelid: assessed by lymphoscintigraphy. Ophthal Plast Reconstr Surg. 2010; 26(4):281–285

21 Chemosis in the Aesthetic Surgery Setting

Farzad R. Nahai and Foad Nahai

Summary

Chemosis can occur after aesthetic eyelid surgery, especially the more invasive lower eyelid procedures. Being able to recognize and treat this condition is very important for patient safety and satisfaction. Chemosis can arise from local trauma, temporary lymphatic blockage, and scleral exposure. Should conservative measures not suffice to treat chemosis, procedural intervention may be necessary. This chapter presents such an example and how it was treated.

Keywords: chemosis, conjuntivectomy, eye patching

21.1 Patient History Leading to the Specific Problem

This patient is a 67-year-old woman who initially presented to the clinic with an interest in facial rejuvenation (▶ Fig. 21.1). She had prior cataract surgery in 2006 and smokes a pack of cigarettes per week. She does not report any symptoms of dry eye. On exam, she demonstrates moderate to severe signs of panfacial aging including dermatochalasis of the upper and lower eyelids. Her eyelid tone was normal. After consultation, a face and neck lift with upper and lower lid blepharoplasty and periorbital and perioral croton oil peel was recommended.

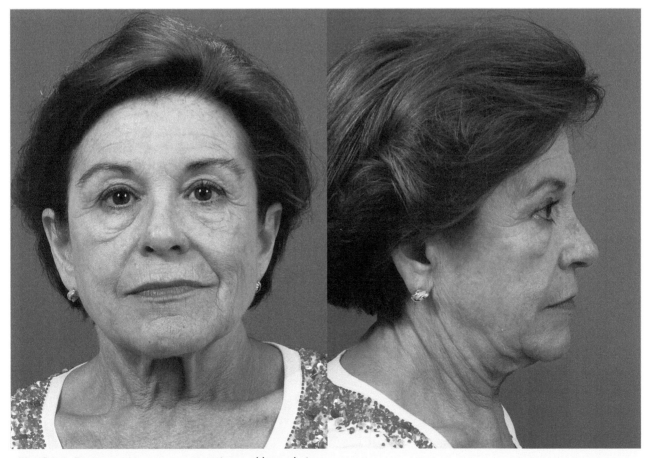

Fig. 21.1 Preoperative anteroposterior and lateral views.

She had an uneventful procedure that included a transpalpebral midface lift, canthopexy, and croton oil peel of the crow's feet (in addition to the face and neck lift and upper lid blepharoplasty). A temporary lateral tarsorrhaphy suture was placed on both sides during the case. After surgery, TobraDex ophthalmic ointment was prescribed. At 1 week postoperation, the temporary tarsorrhaphy suture was removed and the ointment was stopped. At that time, she had no evidence of chemosis.

21.2 Anatomic Description of the Patient's Current Status

At 3 weeks postoperation, delayed chemosis in the right eye was noted on the exam (▶ Fig. 21.2a). Her eyelid closure was normal. The chemosis is evident in the right eye predominantly in the lateral scleral triangle. Chemosis represents fluid collection/edema that appears in the sclera, typically in the lateral triangle, but it can appear medially as well in more severe cases. Anatomically, the edema occurs within the space between the outermost layer of the eye (the reflexion of the conjunctiva from the eyelid) and the underlying bulbar sheath (a.k.a. Tenon's capsule) (▶ Fig. 20.1). It is important to note that the sclera can be as thin as 0.4 mm at the insertion of the rectus muscle about 6 mm behind the corneoscleral junction. The conjunctiva is firmly adherent to the sclera along the entire circumference of the cornea representing a stop point in chemosis formation (▶ Fig. 21.2a, see the right eye between 7 and 8 o'clock positions in the photo).

21.2.1 Recommended Solution to the Problem

- Wetting eye drops.
- Steroid-containing ophthalmic solution or ointment.
- Temporary lateral tarsorrhaphy suture.
- Eye patching at night with or without compression.
- Conjunctivectomy with 24-hour patching.

This case was initially treated with FML (fluorometholone ophthalmic suspension, USP 0.1% sterile) drops. After a week, there was no improvement, so a conjunctivectomy was performed.

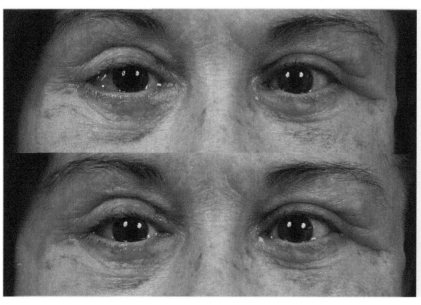

Fig. 21.2 (a) Upper photo demonstrates delayed right-sided chemosis principally involving the lateral scleral triangle. Note that the medial extent of the chemosis is limited by the tissue attachments at the corneoscleral limbus. **(b)** Lower photo is 1 week after conjunctivectomy was performed. Chemosis is completely resolved.

21.3 Technique

The technique for conjunctivectomy is relatively straightforward and simple. With the patient reclined on the exam table, tetracaine (tetracaine hydrochloride ophthalmic solution, USP 0.5% sterile) eye drops are administered for the local anesthetic effect. Under loupe magnification, the conjunctiva overlying the area of chemosis is grasped with a fine single-tooth forceps and tented upward away from the sclera. Next, a horizontally oriented laceration is made with Westcott scissors until the fluid is expressed. Once the conjunctivectomy is made, a small amount of bleeding may occur. Generally, a steroid-containing antibiotic solution or ointment is applied to the area and then a 24-hour eye-patch is applied. In more severe cases of the chemosis and/or in the presence of lagophthalmos, the conjunctivectomy may need to be repeated if it recurs.

21.4 Postoperative Photographs and Critical Evaluation of Results

The postoperative photo demonstrates resolution of the chemosis after a single conjunctivectomy was performed (▶ Fig. 21.2b). In the absence of lagophthalmos, generally a single procedure is needed, as was the case here. In more severe cases of chemosis or if lagophthalmos is present, sometimes a second conjunctivectomy is needed. A long-term postoperative photo demonstrates the result of the blepharoplasty (▶ Fig. 21.3).

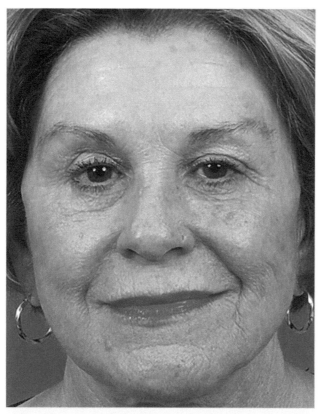

Fig. 21.3 Anteroposterior view at long-term follow-up at more than 1 year demonstrating the results of the blepharoplasty.

21.5 Teaching Points

- Chemosis in the aesthetic setting can be the result of any, or a combination, of the following: thermal and/or environmental exposure of the cornea, poor lid closure, and disruption of the lower lid lymphatics.
- In general, the more invasive the lower eyelid procedure, the more likely chemosis will occur.
- Preventative measures for chemosis include protection of the sclera during surgery, temporary tarsorrhaphy suture, pretreatment with steroid-containing ophthalmic ointment, and minimizing short-term postoperative lagophthalmos.
- Treatment strategies for chemosis include wetting eye drops, steroid-containing ophthalmic drops or ointment, patching the eyelid closed, and conjunctivectomy.

Suggested Reading

[1] Cole HP III, Wesley RE. Conjunctiva: structure and function. In: Bosniak S, ed. Principles of Ophthalmic Plastic and Reconstructive Surgery. Philadelphia, PA: Saunders; 1996:159–163
[2] Enzer YR, Shorr N. Medical and surgical management of chemosis after blepharoplasty. Ophthal Plast Reconstr Surg. 1994; 10(1):57–63
[3] Jones YJ, Georgescu D, McCann JD, Anderson RL. Snip conjunctivoplasty for postoperative conjunctival chemosis. Arch Facial Plast Surg. 2010; 12(2):103–105
[4] Kakizaki H. Tip for preventing chemosis after swinging eyelid procedure. Orbit. 2011; 30(2):82
[5] McCord CD, Kreymerman P, Nahai F, Walrath JD. Management of postblepharoplasty chemosis. Aesthet Surg J. 2013; 33(5):654–661
[6] Patrocinio TG, Loredo BAS, Arevalo CEA, Patrocinio LG, Patrocinio JA. Complications in blepharoplasty: how to avoid and manage them. Rev Bras Otorrinolaringol (Engl Ed). 2011; 77(3):322–327
[7] Thakker MM, Tarbet KJ, Sires BS. Postoperative chemosis after cosmetic eyelid surgery: surgical management with conjunctivoplasty. Arch Facial Plast Surg. 2005; 7(3):185–188
[8] Weinfeld AB, Burke R, Codner MA. The comprehensive management of chemosis following cosmetic lower blepharoplasty. Plast Reconstr Surg. 2008; 122(2):579–586

Part V

Lower Lid

22 Lower Lid: Clinical Overview

Ted H. Wojno

Summary

The lower lid is more prone to complications as compared to the upper eyelid. The following chapters will discuss in detail the management of these vexing problems.

Keywords: ectropion, canthal rounding, lagophthalmos, retraction, lid laxity

22.1 Introduction

There are considerably more chapters in this book devoted to lower eyelid surgery. The reason is simple. Surgery on the lower lid can be more complex and fraught with more complications. Although the position of the upper eyelid with respect to the corneoscleral limbus is principally determined by the levator muscle, lower lid position is influenced by the lower lid retractors (capsulopalpebral fascia and the inferior tarsal muscle), the tension along the tarsal plate, integrity of the medial and lateral canthal tendons, and the degree of relative exophthalmos of the globe. Make a change in any of these parameters and the level and shape of the lower lid may be noticeably altered.

Vertical tension in the lower lid is mainly due to the lower lid retractors (▶ Fig. 22.1). The capsulopalpebral fascia (analogous to the levator muscle in the

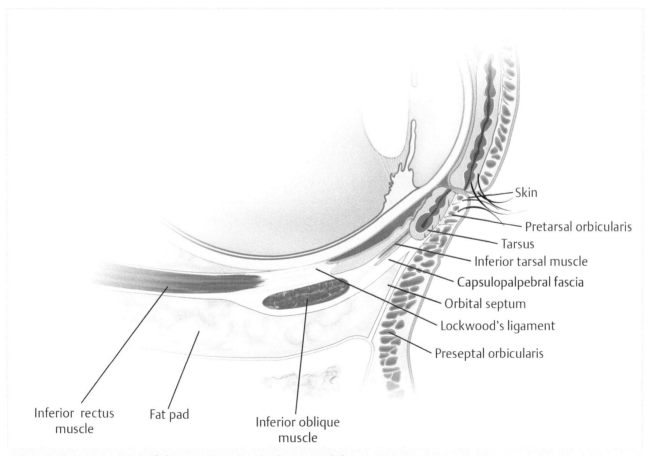

Fig. 22.1 Sagittal view of the structures in the lower eyelid.

Skin

Pretarsal orbicularis

Tarsus

Inferior tarsal muscle

Capsulopalpebral fascia

Orbital septum

Lockwood's ligament

Preseptal orbicularis

Inferior rectus muscle

Fat pad

Inferior oblique muscle

upper eyelid) arises from the inferior rectus muscle and inserts along the lower border of the tarsal plate. Unlike the levator, there are no striated muscle fibers in this structure. The inferior tarsal muscle (analogous to Müller's muscle) arises from the capsulopalpebral fascia and also inserts into the inferior border of the tarsal plate. Often, the inferior tarsal muscle is no more than scattered smooth muscle fibers within the capsulopalpebral fascia. The lower lid retractors function to depress the level of the lower lid in downgaze. As the inferior rectus contracts when looking down, the pull on the retractors is transmitted to the tarsal plate and the eyelid moves inferiorly to permit unobstructed vision. Surgical release of the lower lid retractors allows the lid margin to rise superiorly on the globe, while tightening them is frequently performed in repair of involutional entropion.

Horizontal tension along the globe is maintained by the tarsus and the medial and lateral canthal tendons and is often referred to as the "tarsoligamentous sling." These structures become lax with age, necessitating surgical modification in lower eyelid surgery. Reconstruction of the lateral canthus can be difficult, and any variation from the normal position and shape is immediately obvious and often a source of cosmetic dissatisfaction to patients. Surgery on the medial canthal tendon can damage the inferior canaliculus and lacrimal sac, resulting in excessive tearing or dacryocystitis.

The degree of projection of the globe as measured by various exophthalmometry devices is also critical in surgical planning. This situation has classically been compared to the man with a large belly who tightens his belt. The more he tightens his belt, the greater the overhang of his belly. Similarly, when the globe is relatively exophthalmic, surgical horizontal lid tightening may cause the lid margin to slip inferiorly on the globe, resulting in cosmetically objectionable lid retraction. This is often remedied by releasing the lower eyelid retractors and interposing a spacer graft between the cut edge of the retractors and the inferior border of the tarsal plate to effectively lengthen the retractors and add support to the lower eyelid. Hirmand et al found that exophthalmometry readings of 18 or greater anatomically predisposed patients to retraction and developed protocols for surgical correction. I have found that this measurement is important when doing lower eyelid surgery.

Lower lid malposition after eyelid surgery can be conceptualized according to ▶ Box 22.1.

It is important to realize that retraction, lateral canthal rounding, ectropion, and lagophthalmos can exist by themselves or in any combination. It is also important to distinguish between lower lid retraction (where the lid margin is still positioned against the globe but in a lower than normal level) and frank ectropion (displacement of the lid margin away from the eye). Entropion (inward rotation of the eyelid margin resulting in lashes rubbing on the globe) must also be distinguished from trichiasis (posterior misdirection of the lashes from a normally positioned lid margin). Both entropion and trichiasis are very unusual complications of eyelid surgery.

Box 22.1 Lower Lid Malposition after Eyelid Surgery

- Retraction (scleral show).
- Lateral canthal rounding (round eye deformity).
- Ectropion.
- Lagophthalmos.
- Entropion.
- Trichiasis.

- Lid margin and canthal laxity.
- Heavy jowls.
- Midface ptosis.
- Flat malar eminence.
- Actual and relative exophthalmos.
- Excess skin excision.
- Middle lamellar scarring.

Factors that predispose to lower lid malposition are listed in ▶ Box 22.2.

Again, any of these factors can exist in isolation or may occur in multiple combinations.

There are two classic tests for excess lower lid laxity that are performed in the preoperative patient assessment. In the "lid distraction test" ("pull-away test"), the examiner grasps the lower lid just below the lid margin and pulls it away from the globe (▶ Fig. 22.2). A separation of greater than 10 mm from the globe indicates that the eyelid is at high risk for postoperative lower lid malposition. Lesser measurements indicate a decreasing degree of risk down to 5 mm, which may be considered normal and thus very low risk. The second test is the "snap back test" (▶ Fig. 22.3). The examiner pulls the lower lid inferiorly toward the orbital rim and quickly releases it. A normal lid will "snap back" into position quickly and cleanly, while a lid with excess laxity will take longer to do so and may even remain in a position of ectropion until the next blink.

If ectropion/lid retraction occurs in the postoperative period, one can perform a "two-finger test" as outlined by Patipa to determine the etiology of the problem. In the first step of this test, the examiner places the index

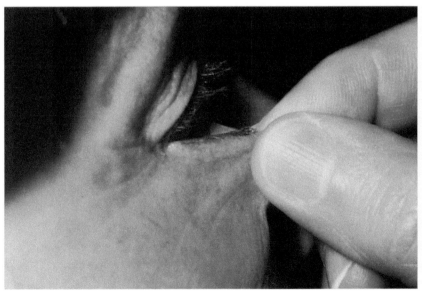

Fig. 22.2 In the "lid distraction test," the examiner pulls the lower eyelid away from the globe with the thumb and forefinger.

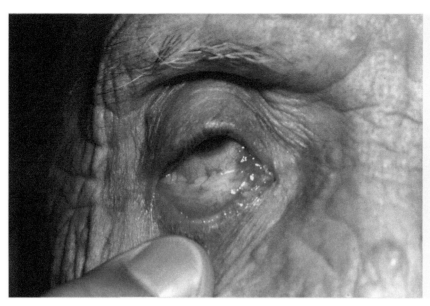

Fig. 22.3 In the "snap back test," the examiner pulls the lower eyelid inferiorly and quickly releases it.

finger against the lateral, lower eyelid and pushes it toward the lateral orbital rim (effectively performing a horizontal tightening of the lower lid). If the ectropion/retraction is corrected with this maneuver, horizontal shortening of the lower eyelid is indicated (▶ Fig. 22.4). It is important to only push the eyelid laterally and not superiorly. If the ectropion remains, the examiner then pushes superiorly with the middle finger in the middle third of the eyelid. If the ectropion/retraction is eliminated by this additional step, a posterior lamellar or middle lamellar graft may be needed (▶ Fig. 22.5). Some have added an additional step with a "three-finger test" in which a third finger is used to push skin up from the midface. Here, if the ectropion/retraction is now reduced, a skin graft or midface lift may additionally be required indicating a relative skin shortage in the eyelid.

Perhaps, the greatest paradigm shift in lower eyelid aesthetic surgery has been the change from fat excision to fat repositioning. This was originally

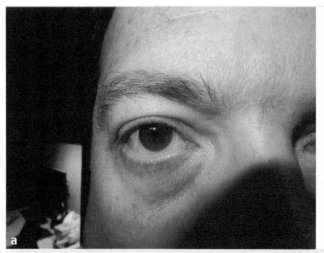
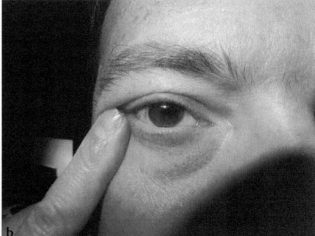

Fig. 22.4 (a) A case of postoperative lower eyelid retraction. **(b)** In the first step of the "two-finger test," the examiner pushes the lower eyelid toward the lateral orbital rim with the index finger effectively relieving the retraction seen in (a).

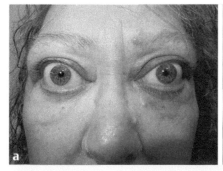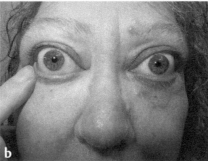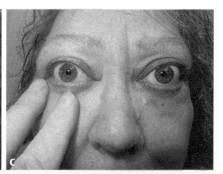

Fig. 22.5 **(a)** A case of lower eyelid retraction in a patient with thyroid eye disease. **(b)** In the first step of the "two-finger test," the examiner pushes the lower eyelid toward the lateral orbital rim but, in this case, the retraction remains. **(c)** In the second step of the "two-finger test," the examiner now additionally pushes superiorly with the middle finger in the middle third of the lower eyelid. The retraction is now eliminated and indicates that a posterior lamellar graft will likely be needed for correction.

conceived by Loeb and then Hamra and has been elaborated on by numerous authors. Appreciation for the anatomy of the "tear trough," which is the junction between the lower eyelid and the cheek, has spurred the development of a variety of surgical and nonsurgical treatments that have improved our abilities to contour this area with excellent cosmetic results. I believe that lower lid fat repositioning and augmentation not only improves the aesthetics of this area but also increases the longevity of our surgical interventions much to the benefit of our patients.

Suggested Reading

[1] Hamra ST. Arcus marginalis release and orbital fat preservation in midface rejuvenation. Plast Reconstr Surg. 1995; 96(2):354–362

[2] Hirmand H, Codner MA, McCord CD, Hester TR, Jr, Nahai F. Prominent eye: operative management in lower lid and midfacial rejuvenation and the morphologic classification system. Plast Reconstr Surg. 2002; 110(2):620–628, discussion 629–634

[3] Loeb R. Naso-jugal groove leveling with fat tissue. Clin Plast Surg. 1993; 20(2):393–400, discussion 401

[4] Patel MP, Shapiro MD, Spinelli HM. Combined hard palate spacer graft, midface suspension, and lateral canthoplasty for lower eyelid retraction: a tripartite approach. Plast Reconstr Surg. 2005; 115(7):2105–2114, discussion 2115–2117

23 The Dry Eye

Ted H. Wojno

Summary

The etiology of "dry eye" is often difficult to determine and is frequently multifactorial. This chapter will delineate the common causes of this complaint and instruct the surgeon to diagnose and manage such complaints, especially in the postoperative period of eyelid surgery.

Keywords: dry eye, keratoconjunctivitis sicca, precorneal tear film, meibomian gland dysfunction, basic secretion tear test, keratitis, artificial tears

23.1 Patient History Leading to the Specific Problem

The patient is a 60-year-old white woman who underwent four-lid blepharoplasty and returns 1 month after the surgery complaining of severe irritation and burning of both eyes (▶ Fig. 23.1). This is accompanied by fluctuation of vision and intermittent tearing from both eyes. She has been using cold compresses and over-the-counter artificial tears several times a day with no relief. Her past eye history is negative for ophthalmologic problems other than wearing bifocals. Her past medical history reveals no systemic or ocular allergies. She is otherwise completely healthy.

23.2 Anatomic Description of the Patient's Current Status

This patient's complaints are common after blepharoplasty surgery. The etiology of postblepharoplasty "dry eye" is multifactorial. From an ophthalmic standpoint, dry eye is due to either reduced tear production or increased tear evaporation. The patient typically complains of irritated, red eyes and intermittent blurred vision. When severe, dry eye can significantly affect the quality of life.

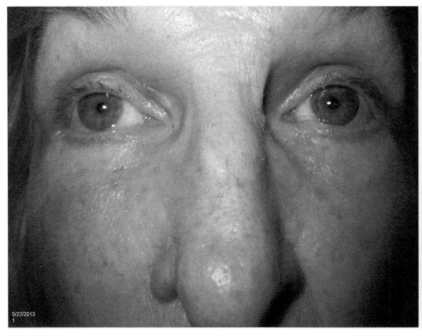

Fig. 23.1 A 60-year-old woman 1 month after four-lid blepharoplasty with ocular discomfort and erythema.

The tear film can be conceptualized as a three-layered sandwich (►Fig. 23.2). The inner mucin layer is produced by conjunctival goblet cells. It functions to protect the ocular surface and provide a smooth surface for the adherence of the overlying aqueous layer. The middle aqueous layer is produced by the basic secretory glands of Wolfring and Krause scattered throughout the palpebral conjunctiva and the main and accessory lacrimal glands. The outer lipid layer is mainly produced by the meibomian glands of the eyelids and prevents evaporation of the aqueous layer. Disruption in any of these three layers leads to dry eye symptoms.

Reduced tear production (aqueous layer deficiency) is the most common cause of dry eye. It is more common in women older than 40 years and the incidence increases with age. It is worsened by diuretics, antihistamines, anticholinergics, antidepressants, connective tissue disorders, previous LASIK surgery, low-humidity environments, and other causes. About 10% of patients with aqueous tear deficiency will have Sjögren's syndrome. There is no evidence that blepharoplasty itself causes a change in the basic secretion of the aqueous component of tears, but it is very common for symptoms to manifest after surgery. It is typically managed by supplementation with

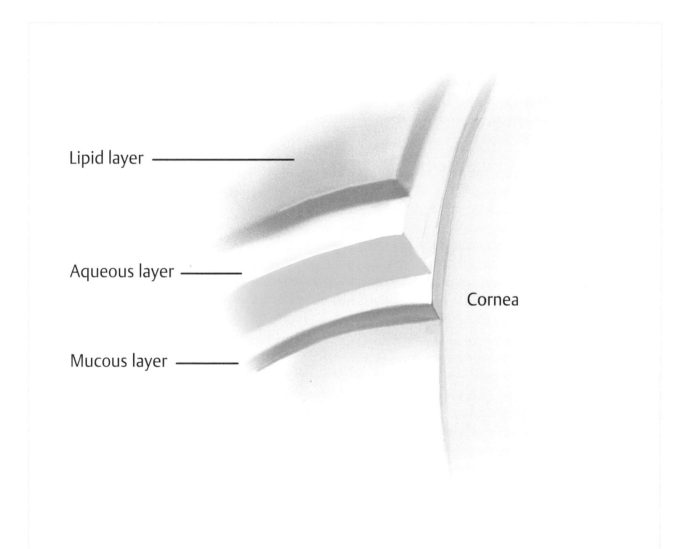

Lipid layer

Aqueous layer

Mucous layer

Cornea

Fig. 23.2 Diagrammatic demonstration of the precorneal tear film layers.

over-the-counter artificial tear drops and ointments. Frequent use of tear supplements will suffice for most patients. Severe cases may require placement of silicone punctal plugs (to slow the removal of tears from the ocular surface), cyclosporine ophthalmic drops (Restasis) to increase aqueous tear production, and sometimes topical ophthalmic steroid drops (which can cause cataract and elevate intraocular pressure) to reduce inflammation.

Evaporative dry eye (lipid layer instability) is typically caused by meibomian gland dysfunction, which is especially common in patients with rosacea. Redness of the lid margins, midface telangiectasis, rhinophyma, a history of chalazia, and northern European ancestry are suggestive of underlying rosacea. This author's clinical impression from over 33 years of practice is that eyelid surgery may worsen the symptoms of rosacea and increase meibomian gland dysfunction in those patients so predisposed. Meibomian gland dysfunction is typically managed by warm compresses and eyelid hygiene with baby shampoo lid scrubs or over-the-counter eyelid scrub preparations. More recalcitrant cases will usually respond to a 2-month course of oral tetracycline, 50 mg daily, to normalize meibomian secretion.

Evaporative dry eye is also due to mechanical disorders of the eyelids such as lagophthalmos, lid retraction, and ectropion. Even a minimal amount of corneal exposure will lead to significant symptoms with findings of exposure keratitis on microscopic exam of the eyes. Likewise, exposure of the palpebral conjunctiva in ectropion will cause enough discomfort to generate complaints from affected patients. Mild degrees of ectropion, lid retraction, and lagophthalmos will usually resolve with time and conservative therapy such as eyelid massage. Persistent and severe lid position abnormalities will require additional surgery and in worst cases may need skin grafting.

23.3 Recommended Solution to the Problem

- Examine the ocular surface with fluorescein and a penlight.
- Perform a basic secretion tear test with a topical ophthalmic anesthetic eye drop.
- Examine the eyelids for evidence of ectropion, retraction, and/or lagophthalmos.
- Push on the eyelids to examine the meibomian secretions.
- Look for evidence of rosacea on the patient's face.

23.4 Technique

The most reliable way to examine the ocular surface is with the slit-lamp biomicroscope. Given that this instrument is not typically found in the office of plastic surgeons, one can still easily assess for the presence of keratitis by placing a drop of fluorescein from a tap water–moistened strip into the patient's inferior cul-de-sac (▶ Fig. 23.3; ▶ Fig. 23.4). These strips are easily purchased from a variety of medical suppliers. A moderate to severe keratitis can be observed with the aid of a penlight (▶ Fig. 23.5). If available, a cobalt blue penlight will greatly aid in the diagnosis by showing typical green fluorescence. Fluorescein staining of the cornea is suggestive of dry eye syndrome of any etiology.

The basic secretion tear test can be performed by instilling a drop of an ophthalmic topical anesthetic such as proparacaine 0.5%, followed by a drop

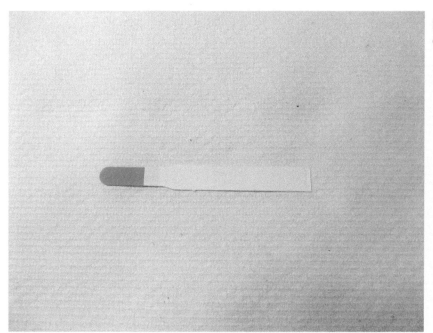

Fig. 23.3 A fluorescein-impregnated ophthalmic strip.

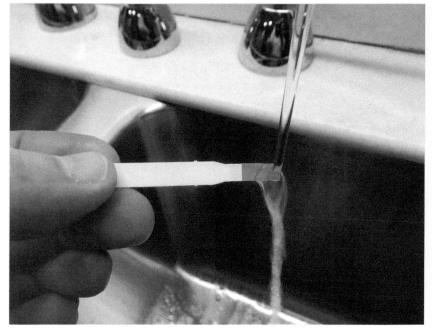

Fig. 23.4 Wetting the fluorescein strip in tap water.

of 1 or 2% lidocaine for more complete ocular surface anesthesia. Dry the eye with a tissue and place a strip of the Schirmer paper (again, available from a variety of suppliers) onto the lower lid near the lateral canthus as shown and wait for 5 minutes (▶Fig. 23.6; ▶Fig. 23.7). Wetting of less than 10 mm is suggestive of aqueous deficiency dry eye (▶Fig. 23.8).

Visually assess the eyelids for the presence of ectropion and lid retraction. A penlight may be helpful to reveal subtle displacement of the lower lid from the ocular surface. The lower lid position should normally be at or just above the inferior corneal limbus. The presence of inferior or superior scleral show is usually abnormal. Ask the patient to gently close the eyes to

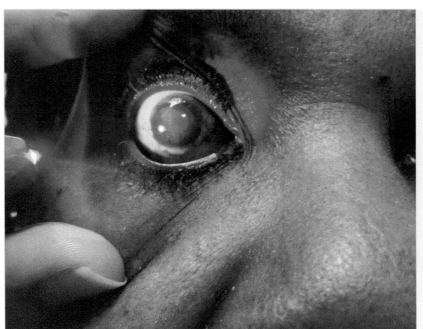

Fig. 23.5 Cobalt blue penlight illumination of the cornea after application of fluorescein demonstrating keratitis.

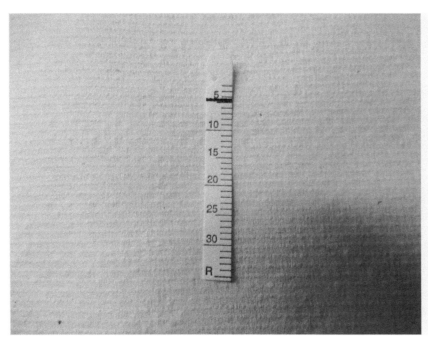

Fig. 23.6 Schirmer tear strip used to measure tear production.

check for lagophthalmos. Again, a penlight is often helpful. Ectropion, lid retraction, and lagophthalmos may indicate that too much skin was removed in the surgery or that excess horizontal lower lid laxity was not addressed.

To examine the meibomian glands, place a finger on the lower lid just below the lid margin and gently compress the eyelid against the globe (▶ Fig. 23.9). Perform the same maneuver on the upper eyelids. Normally, a tiny amount of clear oil can be observed coming from the orifices of the meibomian glands just posterior to the lash follicles. In meibomian gland dysfunction, thick, yellow oil can be observed coming from the glands, while, in severe cases, thick, cheeselike secretion is noted.

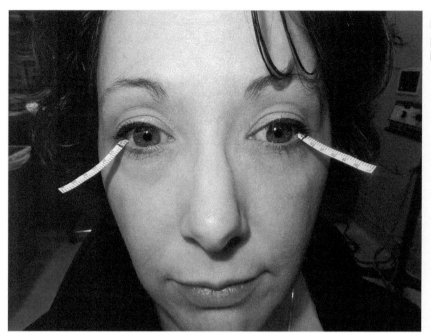

Fig. 23.7 The Schirmer tear strips in place at the lateral corners of both lower lids.

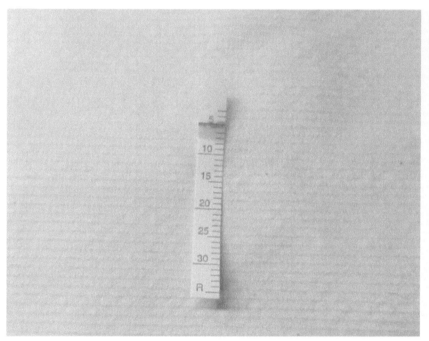

Fig. 23.8 The Schirmer tear strip after removal at 5 minutes demonstrating minimal tear production.

Look for the typical findings of rosacea such as midface telangiectasis, rhino-phyma, and small pustules. Look for evidence of redness of the lid margins and chalazia on the tarsal conjunctiva as is often seen in rosacea.

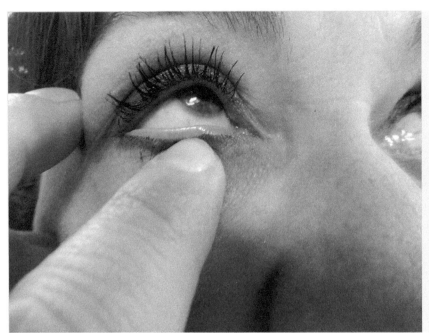

Fig. 23.9 Gentle compression of the lower eyelid to assess for the quality of meibomian secretions.

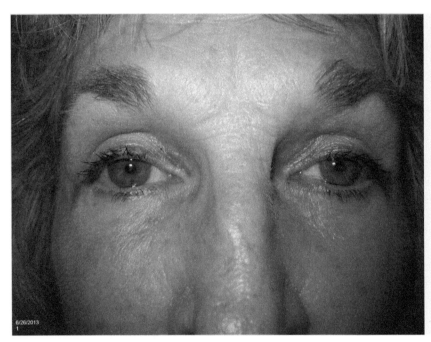

Fig. 23.10 The same patient as shown in ▸ Fig. 23.1 after a 2-month course of oral doxycycline with resolution of signs and symptoms of ocular irritation.

23.5 Postoperative Photographs and Critical Evaluation of Results

This patient had no evidence of keratitis with fluorescein staining and a normal basic secretion tear test (over 10 mm of wetting of the Schirmer strip at 5 minutes). There was no sign of ectropion, lid retraction, or lagophthalmos on exam. Pressure on the upper and lower lids reveals thick and cheesy secretions from the meibomian glands. Exam of the midface shows numerous telangiectatic blood vessels indicative of underlying rosacea. The patient is of northern European ancestry and has a family history of rosacea. She responded nicely to a 2-month course of 50 mg/day of doxycycline, with resolution of symptoms of ocular redness and irritation. She also reports that her midface telangiectasis, which she previously thought was normal, has significantly improved (▸ Fig. 23.10).

23 The Dry Eye

23.6 Teaching Points

- Dry eye syndrome is common after blepharoplasty.
- Dry eye syndrome is multifactorial in origin.
- The most common causes of dry eye syndrome can be easily diagnosed and managed by the surgeon.
- If nonresponsive to basic therapy, patients will benefit from referral to an ophthalmologist.

Suggested Reading

[1] Akpek EK, Klimava A, Thorne JE, Martin D, Lekhanont K, Ostrovsky A. Evaluation of patients with dry eye for presence of underlying Sjögren syndrome. Cornea. 2009; 28(5):493–497
[2] American Academy of Ophthalmology Cornea/External Disease Panel. Preferred Practice Pattern Guidelines. Dry Eye Syndrome. San Francisco, CA: American Academy of Ophthalmology; 2013. Available at www.aao.org/ppp
[3] Schiffman RM, Walt JG, Jacobsen G, Doyle JJ, Lebovics G, Sumner W. Utility assessment among patients with dry eye disease. Ophthalmology. 2003; 110(7):1412–1419

24 Prevention and Treatment of Irregularities of the Lower Eyelids following Fat Grafts

Juan Diego Mejia and Foad Nahai

Summary

The periorbital region is greatly affected by atrophy through the aging process. Since most of the atrophy is attributable to subcutaneous fat loss, if required, autologous fat is the ideal soft tissue filler. However, transfer of fat into the lower eyelid is not without complications. Even surgeons with vast experience state that the lower eyelid is one of the most difficult areas for structural fat grafting because of the possibility of irregularities and lump formation. Even though there are guidelines that have reduced their incidence, postoperative irregularities are still the most common complication after fat grafting to the lower eyelids. Preventive measures are best to avoid these irregularities. The injection of small quantities of fat, the placement of the fat in a deep plane, and avoiding overcorrection can help achieve an optimal result free of complications. If postoperative irregularities develop, the characteristics of the lumps and patient preference will help define the best treatment option.

Keywords: fat transfer, periorbital fat grafting, periorbital hollows, periorbital rejuvenation, lower eyelids, irregularities

24.1 Introduction

Volume loss is one of the hallmarks of facial aging. It involves the eyelids and cheeks, in addition to changes in lid tone and skin, and accounts for the visible changes. Options for restoration of the volume include fillers, dermis fat grafts, and fat. Since most of the volume loss with age is secondary to fat loss, it is appropriate that autologous fat be grafted to replace this volume. Though fat atrophy occurs most commonly with advancing age, it can also be drug-induced, iatrogenic, or idiopathic. The periorbital hollows are very susceptible to this change and can become very apparent. Autologous fat transfer to these hollows is an important step in the process of periorbital rejuvenation. It can be performed in isolation or as an adjunct to lower lid blepharoplasty in patients with significant nasojugal grooves and tear troughs. Fat transfer alone will improve the nasojugal groove, the tear trough, and the skeletonization of the lid–cheek junction in patients with no excess skin and minimal or no eyelid bags. However, patients with excess skin and herniated fat pads are better candidates for a lower blepharoplasty. Besides acting as the ideal filler, autologous fat has other applications. Infiltration of fat into the lower lid can provide structural support, thereby correcting mild cases of scleral show. Patients with thin, wrinkled lower lid skin will also see an improvement in the quality of their skin after fat grafting. One of the concerns is that placement of the fat must be superficial, which makes the patient more susceptible to postoperative irregularities. Fat transfer can improve dark circles around the lower eyelids. This is achieved by adding volume to concave areas and producing smoother transition lines, thereby reducing eyelid shadows.

However, transfer of fat into the lower eyelid is not without complications. Even surgeons with vast experience in this area claim that the lower eyelid is one of the most difficult areas for fat grafting because of the possibility of irregularities and lumping of the fat. Even though there are guidelines to reduce the risk, postoperative irregularities are still the most common complication after fat grafting to the lower eyelids.

24.2 Patient History Leading to the Specific Problem

This patient presented for consultation after injections of excessive amounts of autologous fat into the lower periorbital area (▶ Fig. 24.1). The injections were at all levels. In addition to the obvious overinjection of fat, she has lid retraction more noticeable on the right than the left. Given the unpredictability of the survival of the grafted fat, this is not an uncommon occurrence. In most patients, transconjunctival and transcutaneous fat removal have proven to be a relatively straightforward and effective procedure for correction of this problem. However, we have encountered patients in whom excessive fat infiltration into the orbicularis has proven challenging to remove.

In this patient, the transcutaneous approach was chosen so that her lid retraction and skin excess could also be addressed, along with removal of

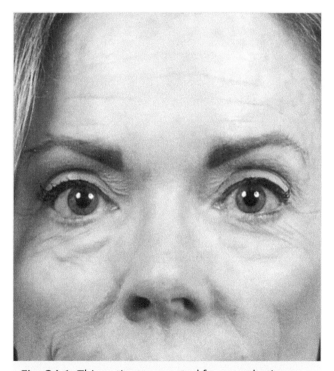

Fig. 24.1 This patient presented for consultation after injections of excessive amounts of autologous fat into the lower periorbital area. The injections were at all levels. In addition to the obvious overinjection of fat, she has lid retraction more noticeable on the right than the left.

excess injected fat. The injected fat bears little resemblance to the periorbital fat and maintains the appearance and morphologic character of the area from which it was harvested (▶Fig. 24.2). Typically, the fat is whiter in color and very fibrous. In this patient, most of the offending fat was deep to the orbicularis and relatively easy to remove. In addition to the removal of the fat, the patient underwent a canthal reanchoring and subperiosteal midface lift (▶Fig. 24.3).

As removal of the excess fat can be challenging, preventive measures should always be taken when transferring fat to the periorbital region to avoid postoperative irregularities (▶Fig. 24.4). These measures include the following:

- *Injection of small quantities of fat with every withdrawal (0.03–0.05 mL)*: In the rest of the face, 0.1 mL of fat with every withdrawal is accepted. Due to the thin skin of the lower lid, this amount of fat can leave visible lumps. To prevent this, half to one-third of this amount (0.03–0.05 mL) should be injected with every pass through the periorbital hollows.
- *Placement of the fat in a deep plane (suborbicularis, against the periosteum)*: The lower eyelid skin contains a very thin dermis and the subcutaneous compartment is practically inexistent. The only true protective layer against visible lumps is the orbicularis muscle. The placement of fat in the submuscular plane decreases the chances of postoperative irregularities.
- *Do not overcorrect*: Since the lower periorbital area has very little movement, most of the fat that is transferred to this region survives. For the lower eyelids, 1 to 3 mL of fat is usually enough for each side.
- *If visible lumps are seen after infiltration, take immediate measures to correct this*: If lumps are noticed immediately after infiltration, digital pressure is usually effective. However, fat should never be placed with the idea that pressure can change the lid shape after transfer. Big lumps that do not flatten easily might need liposuction.
- *For superficial injection, consider nanofat grafts*, which consist of further processing, emulsification, and filtering of the lipoaspirate. These samples have low adipocyte viability but are rich in adipose-derived stem cells, which account for its positive effects on skin rejuvenation.

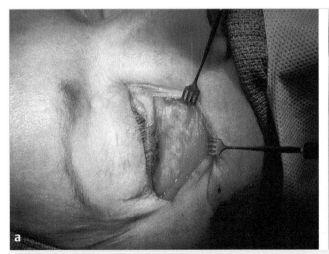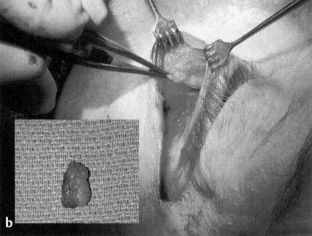

Fig. 24.2 (a,b) In this patient, the transcutaneous approach was chosen so that her lid retraction and skin excess could also be addressed, along with removal of excess injected fat. As seen above, the injected fat bears little resemblance to the periorbital fat and maintains the appearance and morphologic character of the area from which it was harvested. Typically, the fat is whiter in color and very fibrous. In this patient, most of the offending fat was deep to the orbicularis and relatively easy to remove. In addition to the removal of the fat, the patient underwent a canthal reanchoring and subperiosteal midface lift.

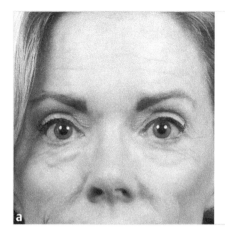
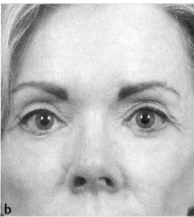

Fig. 24.3 **(a)** Before and **(b)** after removal of fat grafts, canthopexy orbicularis redraping, and midface lift through skin muscle approach.

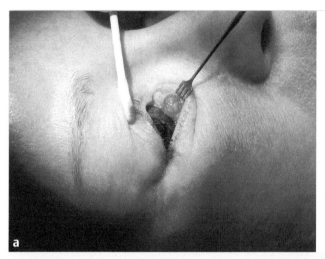
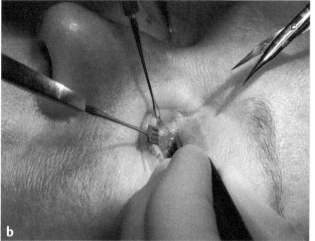

Fig. 24.4 **(a,b)** Patient with overinjection of fat grafts medially. In this case as the excess fat was well defined, limited to the medial part of the lid and deep to the orbicularis, the transconjunctival approach was chosen for bilateral removal. Additionally, as there was no excess skin, the transconjunctival approach was our choice.

24.3 Treatment of Postoperative Irregularities

There are several reported options for dealing with irregularities, lumping, and overgrafting of fat in the lower eyelid. We have had experience with all. In our experience, surgical removal has proven to be the most effective.

- *Massage*: When the lumps are small and diffuse, immediate postoperative massage can soften and reposition the excess fat. The lump should be massaged in a rolling motion against the underlying bone to allow enough pressure to be exerted. Coleman recommends performing the massage for 30 seconds, four to six times per day for a few weeks.
- *Steroid injection*: The injection of steroids such as triamcinolone into the lumps can help decrease their volume. However, this is unpredictable in the sense that it can also lead to thinning of the skin, excessive atrophy of the subcutaneous tissue, hyperpigmentation, visible crystals under the skin, and the appearance of telangiectasia. Thinning of the skin and the subcutaneous tissue can actually make the lumps more visible. In addition, the effect on the fat grafts can be temporary, and when the lumps return, they can rebound to a larger volume.

- *Liposuction*: Liposuction of the excess grafted fat is a simple and minimally invasive solution. The same cannula used to infiltrate the fat can be applied to suction it. Before liposuction, Coleman recommends perforating the capsule around the fatty collection to gain access to the fat. More suction than expected might be necessary and the surgeon should stop and evaluate the lower lid several times during the process. The look and feel of the lower lid will indicate the surgeon when enough fat has been removed. The surgeon should be prepared to perform some additional fat grafting as an adjunct to the liposuction to achieve optimal results. The patient must be informed that the correction of the problem may require more than one procedure. In our experience, the fat is firm, tough, and not readily suctioned.
- *Direct excision*: When the lumps are small and easily identifiable, these can be excised through a small incision through the skin directly above the fat graft. However, the presence of multiple irregularities can make the various skin incisions aesthetically unpleasing. The same can be said for larger lumps that may require a longer incision. In these cases, liposuctioning or excision of the fat through a blepharoplasty approach might be a better option, keeping in mind the possible complications that can occur with the latter (lower lid malposition). Again, the patient must be warned that two or three sessions might be needed to achieve optimal results.
- *Other chemical agents*: Lipolysis of the excess fat grafts can also be a potential solution for postoperative irregularities. Substances marketed under names such as "Lipodissolve" and "Lipostabil" (Artesan Pharma, Lüchow, Germany) contain phosphatidylcholine solubilized in sodium deoxycholate. Many clinical studies have shown its clinical effect by a decrease in adipose tissue volume after subcutaneous injections. One, however, failed to see any improvement in lower eyelid fat pads after multiples injections of phosphatidylcholine and deoxycholate in a randomized, double-blind, placebo-controlled study in 45 healthy adults. Phosphatidylcholine and deoxycholate seem to decrease fat cell volume due to changes in the cell membrane integrity, adipocyte dysfunction, and cell necrosis. Their lipolytic effect is not related to an induction of a lipolytic pathway. Recent studies have concluded that phosphatidylcholine is not the active substance in these solutions; rather, the changes in cell membrane integrity are more likely attributable to the detergent effect of deoxycholate. It is important to note that the effect of these substances may not be specific for fat cells, and further studies need to be conducted to determine their effect on surrounding tissues. Although usually well tolerated after injection, local inflammatory reactions such as erythema, pain, and edema can be seen in the patient.

24.4 Teaching Points

- The treatment of periorbital hollows with autologous fat grafting is effective but not problem free. Although the consensus is that not all the grafted fat will take, postoperative irregularities continue to be a frustrating complication.

- Preventive measures are the best treatment. The injection of small quantities of fat with every withdrawal, the placement of the fat in a deep plane, and avoiding overcorrection can help achieve an optimal result free of complications.
- Although not all the fat will take, it is best to avoid overgrafting.
- If postoperative irregularities develop, the characteristics of the lumps and patient needs will guide options for treatment.
- In our experience, surgical resection has proven effective and safe.

Suggested Reading

[1] Ablon G, Rotunda AM. Treatment of lower eyelid fat pads using phosphatidylcholine: clinical trial and review. Dermatol Surg. 2004; 30(3):422–427, discussion 428

[2] Codner MA, Nahai F, Hester TR, McCord C, Day CR. Role of fat in the lower eyelid. Perspect Plast Surg. 2001; 15:1

[3] Carraway JH, Coleman S, Kane MAC, Patipa M. Periorbital rejuvenation. Aesthet Surg J. 2001; 21(4):337–343

[4] Coleman SR, ed. Infraorbital and cheek regions. In: Structural Fat Grafting. St. Louis, MO: Quality Medical Publishing; 2004:293

[5] Coleman SR. Structural fat grafting: more than a permanent filler. Plast Reconstr Surg. 2006; 118(3, Suppl):108S–120S

[6] Coleman SR. Revisional fat grafting of the cheek and lower eyelid. In Grotting JC, ed. Reoperative Aesthetic and Reconstructive Plastic Surgery. 2nd ed. St. Louis, MO: Quality Medical Publishing; 2006:403

[7] Coleman SR. Facial augmentation with structural fat grafting. Clin Plast Surg. 2006; 33(4):567–577

[8] Kranendonk S, Obagi S. Autologous fat transfer for periorbital rejuvenation: indications, technique, and complications. Dermatol Surg. 2007; 33(5):572–578

[9] Reeds DN, Mohammed BS, Klein S, Boswell CB, Young VL. Metabolic and structural effects of phosphatidylcholine and deoxycholate injections on subcutaneous fat: a randomized, controlled trial. Aesthet Surg J. 2013; 33(3):400–408

[10] Rittes PG. The use of phosphatidylcholine for correction of localized fat deposits. Aesthetic Plast Surg. 2003; 27(4):315–318

[11] Salti G, Ghersetich I, Tantussi F, Bovani B, Lotti T. Phosphatidylcholine and sodium deoxycholate in the treatment of localized fat: a double-blind, randomized study. Dermatol Surg. 2008; 34(1):60–66, discussion 66

[12] Spector JA, Draper L, Aston SJ. Lower lid deformity secondary to autogenous fat transfer: a cautionary tale. Aesthetic Plast Surg. 2008; 32(3):411–414

[13] Stutman RL, Codner MA. Tear trough deformity: review of anatomy and treatment options. Aesthet Surg J. 2012; 32(4):426–440

[14] Treacy PJ, Goldberg DJ. Use of phosphatidylcholine for the correction of lower lid bulging due to prominent fat pads. J Cosmet Laser Ther. 2006; 8(3):129–132

[15] Tawfik HA, Zuel-Fakkar N, Elmarasy R, Talib N, Elsamkary M, Abdallah MA. Phosphatidylcholine for the treatment of prominent lower eyelid fat pads: a pilot study. Ophthal Plast Reconstr Surg. 2011; 27(3):147–151

[16] Tonnard P, Verpaele A, Peeters G, Hamdi M, Cornelissen M, Declercq H. Nanofat grafting: basic research and clinical applications. Plast Reconstr Surg. 2013; 132(4):1017–1026

[17] Tonnard PL, Verpaele AM, Zeltzer AA. Augmentation blepharoplasty: a review of 500 consecutive patients. Aesthet Surg J. 2013; 33(3):341–352

25 Autogenous Tissue Augmentation: Lower Eyelid Malposition

Glenn W. Jelks and Elizabeth B. Jelks

Summary

Thorough zonal physical examination of the eyelids and contiguous periorbital areas with a seven-parameter sequence enhances successful management of autogenous tissue augmentation–related lower eyelid deformities. Computer-assisted composite photographic techniques aid in documentation, evaluation, and management of eyelid and periorbital deformities.

Keywords: lower eyelid malposition, lower eyelid fat graft deformity, complication of fat grafting, zonal analysis of periorbital deformities, composite photographic analysis

25.1 Patient History Leading to the Specific Lower Eyelid Problem

This 35-year-old man had a previous autogenous tissue injection 1 year earlier into both nasojugal interfaces for treatment of the "tear trough deformity" (▶Fig. 25.1a). Tissue was harvested from the abdomen by syringe suction after saline and lidocaine solution infiltration. Fatty tissue was obtained by gravity separation, and 2 mL was injected into the subcutaneous tissues of each nasojugal interface with a 1 mL syringe and 21-gauge needle. Over the last year, the patient developed a painful, tender, and firm 2 cm by 1 cm mass on the right nasojugal region (▶Fig. 25.1b).

He also complained of tearing and right eye "irritation." He desired removal of the mass and alleviation of his discomfort. He was concerned about eyelid asymmetry, scars, lower eyelid malposition, corneal exposure, tearing, and impaired vision. He had no significant other medical issues. Brain, orbits, and paranasal computed tomographic radiography without contrast revealed "diffuse thickening of right inferior lid extending from the medial canthus region laterally. This is an infiltrative process, most likely inflammatory, please clinically correlate. The adjacent osseous structures and adjacent paranasal sinus cavities are clear."

25.2 Anatomic Description of the Patient's Current Status with Anatomical Analysis

This patient demonstrates one of the most problematic situations of a persistent mass in an area previously augmented with injected "filler" material (▶Fig. 25.1b). This is a complex problem and requires thoughtful evaluation. Documentation and prevention of lower eyelid malposition is essential.

The recommended methods for evaluation are as follows:
- Computer-assisted composite photographs, which document symmetry, deformity, and severity (▶Fig. 25.2).
- Zonal anatomical analysis, which defines the region of involvement (▶Fig. 25.3).
- A seven-step physical examination, which predicts the level of involvement (▶Fig. 25.4).

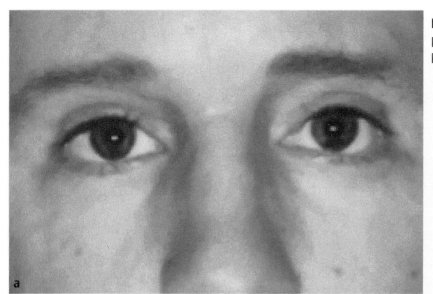

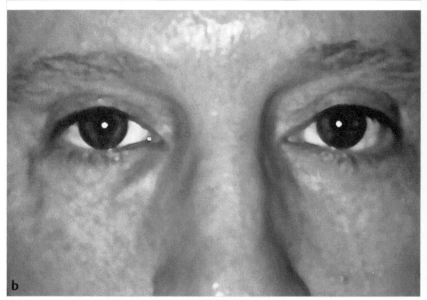

Fig. 25.1 **(a)** Seven years preinjection. **(b)** One year postinjection.

25.2.1 Composite Photographic Analysis

(▶Fig. 25.2)

   Note the following:
   • Asymmetry of compartmental midfacial volume loss.
   • Right lower eyelid 1 mm higher than left lower eyelid.
   • Minimal lower eyelid skin excess or rhytides.

25.2.2 Zonal Analysis

(▶Fig. 25.3a)

25.2.3 Zonal Anatomy

(▶Fig. 25.3b,c)

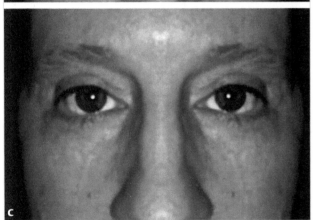

Fig. 25.2 Computer-assisted composite photographic analysis. **(a)** Right composite image. **(b)** Image of patient 1 year postinjection. **(c)** Left composite image. Note: asymmetry of midfacial compartmental volume and right lower eyelid vertical displacement. Technique for creating composite photographic images for facial analysis: define the midline of the facial image of regard **(a)**; divide the face into halves; make copies of right and left halves; flip horizontally and then merge to created right composite **(b)** and left composite images **(c)**.

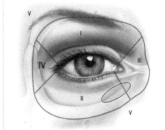

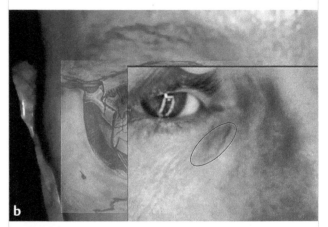

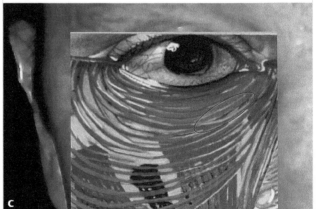

Fig. 25.3 (a) Zonal analysis. **Zone I**, upper eyelid: normal; **Zone II**, lower eyelid: vertical displacement, mass; **Zone III**, medial canthus: elevated lid margin, mass; **Zone IV**, lateral canthus: normal; **Zone V**, periorbital: nasojugal, midface, cheek mass. **(b)** Photograph and anatomy overlay with mass outlined. **(c)** Anatomy overlay with mass outlined.

25.2.4 Seven-Step Analysis

(▶ Fig. 25.4)

25.3 Recommended Solution to the Problem/Technique

- Skin incision at the superior margin of mass (▶ Fig. 25.5a).
- Surgical dissection of mass from subcutaneous tissue and orbicularis oculi muscle to level of orbital septum (▶ Fig. 25.5b–d).

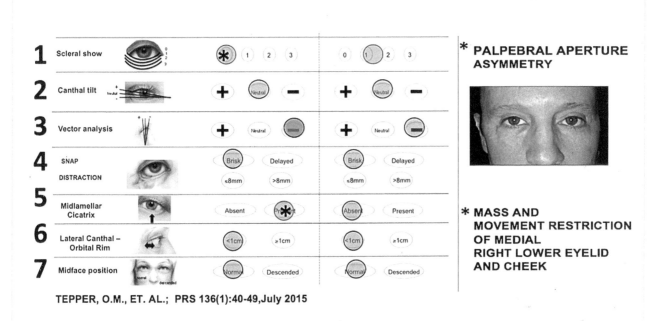

Fig. 25.4 Seven-step physical examination analysis. Palpebral aperture asymmetry, mass in Zone II, III, and V, movement restriction of medial right lower eyelid, medial canthus and cheek.

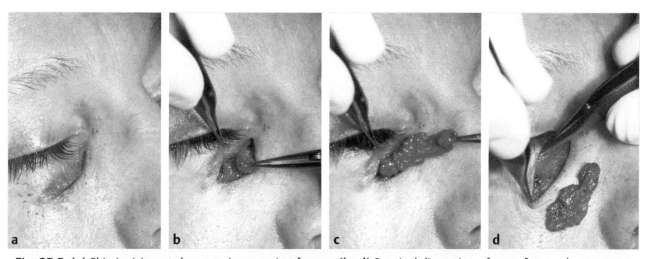

Fig. 25.5 **(a)** Skin incision at the superior margin of mass. **(b–d)** Surgical dissection of mass from subcutaneous tissue and orbicularis oculi muscle to level of orbital septum.

- Release of lower eyelid and cheek movement restrictions with lysis of adhesions and resection of scar tissue.
- Excision of mass with portions of preseptal and orbital orbicularis oculi muscle.
- Suture approximation of orbicularis oculi muscle.
- Suture closure of skin wound.
- Gross examination of mass:
  - 2 cm × 1 cm × 1 cm irregular tissue with encapsulated 3-mm spherical masses of firm yellow material (▶ Fig. 25.6).
- Histological pathology results: Marked inflammatory lymphocytic, leukocytic, and monocyte cellular proliferation. Cellular vacuolation of lipid material within skeletal muscle.

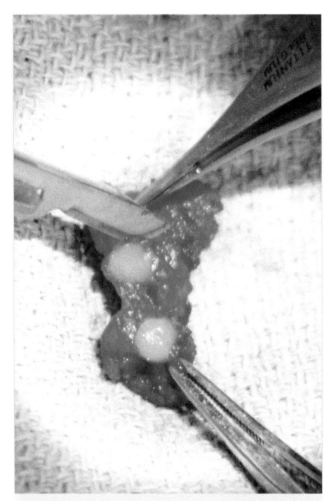

Fig. 25.6 Gross examination of mass: 2 cm × 1 cm × 1 cm irregular tissue with encapsulated 3-mm spherical masses of firm yellow material. Histological pathology results: marked inflammatory lymphocytic, leukocytic, and monocyte cellular proliferation, cellular vacuolation of lipid material within skeletal muscle.

25.4 Postoperative Photographs and Critical Evaluation of Results

The postoperative photographs of this patient at 9 months and 2 years show the removal of the medial right lower eyelid mass and improvement in medial canthal, lower eyelid, and cheek position. Five years postoperative, both lower eyelid positions have descended to reveal less than 1 mm of scleral show.

The depression of the right nasojugal region and contour irregularity of the right lower eyelid, cheek, and midface are present in all postoperative photographs (▶Fig. 25.7; ▶Fig. 25.8a–i).

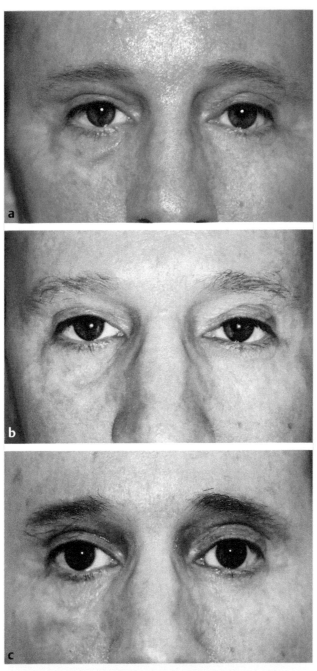

Fig. 25.7 (a) Postoperative situation at 9 months.
(b) Postoperative situation at 2 years.
(c) Postoperative situation at 5 years.

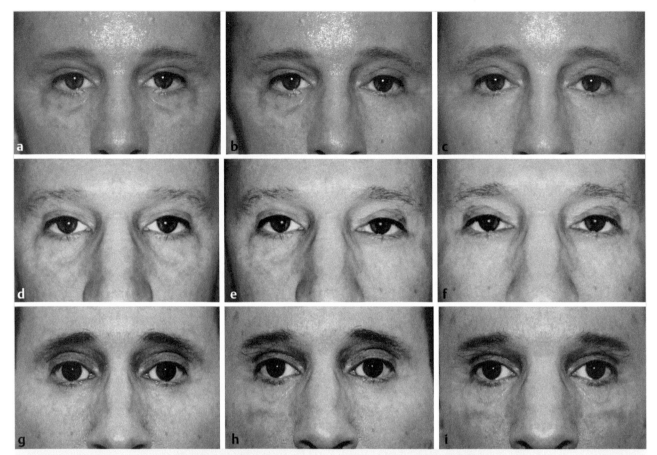

Fig. 25.8 **(a)** Right **composite at 9 months postoperative. (b)** Nine months postoperative. **(c)** Left composite at 9 months postoperative. **(d)** Right composite at 2 years postoperative. **(e)** Two years postoperative. **(f)** Left composite at 2 years postoperative. **(g)** Right composite at 5 years postoperative. **(h)** Five years postoperative. **(i)** Left composite at 5 years postoperative.

Composite computer-assisted photographic analysis documented surgical results and the influence of compartmental facial volume loss.

25.5 Teaching Points

- A complete, accurate history of any previous treatment, trauma, infection, or congenital deformity of the involved area is required to determine any preexisting or contributory conditions. Preoperative photographs are very helpful.
- Computer-assisted composite photographic analysis provides a valuable tool for documentation of the evaluation and management of the problem. The surgical intervention caused a depression of right nasojugal area and did not improve contour irregularities of the right cheek and midface. Surgery removed the tumor and functional impairment of involved periorbital tissue; however, contour irregularities of the right cheek, midface, and nasojugal areas persist. Volume replenishment to submuscular facial compartments may be beneficial.
- Zonal analysis was performed to determine extent of anatomical involvement and functional consequences, such as: lagophthalmos and impaired lower eyelid closure (Zone II); tearing and lacrimal drainage

impairment (Zone III); lateral canthal malposition (Zone IV); and cheek, midface, nasojugal, and temporal deformities (Zone V).

- A thorough physical examination of the eyelids and periorbital area is performed with a proven seven-parameter sequence that provides information to determine preexisting or potential lower eyelid or lateral canthal malpositions.

Suggested Reading

[1] Cotofana S, Schenck TL, Trevidic P, et al. Midface: clinical anatomy and regional approaches with injectable fillers. Plast Reconstr Surg. 2015; 136(5, Suppl):219S–234S

[2] Jelks GW, Jelks EB. Prevention of ectropion in reconstruction of facial defects. Clin Plast Surg. 2001; 28(2):297–302, viii

[3] McCord CD, Jr. The correction of lower lid malposition following lower lid blepharoplasty. Plast Reconstr Surg. 1999; 103(3):1036–1039, discussion 1040

[4] Spinelli HM, Jelks GW. Periocular reconstruction: a systematic approach. Plast Reconstr Surg. 1993; 91(6):1017–1024, discussion 1025–1026

[5] Jelks GW, Jelks EB. The influence of orbital and eyelid anatomy on the palpebral aperture. Clin Plast Surg. 1991; 18(1):183–195

[6] Rzany B, DeLorenzi C. Understanding, avoiding, and managing severe filler complications. Plast Reconstr Surg. 2015; 136(5, Suppl):196S–203S

[7] Tepper OM, Steinbrech D, Howell MH, Jelks EB, Jelks GW. A retrospective review of patients undergoing lateral canthoplasty techniques to manage existing or potential lower eyelid malposition: identification of seven key preoperative findings. Plast Reconstr Surg. 2015; 136(1):40–49

[8] Zide Barry M, Jelks GW. Surgical Anatomy of the Orbit. New York, NY: Raven Press; 1986

26 Lower Eyelid Malposition following Aesthetic Surgery

Richard D. Lisman and Alison B. Callahan

Summary

The most common complication of lower eyelid blepharoplasty is lower eyelid retraction. This is best understood as the result of an imbalance in lower eyelid forces in which negative, downward vectors prevail over the lower eyelid's upward support. It is important to determine which negative vectors are contributing to the retraction in order to properly address them in surgical repair. This chapter describes the assessment of lower eyelid retraction following lower eyelid blepharoplasty and its surgical repair with full-thickness skin grafts when anterior lamellar deficiency is deemed the primary force of retraction.

Keywords: eyelid retraction, blepharoplasty, skin graft, transcutaneous, overresection, Frost, anterior lamella

26.1 Patient History Leading to the Specific Eyelid Problem

This 55-year-old woman had a prior facelift with four-eyelid blepharoplasty (▶Fig. 26.1). Postoperatively, she developed progressive lower eyelid malposition. She was referred to our care, expressing concern over both the appearance of her lower eyelids and ocular surface discomfort. When attempting to manually elevate the eyelid with a finger, the eyelid had minimal upward mobility.

26.2 Anatomic Description of the Patient's Current Status

The patient demonstrates the most common complication of lower eyelid blepharoplasty: lower eyelid retraction. It is best understood as the result of an imbalance in lower eyelid forces in which negative, downward vectors

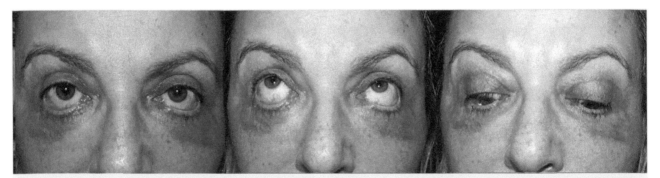

Fig. 26.1 Bilateral lower eyelid retraction following transcutaneous lower eyelid blepharoplasty, demonstrated in **(a)** primary gaze, **(b)** upward gaze, and **(c)** downward gaze.

prevail over the lower eyelid's upward support. Commonly encountered abnormal negative vectors that are found following aesthetic lower eyelid surgery include excessive skin resection, cicatrization of the anterior and middle lamellae, and lateral canthal dystopia/laxity. In addition to a suboptimal aesthetic, lower eyelid malposition and eyelid retraction can cause decompensation of the ocular surface through poor eyelid closure and excess exposure.

When clinically assessing lower eyelid retraction after blepharoplasty and deciding on a restorative approach, it is important to determine which of the three common negative vectors mentioned above (excessive skin resection, cicatrization of the anterior and middle lamellae, and lateral canthal laxity) are contributing to the retraction. This can be assessed by attempting to elevate the lower eyelid with a finger pushing upward, first at the lateral canthus and then at the central eyelid position (▶ Fig. 26.2).

If, with upward pressure at the lateral canthus, the eyelid elevates to a sufficiently high position without bowstringing under the globe or inducing an unnatural bowing of the central or medial eyelid, then lateral canthal laxity is likely the predominant pathology and a simple tarsal resuspension should be sufficient to correct the malposition. However, if one meets significant resistance or if the eyelid creates a bowing deformity, additional negative vectors are likely at play and a simple tarsal resuspension is likely to fail.

One should next attempt to elevate the lower eyelid with a finger at the central lid position. If the lid elevates easily without resistance to a sufficient

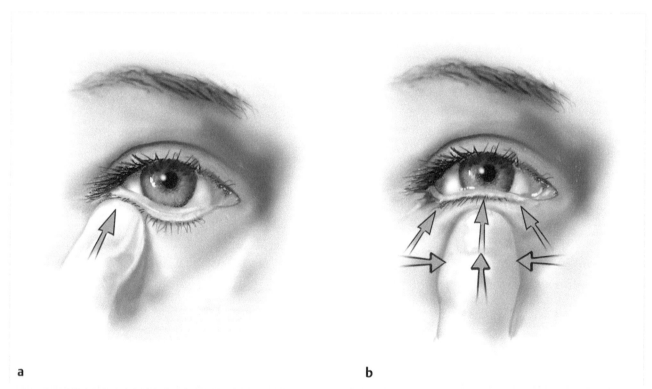

a   b

Fig. 26.2 Attempted elevation of the lower eyelid with upward digital pressure at **(a)** the lateral canthus and **(b)** central eyelid.

height, then middle lamellar scarring is the predominant vector that must be overcome, and a posterior lamellar spacer graft with canthoplasty will be the recommended surgical intervention. We prefer to use hard palate, though ear cartilage and acellular dermis are also commonly used with success as posterior lamellar spacer grafts to help correct lower eyelid retraction following blepharoplasty.

As was the case in the patient presented here, when upward pressure in any location across the lower eyelid fails to elevate the lower eyelid to a suitable position, it may be interpreted that a true anterior lamellar deficiency exists. Excessive skin resection resulted in a foreshortened anterior lamella that is now pulling the lower eyelid downward and outward, creating an ectropion. In these cases, one may also observe lower eyelid movement/retraction upon opening of the mouth. Chronic exposure of the ocular surface to the environment leads to dry eye, exposure keratopathy, and epiphora, and, if left untreated these can lead to more serious corneal decompensation. Unfortunately, with true anterior lamellar deficiency, neither a simple tarsal resuspension nor posterior lamellar lengthening surgery will sufficiently address the pathology.

26.2.1 Analysis of the Problem

Using the methodology outlined above will guide you toward the appropriate surgical intervention. If excessive skin resection is recognized, steps should be taken to rectify the shortage. If recognized early in the postoperative period, sutures can be removed on day 2 or 3 and the wound gaped to allow for subsequent granulation. Massage is needed throughout granulation to counter the inherent forces of contracture. Unfortunately, most anterior lamellar deficiencies become evident in the late postoperative period. At this juncture, with such significant anterior lamellar deficiency, one must replenish the length with a skin graft in order to restore the eyelid's natural structure and function. This may be accomplished by harvesting skin from any number of locations, but we firstly recommend the posterior auricular skin as it most closely resembles the thin eyelid skin; supraclavicular or inner arm skin are other good alternatives. In other settings, skin from the ipsilateral upper eyelid provides an excellent match; however, when addressing lower eyelid retraction and impaired closure, we would advise against further jeopardizing closure by taking upper eyelid skin. To more closely match the extremely thin eyelid skin, we recommend heavily debulking any full-thickness graft from the posterior surface, rendering it more akin to a split-thickness graft while avoiding the sheen known to occur with true split-thickness grafts.

26.3 Recommended Solution to the Problem

Full-thickness skin graft with lateral canthal support:
- Release anterior lamella.
- Resuspend lower eyelid with tarsal strip.
- Replenish deficient anterior lamella with (thinned) full-thickness skin graft.
- Place skin graft and lower eyelid on stretch with posterior compression via modified Frost suture.

26.4 Technique

Using a #15 blade, a lateral canthal incision (crow's foot) is made and then extended subciliary with iris/small sharp blepharoplasty scissors. The epidermis is then freed from any underlying cicatrix with sharp dissection while lifting the inferior edge of the wound with a skin hook and placing the adjacent skin on traction away from your dissection. Bands of cicatrix are strummed with the scissors and incised as the dissection is carried inferiorly to the inferior orbital rim.

One then continues on to the tarsal suspension canthoplasty, firstly performing a canthotomy and cantholysis. The anterior and posterior lamellae are separated and mucocutaneous junction excised with (authors' preference) a #30 blade. A pocket for the tarsal strip is created along the lateral orbital rim with a #15 blade and/or Colorado-tipped cautery. Having released the downward forces of the skin shortage previously and any accompanying cicatrix, the lower lid should now be able to freely elevate to the desired position. Any number of suture choices exist for tarsal resuspension, but the authors' preference is to use a double-armed 4–0 Polydek placed superiorly and inferiorly through the tarsal strip and then secured to the inner aspect of the lateral orbital rim through two periosteal passes. We also place a 4–0 PDS suture through the lateral soft tissue edge of the tarsal strip to the periosteum, thus further bolstering the suspension and covering the underlying Polydek knot to prevent suture cysts. The lateral canthal angle is then reapproximated with two 6–0 chromic sutures and re-enforced with one 6–0 silk.

With the lower eyelid now at its desired position, the true size of the anterior lamellar deficiency (i.e., skin shortage) is now revealed. One then harvests a full-thickness skin graft from the surgeon's site(s) of choice. Again, we would recommend utilizing, if available, a posterior auricular skin. It is imperative to thin the graft from the posterior surface as much as possible without buttonholing to help achieve a thickness more suitable for eyelid skin replacement. This may be accomplished by placing the inverted graft on stretch over a finger and excising excess subcutaneous tissue with a curved Steven's scissors.

Each graft may then be sutured into place, making sure to slightly oversize to combat anticipated contracture. We prefer the slight inflammation achieved with 6–0 silk to facilitate take of the graft. Of subtler note, one of the 6–0 silk sutures at the lateral canthus should include a deeper pass through muscle to drive the crease posteriorly, eliminating webbing at the lateral canthus (▶ Fig. 26.3).

Finally, and perhaps most importantly, the skin graft and lower eyelid should be stretched superiorly to the brow via a Frost suture with underlying bolster compression pushing the graft posteriorly. This will both facilitate vascular supply to the posterior surface of the skin graft and counter cicatricial forces that will pull the eyelid downward during wound healing. To do so, one places three double-armed 6–0 silk sutures across the skin graft and through the upper eyelid and then to the brow in a modified Frost suture. Passes should be taken first of the inferior skin graft margin, then superior graft margin exiting the gray line, then upper eyelid gray line exiting anteriorly, and then to the brow. Prior to securing each suture over a bolster at the inferior skin graft margin and superior brow, a bolster is placed over the skin graft (but under the sutures), thus compressing the bolster posteriorly upon tightening of the sutures (▶ Fig. 26.4).

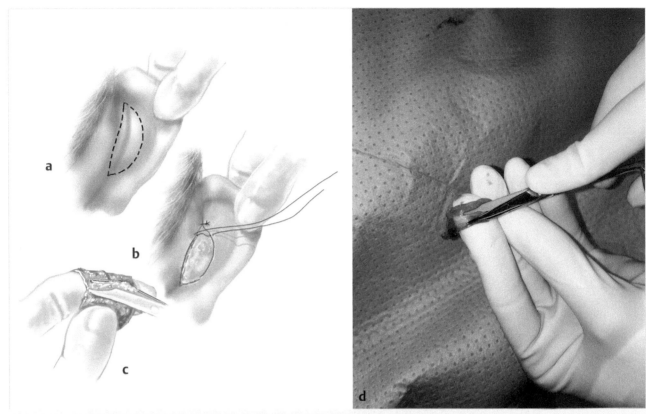

Fig. 26.3 Technique for harvesting posterior auricular skin graft. **(a)** Location of donor graft, **(b)** closure of donor site, and **(c and d)** thinning the graft's posterior (subcutaneous) tissue.

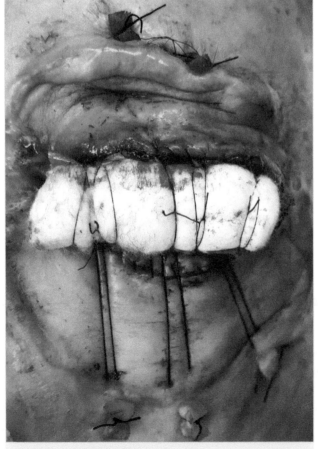

Fig. 26.4 Modified Frost suture.

26.5 Postoperative Photographs and Critical Evaluation of Results

At 1 year postoperatively, one can readily see the improved lower eyelid height, contour, and orientation with regard to the globe. The eyelids still have a small degree of discoloration and irregularity, which will continue to fade and improve with time and/or secondary interventions (▶ Fig. 26.5).

Skin grafts pose an aesthetic challenge to the surgeon and require significant patience on the part of both the patient and the surgeon to allow for time to smooth over the contours and transitional edges. With sufficient time, however, they often blend nicely into the surrounding tissue without need for further intervention. To hasten or improve this process, dermabrasion, lasers, and, more recently, 5-fluorouracil have been used with success to smooth the appearance of skin grafts in the eyelids. Still, expectations must be set a priori with the patient, in terms of both the time required for good aesthetic result and the possibility of additional cosmetic interventions.

To further illustrate the use of this technique as well as contrast it to the approaches for other causes of secondary lower eyelid retraction after blepharoplasty, we have included additional images of long-term postoperative results (▶ Fig. 26.6).

26.6 Teaching Points

- Eyelid retraction is the most common complication following lower eyelid blepharoplasty.
- A transconjunctival approach circumvents many complications by avoiding an anterior and/or middle lamellar wound prone to contracture.
- Preoperative identification of patients at risk for developing lower eyelid retraction is crucial.
- When present, laxity should be addressed at the time of surgery with a lateral canthal tightening procedure and conservative skin resections.
- Taking a systematic approach to the evaluation of lower eyelid retraction will enable you to minimize the extent of surgery required.
- If the eyelid does not easily elevate with digital pressure, anterior lamellar deficiency is the strongest component of retraction, and a skin graft is likely required for its repair.

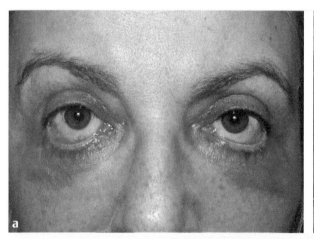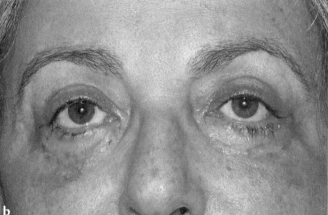

Fig. 26.5 (a) Preoperative and (b) postoperative (1 year) comparison.

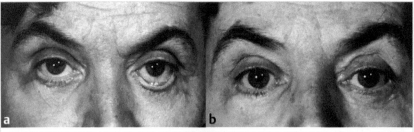

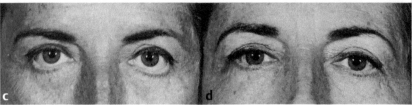

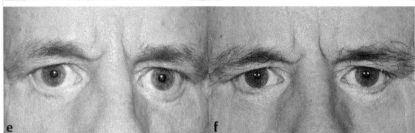

Fig. 26.6 (a,b) Before and after full-thickness skin graft to the left lower eyelid (for retraction after blepharoplasty).
(c,d) Before and after bilateral tarsal suspension (lower lid laxity).
(e,f) Before and after hard palate graft (middle lamellar scar).

- Superb outcomes are possible when this technique is performed well with appropriate patient counseling as to the length of time required for the desired outcome.

Suggested Reading

[1] Baylis HI, Perman KI, Fett DR, Sutcliffe RT. Autogenous auricular cartilage grafting for lower eyelid retraction. Ophthal Plast Reconstr Surg. 1985; 1(1):23–27

[2] Baylis HI, Long JA, Groth MJ. Transconjunctival lower eyelid blepharoplasty. Technique and complications. Ophthalmology. 1989; 96(7):1027–1032

[3] Belinsky I, Patel P, Charles NC, Lisman RD. Ointment granulomas following sutureless transconjunctival blepharoplasty: diagnosis and management. Ophthal Plast Reconstr Surg. 2015; 31(4):282–286

[4] Eberlein A, Schepler H, Spilker G, Altmeyer P, Hartmann B. Erbium:YAG laser treatment of post-burn scars: potentials and limitations. Burns. 2005; 31(1):15–24

[5] Li TG, Shorr N, Goldberg RA. Comparison of the efficacy of hard palate grafts with acellular human dermis grafts in lower eyelid surgery. Plast Reconstr Surg. 2005; 116(3):873–878, discussion 879–880

[6] Lelli GJ, Jr, Lisman RD. Blepharoplasty complications. Plast Reconstr Surg. 2010; 125(3):1007–1017

[7] McCord CD, Miotto GC. Dynamic diagnosis of "fishmouthing" syndrome, an overlooked complication of blepharoplasty. Aesthet Surg J. 2013; 33(4):497–504

[8] McKinney P, Zukowski ML, Mossie R. The fourth option: a novel approach to lower-lid blepharoplasty. Aesthetic Plast Surg. 1991; 15(4):293–296

[9] Pacella SJ, Nahai FR, Nahai F. Transconjunctival blepharoplasty for upper and lower eyelids. Plast Reconstr Surg. 2010; 125(1):384–392

[10] Perkins SW, Dyer WK, II, Simo F. Transconjunctival approach to lower eyelid blepharoplasty. Experience, indications, and technique in 300 patients. Arch Otolaryngol Head Neck Surg. 1994; 120(2):172–177

[11] Yoo DB, Azizzadeh B, Massry GG. Injectable 5-FU with or without added steroid in periorbital skin grafting: initial observations. Ophthal Plast Reconstr Surg. 2015; 31(2):122–126

27 Round Eye Deformity

Gabriele Cáceres Miotto and Clinton McCord

Summary

Round eye deformity is the unpleasing eye shape that develops either due to aging and laxity of the lateral canthus or secondarily due to stretching, damaging, or scarring of the lateral canthal tendon after previous surgery or trauma. The lateral scleral triangle becomes rounder and distorted due to loss of integrity or strength of the lateral canthal tendon. Besides the unpleasing aesthetic shape of the eyes, many patients report poor blinking and constant tearing of the eyes, lack of complete eye closure at night, and many nonspecific complaints related to abnormal eye position and lubrication. Severe cases present with scleral show and/or lower lid retraction. Patients who present with round eye deformity can be treated effectively with lower lid skin muscle blepharoplasty for soft tissue repositioning and recruitment associated with canthopexy or canthoplasty to restore the lateral canthal tendon support and position. Sometimes, a drill hole canthopexy or canthoplasty is necessary to give adequate support to the lateral canthus and restore the optimal function of the blinking mechanism. The use of lower lid spacers may also be necessary to correct severe cases of round eyes with lower lid retraction.

Keywords: Round eye, fishmouthing syndrome, canthal dehiscence, blepharoplasty, dry eyes, canthoplasty, canthopexy

27.1 Patient History Leading to the Specific Problem

A normal eye fissure has visible sclera on either side of the cornea, known as the medial and lateral scleral triangles. Round eye deformity is present when the lateral scleral triangle becomes rounder and distorted due to loss of integrity or strength of the lateral canthal tendon. Round eye deformity can be primary due to aging and laxity of the lateral canthus, or secondary to stretching, damaging, or scarring of the lateral canthal tendon due to surgery or trauma.

Patients with round eye deformity usually present with the following symptoms:

- Poor blinking mechanism leading to chronic dry eyes that do not subside with continuous use of eye drops or eye lubricants.
- Tearing of the eyes.
- Unpleasing aesthetic shape of the eyes or complaints of "small eyes" after eyelid surgery.
- *Fishmouthing* syndrome during blinking.
- Lack of complete eyelid closure.
- Nonspecific symptoms related to abnormal eye position or lubrication.
- Scleral show and/or lower lid retraction.

The patient shown in ▶ Fig. 27.1 presented with round eye deformity after a previous four-lid blepharoplasty performed elsewhere. The major complaints were unpleasing eyelid shape, lack of eyelid closure, and excessive tearing due to poor blinking mechanics. On examination, she presented with unpleasing eye shape, rounding of the lateral scleral triangle, scleral show, and poor eyelid closure.

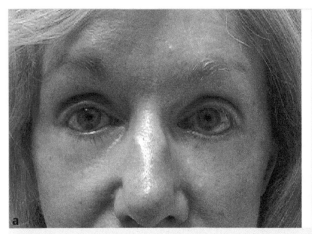
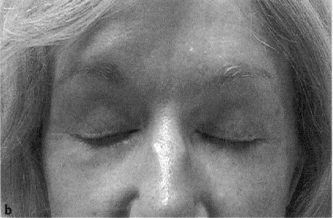

Fig. 27.1 (a,b) A 53-year-old female patient showing canthal dehiscence, small and round lateral scleral triangle, eyelash deformity, and poor closure after previous blepharoplasty.

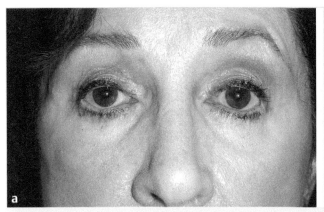
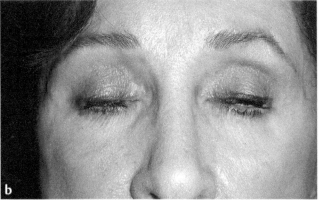

Fig. 27.2 (a,b) A 61-year-old female patient with round eye deformity and incomplete closure of the eyes with blinking after previous blepharoplasty.

The patient shown in ▶ Fig. 27.2 also presented with round eye deformity after a previous four-lid blepharoplasty elsewhere. The major complaints were unpleasing eyelid shape and lack of eyelid closure. On examination, she presented with distortion of the lateral scleral triangle, mild scleral show, and poor eyelid closure. She also had concomitant eyelid ptosis.

27.2 Anatomic Description of the Patient's Current Status

In both cases, the distortion of the lateral scleral triangle is very clear. The normal pointy shape of the most lateral angle of the lateral scleral triangle is blunt, rounded, and displaced inferiorly. The rounding of the lateral scleral triangle makes the eye fissure look unnatural with loss of the natural almond shape of the eyes. This is particularly visible at rest and can be more severe in patients with deep-set eyes. Other problems such as poor eyelid closure and scleral show are also present.

A dynamic distortion often happens in the round eye deformity. During blinking, the lateral canthus is more easily displaced nasally and this abnormal blinking biomechanics causes incomplete eyelid closure with gapping of the eyelids. Patients with round eye deformity can also present with a phenomenon called fishmouthing syndrome. Fishmouthing syndrome is a dynamic deformity of the eyelid during blinking that resembles the concentric movement of a fish mouth. The normal eye blinking happens due to the contracture of the inner canthal orbicularis oculi muscle, a very powerful muscle group. When this strong medial contraction finds lateral resistance or counterpull at the lateral canthus, the eyelids close in a vertical vector. When there is laxity or dehiscence at the level of the lateral canthal tendon, the contraction of the inner orbicularis oculi muscle during blinking causes a strong pull of the eyelids toward the nose, creating a rounded and weak approximation of the eyelids instead (▸Fig. 27.3).

Fishmouthing syndrome also produces medial and downward displacement of the upper lid lashes due lateral canthal tendon weakness. This eyelash deformity is called "cow lashes" deformity and is a sign of the fishmouthing syndrome: straight upper eyelashes pointing nasally and downward (▸Fig. 27.4). This deformity can be seen at rest and is intensified during blinking.

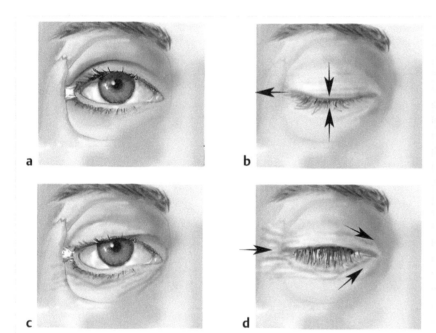

Fig. 27.3 (a–d) Poor blinking mechanism present in the round eye deformity due to weakening of the lateral canthal tendon. From Codner MA, McCord Jr CD. Eyelid & Periorbital Surgery. 2nd ed. New York, NY: Thieme; 2016.)

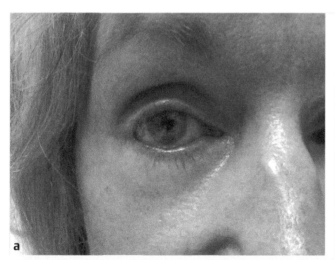
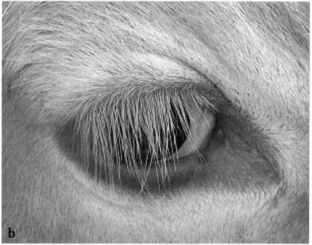

Fig. 27.4 (a,b) "Cow lashes" deformity present in round eye deformity.

27.3 Recommended Solution to the Problem

Patients who present with round eye deformity are treated with lower lid skin muscle blepharoplasty approach for soft tissue repositioning and recruitment, and canthopexy or canthoplasty to restore the lateral canthal tendon support and position.

Recommended treatment to the patient shown in ▶ Fig. 27.1:

- Lower lid skin muscle blepharoplasty approach, subperiosteal release of orbitomalar ligament and periorbital attachments, release of lower eyelid retractors, canthal tendon anchoring through canthopexy, drill hole fixation to the lateral orbital rim, and orbicularis suspension.

Recommended treatment to the patient shown in ▶ Fig. 27.2:

- Lower lid skin muscle blepharoplasty approach, subperiosteal release of orbitomalar ligament and periorbital attachments, horizontal lid shortening due to excessive laxity, canthal tendon anchoring through canthoplasty with drill hole fixation, and orbicularis suspension.

27.4 Technique

A subciliary incision is performed and a skin muscle flap is elevated preserving a strip of pretarsal orbicularis (▶ Fig. 27.5a,b). The orbitomalar ligament and periosteal attachments are released in a subperiosteal plane, freeing the lower lid and upper cheek from the deeper planes (▶ Fig. 27.5c). Then, the lower lid retractors are released to expand the posterior lamella and lift the lower lid if necessary (performed for the patient shown in ▶ Fig. 27.1). When the periosteum of the lateral orbital rim is scared, weakened, or distorted, but there is no lower lid laxity, like in this case shown in ▶ Fig. 27.1, a canthopexy is performed through a drill hole in the lateral orbital rim (▶ Fig. 27.6). When the patient presents with lower lid laxity due to horizontal excess, like in the patient shown in ▶ Fig. 27.2, a canthoplasty with resection of the lower lid excess is performed with a drill hole fixation (▶ Fig. 27.7).

A single drill hole is created at the lateral orbital rim to secure the canthopexy or canthoplasty according to eye prominence and optimal lid positioning. Positioning the inner drill hole well inside the orbital rim is a crucial step to reconstruct the normal anatomy.

For the canthopexy (case 1), a double-armed 4–0 permanent suture such as Mersilene is passed through the lateral canthal tendon. Both arms of the suture pass through the drill hole and are tied to the temporal fascia. Positioning the lateral canthal tendon inside the orbital rim is a crucial maneuver to avoid buckling and distortion of the lateral canthal region. After the canthopexy is performed, the lateral orbicularis oculi muscle is undermined from the skin and used as a handle/sling to reposition the lower eyelid and upper cheek superiorly in an anatomical position. The lateral orbicularis sling is sutured to the deep temporal fascia and the skin is repositioned accordingly and closed with 6–0 nonabsorbable sutures (▶ Fig. 27.8).

For the canthoplasty (case 2), a double-armed 4–0 permanent suture such as Mersilene is passed through the tarsal plate of the lower eyelid and the remaining upper lid canthal tendon. Both arms of the suture pass through the drill hole and are tied to the temporal fascia. Positioning the neocanthus (lower lid tarsal edge) inside the orbital rim is a crucial maneuver to avoid buckling and to reconstruct of the lateral canthal region in an anatomical position.

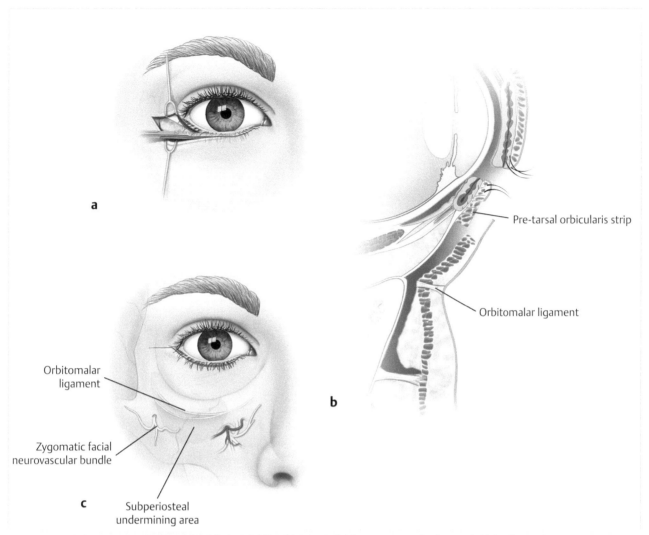

Pre-tarsal orbicularis strip

Orbitomalar ligament

Orbitomalar ligament

Zygomatic facial neurovascular bundle

Subperiosteal undermining area

Fig. 27.5 **(a)** Intraoperative image showing the skin muscle flap incision for lower lid blepharoplasty. **(b)** Intraoperative image showing the skin muscle flap reflected inferiorly and the undermined lateral canthal area. **(c)** The area of subperiosteal dissection (shaded area over zygoma and maxilla) necessary for tissue mobilization and repositioning. This includes the release the orbitomalar ligament in the area.

Lastly, the lateral orbicularis oculi muscle is undermined from the skin and used as a handle/sling to elevate the lower eyelid and upper cheek. The orbicularis is secured to the deep temporal fascia and the skin is repositioned accordingly and closed with nonabsorbable 6–0 sutures (▶ Fig. 27.8).

27.5 Postoperative Photographs and Critical Evaluation of Results

27.5.1 Case 1

Preoperative pictures are given in ▶ Fig. 27.9a,b. The patient presents with rounding of the lateral scleral triangle, scleral show, "cow lashes" deformity, and poor eyelid closure after previous four-lid blepharoplasty.

Postoperative pictures are given in ▶ Fig. 27.9c,d. The patient is shown at 6 months after skin muscle lower lid blepharoplasty approach, lower lid

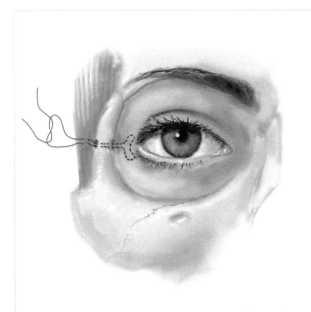

Fig. 27.6 Drill hole fixation of the upper and lower lid tendons with lateral canthopexy, usually done when there is lower lid laxity but no lower lid excess (no need for shortening the lid). From Codner MA, McCord Jr CD. Eyelid & Periorbital Surgery. 2nd ed. New York, NY: Thieme; 2016.)

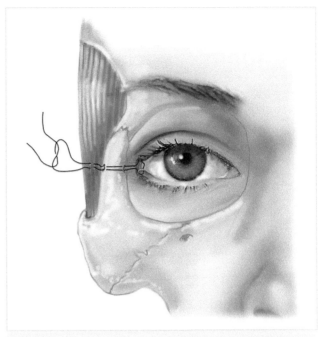

Fig. 27.7 Drill hole fixation of the upper and lower lid tendons with lateral canthoplasty, done when there is lower lid excess. Shortening of the upper lid is performed to provide optimal lid closure and eye shape. From Codner MA, McCord Jr CD. Eyelid & Periorbital Surgery. 2nd ed. New York, NY: Thieme; 2016.)

retractors release, canthopexy using drill hole fixation, and orbicularis suspension. The round eye shape is restored to a pleasant almond shape with normal lateral scleral triangles. Correction of the scleral show and the eye closure deficiency is also achieved. There is also correction of the "cow lashes" deformity. This patient could probably have benefited from a lower lid spacer on her left lower lid for correction of a very subtle residual scleral show, which at the time of surgery was thought not to be necessary.

27.5.2 Case 2

Preoperative pictures are given in ▶Fig. 27.10a,b. The patient presents with distortion of the lateral scleral triangle, mild scleral show, lower lid laxity, and poor eyelid closure after a previous four-lid blepharoplasty. She also had concomitant eyelid ptosis.

Postoperative pictures are given in ▶Fig. 27.10c,d. The patient is shown at 6 months after correction of upper lid ptosis and correction of the round eye deformity through a lower lid skin muscle blepharoplasty approach, lower lid retractors release, lower lid shortening, canthoplasty with drill hole fixation, and orbicularis suspension. The round eye shape is restored to its normal almond shape. There is full correction of the scleral show and eyelid closure deficiency.

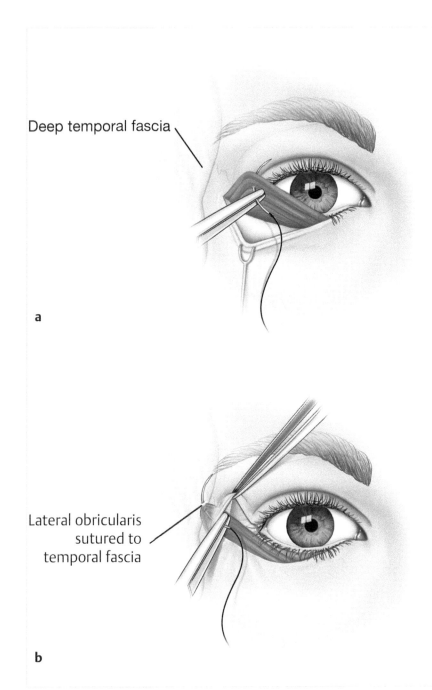

Deep temporal fascia

a

Lateral obricularis
sutured to
temporal fascia

b

Fig. 27.8 (a,b) The orbicularis oculi muscle flap that is used to suspend and support the lower lid. The muscle is sutured to the deep temporal fascia with two to three anchoring stitches for long-term support.

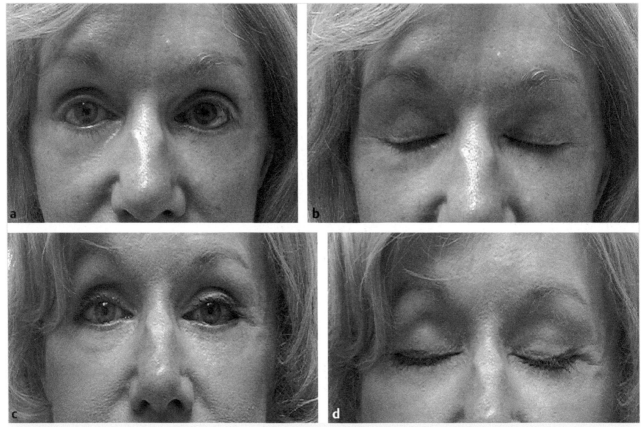

Fig. 27.9 (a,b) A 53-year-old female patient after previous four-lid blepharoplasty presenting with canthal dehiscence, small and round lateral scleral triangle, eyelash deformity, and poor closure. **(c,d)** This is the same patient after lower lid skin muscle blepharoplasty approach, subperiosteal release of orbitomalar ligament and periorbital attachments, release of lower eyelid retractors, canthal tendon anchoring through canthopexy and drill hole fixation to the lateral orbital rim, and orbicularis suspension.

27.6 Teaching Points

- Round eye deformity occurs when there is lack of integrity or loss of strength of the lateral canthal tendon, mainly after previous eyelid surgery.
- Signs and symptoms include mild to severe static and dynamic distortions of the eye shape.
- Recognition of the signs and symptoms associated with the deformity helps to guide the selection of the appropriate treatment.
- The main goal of treatment is to restore lateral canthus integrity though a canthal anchoring procedure.
- Canthopexy or canthoplasty with drill hole fixation is used according to individual particularities, mainly in secondary cases.
- Consider treatment of associated deformities such as lower lid retraction, scleral show, or lagophthalmos when planning the surgical procedure.

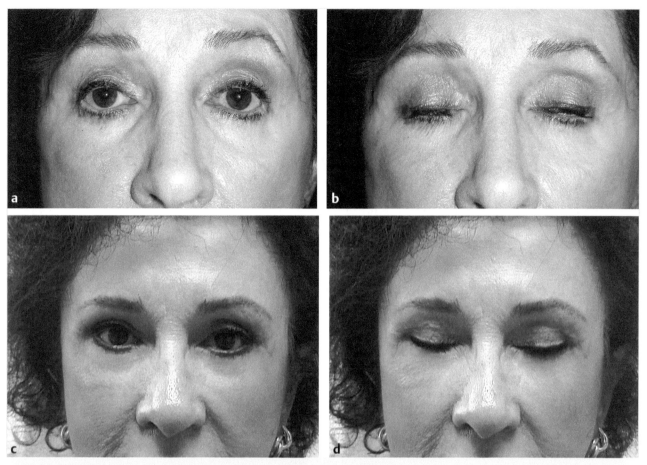

Fig. 27.10 **(a,b)** A 61-year-old woman with round eye deformity after a previous four-lid blepharoplasty elsewhere. She presented with unpleasing eyelid shape and lack of eyelid closure. There is distortion of the lateral scleral triangle, mild scleral show, and poor eyelid closure associated with eyelid ptosis. **(c,d)** This is the same patient after lower lid skin muscle blepharoplasty approach, subperiosteal release of orbitomalar ligament and periorbital attachments, horizontal lid shortening due to excessive laxity, canthal tendon anchoring through canthoplasty with drill hole fixation, and orbicularis suspension.

Suggested Reading

[1] Hirmand H, Codner MA, McCord CD, Hester TR, Jr, Nahai F. Prominent eye: operative management in lower lid and midfacial rejuvenation and the morphologic classification system. Plast Reconstr Surg. 2002; 110(2):620–628, discussion 629–634

[2] McCord CD, Boswell CB, Hester TR. Lateral canthal anchoring. Plast Reconstr Surg. 2003; 112(1):222–237, discussion 238–239

[3] McCord CD, Codner MA. Correction of complications in aesthetic eyelid surgery. In: Eyelid & Periorbital Surgery. 1st ed. St. Louis, MO: Quality Medical Publishing; 2008:269–315

[4] McCord CD, Miotto GC. Dynamic diagnosis of "fishmouthing" syndrome, an overlooked complication of blepharoplasty. Aesthet Surg J. 2013; 33(4):497–504

[5] Muzaffar AR, Mendelson BC, Adams WP, Jr. Surgical anatomy of the ligamentous attachments of the lower lid and lateral canthus. Plast Reconstr Surg. 2002; 110(3):873–884, discussion 897–911

[6] Shorr N. Madame Butterfly procedure with hard palate graft: management of postblepharoplasty round eye and scleral show. Facial Plast Surg. 1994; 10(1):90–118

28 Lateral Canthoplasty: Lateral Canthal Tendon Tightening and Malar Fat Pad Elevation (Mini-Cheek Lift)

Michael Patipa, Michael A. Connor, and Patrick Tenbrink

Summary

The lateral canthal tendon is often overlooked on examination but is one of the most important eyelid structures to evaluate in any patient interested in lower eyelid surgery as well as any patient with tearing symptoms. When lateral canthal tendon laxity is noted preoperatively, tightening the tendon can result in a better cosmetic appearance of the lateral canthal angle, prevent postoperative eyelid malposition, and improve the function of the lower eyelid.

Keywords: lateral canthal tendon, canthoplasty, festoons, midface descent, lower eyelid laxity, lower eyelid retraction, dry eye

28.1 Patient History Leading to the Specific Problem

28.1.1 Case 1

This is a 62-year-old woman with a history of dry eyes (►Fig. 28.1). She had a cosmetic lower eyelid blepharoplasty 3 years prior to evaluation. She had a facelift, endoscopic brow lift, and upper lid blepharoplasty 2.5 years prior to evaluation. She did okay for 2 years and then noted lower eyelid festoons. She was treated with a diuretic without improvement. She saw another physician who recommended filler, which she did not have. She had a negative thyroid workup. She was referred because of her prominent lower eyelid and midface festoons.

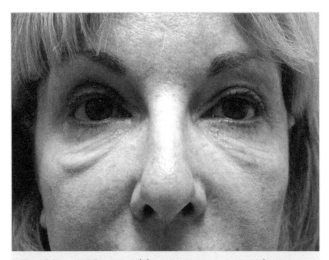

Fig. 28.1 A 62-year-old woman status post lower eyelid blepharoplasty 3 years previously and facelift, brow lift, and upper blepharoplasty 2.5 years ago with dry eye and malar festoons.

28.2 Anatomic Description of the Patient's Current Status

28.2.1 Case 1

This patient demonstrates one of the most common problems encountered following cosmetic lower eyelid surgery (▶Fig. 28.2a–d). She has laxity of her lateral canthal tendons and prominent midfacial festoons, and has significant complaints of dry eye symptoms.

28.2.2 Analysis of the Problem

On examination, the patient has laxity of her lateral canthal tendon. She has mobility of the lateral canthal angle (▶Fig. 28.2a). When a finger is placed at her lateral canthal tendon, it places the lower eyelid back to its normal anatomic position (▶Fig. 28.2b). However, the malar festoons remain. Placing one finger over the lateral canthal angle and one finger over the malar eminence repositions the lower eyelid and midface back to its normal anatomic position (▶Fig. 28.2c). Prior to undertaking surgery, the patient needed an appropriate workup. She had a free T3, free T4, thyroid-stimulating immunoglobulin, and thyroid autoantibodies studies performed. All of those tests were negative. Based on that

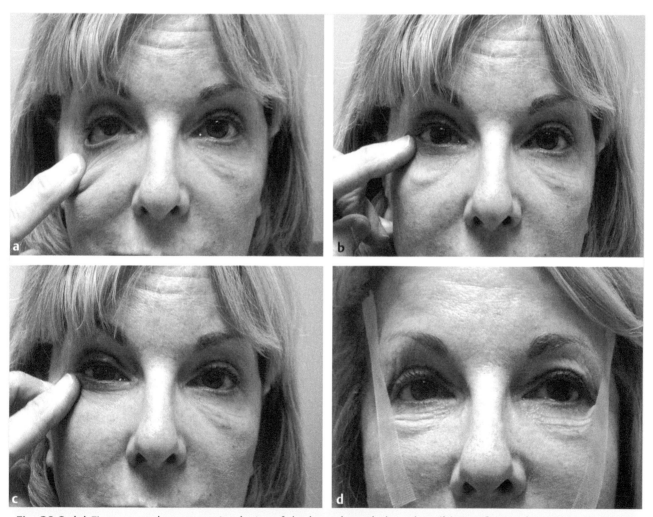

Fig. 28.2 (a) Finger test demonstrating laxity of the lateral canthal tendon. (b) One finger places the tendon back to the lateral orbital rim. (c) Two fingers places the tendon against the orbital rim and lifts the orbitomalar ligament providing vertical support to the lower eyelid. (d) Tape test allows the patient to see and feel what might be achieved after lateral canthal tendon tightening and mini-cheek lift.

evaluation, a lateral canthal tendon tightening and malar fat pad elevation (mini-cheek lift), in conjunction with a cosmetic lower eyelid blepharoplasty, was scheduled. It is intended to place the lower eyelid and midface back to its normal anatomic position and provide an aesthetically pleasing lower eyelid and midface. A 0.5-inch piece of tape placed over the malar eminence and then pulled tightly up to the temple elevates the lower eyelid back to its normal anatomic position, helping the patient preview the shape of the lower eyelids following surgery. The patient needs to understand the redundant or excess lower eyelid skin and folds will not be there after surgery (▶ Fig. 28.2d). The intent of the tape test is simply to illustrate or preview the lower eyelid position.

28.3 Recommended Solution to the Problem

- Cosmetic lower eyelid blepharoplasty with skin muscle flap.
- Tightening of the lateral canthal tendon with reattachment of the lateral tarsus back to the lateral orbital tubercle.
- Malar fat pad elevation with reattachment of the lax orbitomalar ligament to the lateral orbital tubercle.

28.3.1 Dry Eyes, Exposure, Epiphora

Case 2

Here is another clinical presentation with functional complaints that can also be addressed using the same technique described below. This is a 67-year-old woman. She had a cosmetic upper and lower eyelid blepharoplasty elsewhere. She had a subsequent excision and reconstruction of right medial lower eyelid basal cell carcinoma. She was referred for significant dry eyes and excessive reflex tearing due to the dry eyes. She had seen multiple doctors because of her dry eyes. On examination, she had lower eyelid retraction (▶ Fig. 28.3; ▶ Fig. 28.4).

She had laxity of her lateral canthal tendons. She had malar fat pad descent. She had lateral canthal angle mobility and a significantly abnormal snap back test. She underwent a bilateral canthal tendon tightening and malar fat pad elevation (mini-cheek) procedure using a permanent Polydek suture. She stated that her excessive tearing and dry eye symptoms were significantly improved following surgery.

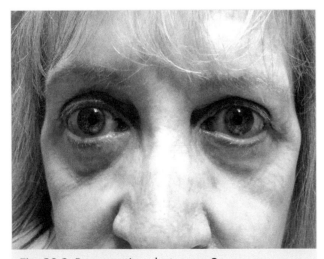

Fig. 28.3 Preoperative photo case 2.

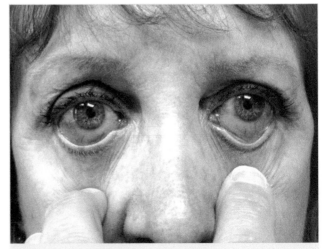

Fig. 28.4 Preoperative distraction test case 2.

28.4 Technique

The malar fat pads are marked (▶ Fig. 28.5a). The procedure is performed through an infraciliary lower eyelid blepharoplasty incision (▶ Fig. 28.5b, c). An infraciliary skin muscle flap is elevated (▶ Fig. 28.5d). A lateral canthotomy is performed, the lower limb of the lateral canthal tendon released, and 0 to 3 mm of lax lateral canthal tendon is resected (▶ Fig. 28.5e, f). A lacrimal rake is inserted and dissection in a preperiosteal plane is performed down to the zygomatic facial vessels without transgressing the vessels, and the malar fat pad is freed up. If the zygomatic facial sensory neurovascular complex is transgressed, this is not a problem as it is a very small sensory nerve and causes no postoperative difficulties (▶ Fig. 28.5g, h). The lower crus of the lateral canthal tendon is completely released.

A 5–0 Vicryl double-armed suture on an S14 needle is used in those cases where there is minimal to moderate laxity of the lateral canthal tendon with only moderate tension from previous cosmetic surgery of the midface. When it is a complicated reoperation, a 4–0 Polydek (braided Mersilene) suture on a half circle-cutting needle is used to reattach the lateral canthal tendon back to the lateral orbital tubercle. The suture is placed in a triple whipstitch fashion through the lateral tarsus. The superior arm of the double-armed suture is placed underneath the upper limb of the superior lateral canthal tendon. The inferior suture is placed 2 to 3 mm below the superior suture. The sutures engage the lateral periorbita, thereby reattaching the lateral canthal tendon back to its insertion at the lateral orbital tubercle (▶ Fig. 28.6). A 6–0 plain suture is then placed through the gray line of the lateral lower eyelid and upper eyelid and tied reforming the lateral canthal angle. The tarsal suture is then tied reattaching the lower lid back to the lateral orbital tubercle.

A skin hook is applied laterally and one arm of the Polydek suture is placed through the orbicularis muscle and malar fat pad going from superior to inferior and it is buried and tied reattaching the malar fat pad back to the lateral orbital tubercle simulating the orbitomalar ligament (▶ Fig. 28.6c–f). When there is redundant skin, two conservative triangles of skin are resected.

A 5–0 Vicryl suture is then placed through the inferior orbicularis muscle in a buried fashion and then through the superior orbicularis muscle engaging

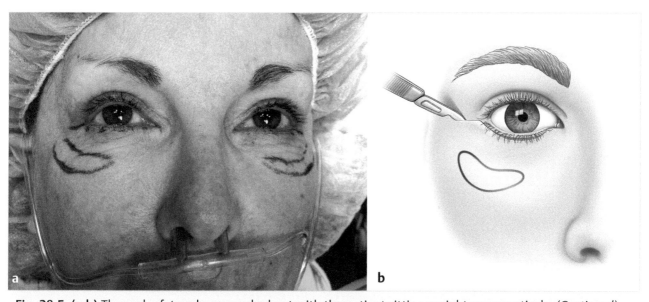

Fig. 28.5 **(a,b)** The malar fat pads are marked out with the patient sitting upright preoperatively. *(Continued)*

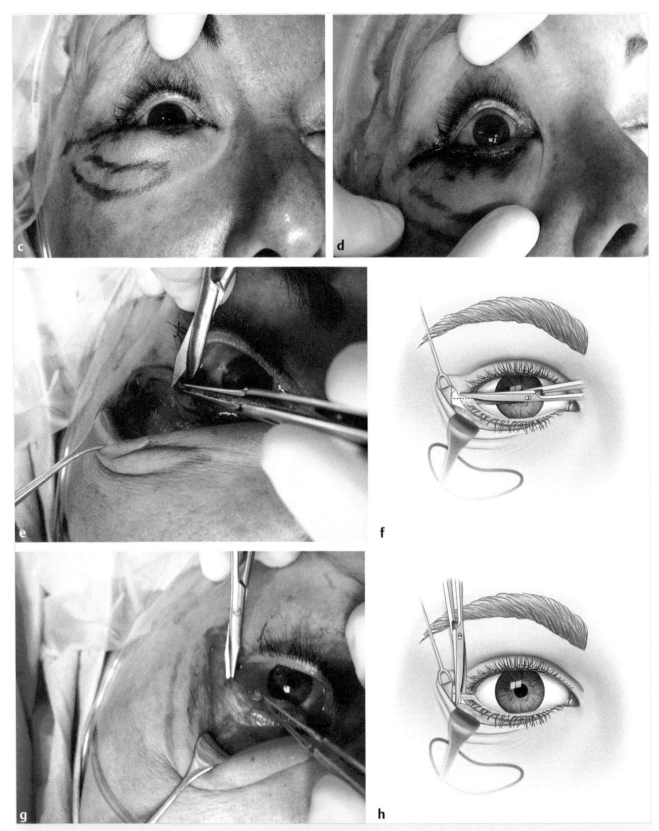

Fig. 28.5 (*Continued*) **(c,d)** A subciliary incision extending into a lateral canthotomy incision is made using a #15 blade. **(e,f)** An inferior cantholysis is performed. **(g,h)** The lower crus of the lateral canthal tendon is completely released.

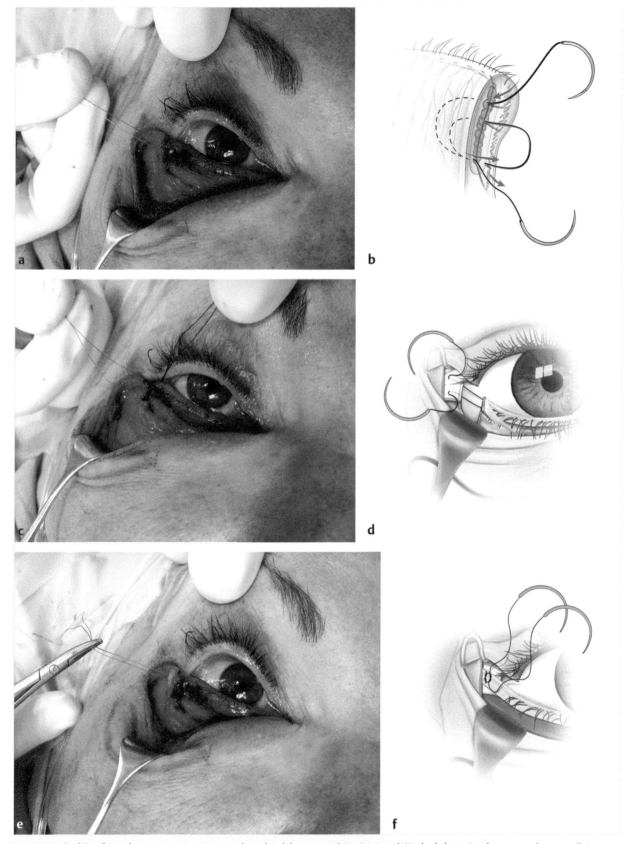

Fig. 28.6 **(a,b)** After the tarsus is trimmed, a double-armed 5–0 Vicryl (Polydek or Prolene can be used) is placed vertically through the tarsus in a whipstitch. The two arms of the suture are placed through the lateral orbital tubercle, inside the orbital rim. **(c-f)** The suture is tied in square knots over the periosteum. *(Continued)*

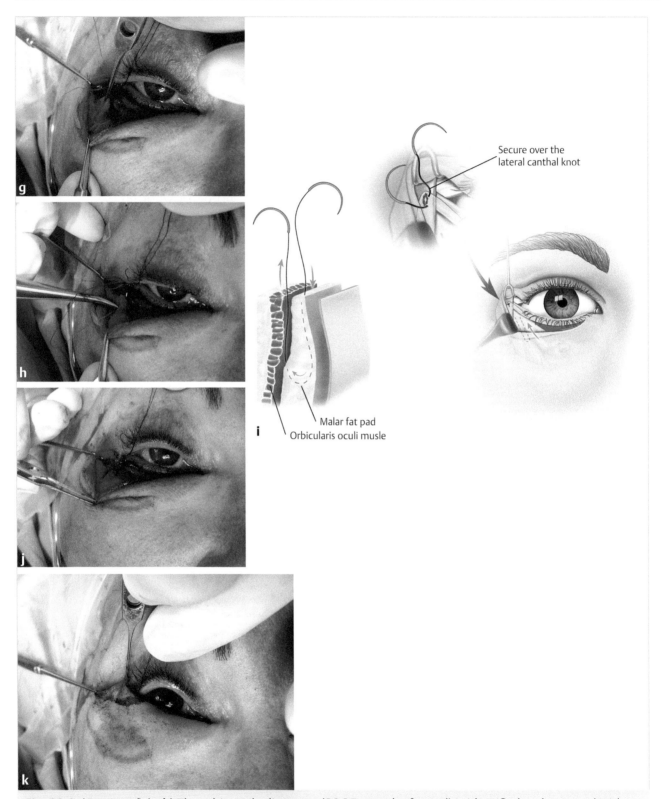

Fig. 28.6 (*Continued*) **(g-k)** The orbitomalar ligament (SOOF or malar fat pad) is identified and engaged with the needle used to reattach the lateral canthal tendon. The suture is tied, securing the orbitomalar ligament to periosteum at the level of the lateral canthal angle. The excess skin and orbicularis is marked out and excised.

the periosteum of the lateral orbital rim and is tied in a buried fashion. This suture tightens the orbicularis muscle sling and also forms a pocket of orbicularis muscle over the lateral orbital tubercle minimizing infections of the lateral canthal tendon Polydek suture. The skin incision is then closed with the 6–0 plain catgut suture (▶Fig. 28.7).

A 5–0 Prolene double-armed suture is then placed through the lateral lower eyelid and lateral brow as a Frost suture. When a skin muscle flap has been elevated, this Frost suture is placed on a bolster in the lower lid (▶Fig. 28.8). When there is no infraciliary incision, the Prolene suture is placed through the gray line of the lower lid margin and then through the lateral brow and tied over a cotton bolster. The patient is treated with antibiotic ophthalmic ointment twice a day to the suture line and fluorometholone drops four times a day for 1 week. Cold compresses are used in a traditional manner.

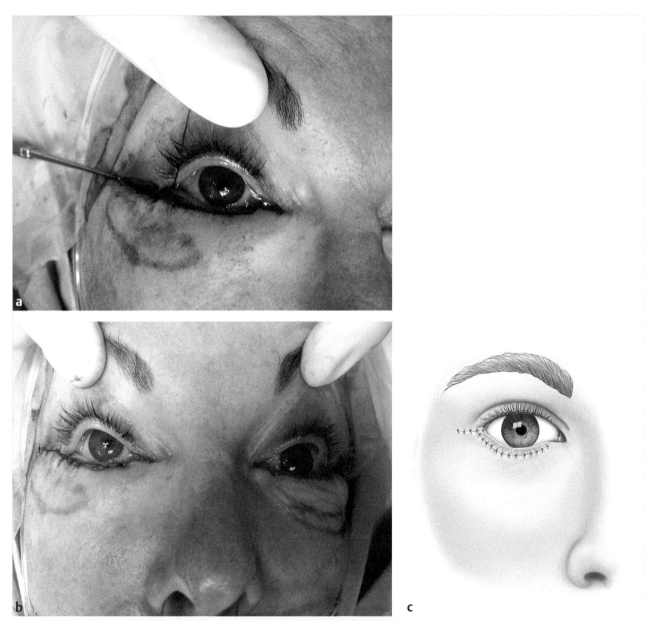

Fig. 28.7 (a-c) A skin hook is placed in the lateral aspect of the wound and the incision is closed with a running 6–0 fast-absorbing plain gut suture.

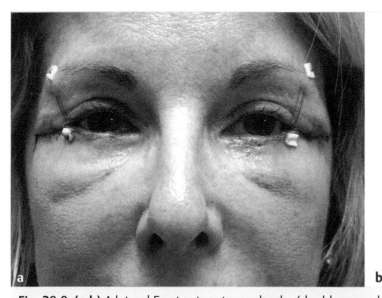
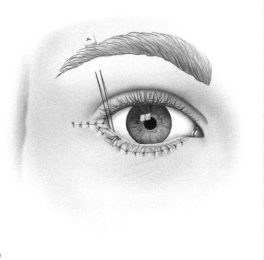

Fig. 28.8 (a,b) A lateral Frost suture tarsorrhaphy (double-armed 5–0 Prolene) is placed to keep the lower eyelid on vertical stretch.

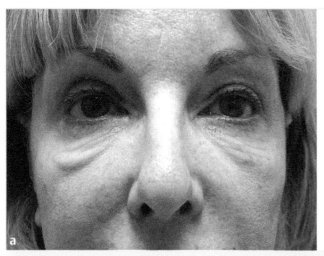
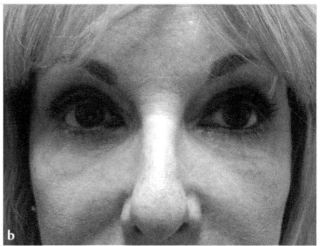

Fig. 28.9 (a) Preoperative photograph demonstrating rounding of the lateral canthus and malar festoons. **(b)** One month postoperative photograph demonstrating an excellent cosmetic result.

28.5 Postoperative Photographs and Critical Evaluation of Results

28.5.1 Case 1

The patient is seen postoperatively showing resolution of the malar festoons and an aesthetically pleasing and functionally appropriate lower lid and midface position (▶ Fig. 28.9).

28.5.2 Additional Applications

Tightening the lateral canthal tendon and elevating the malar fat pad back to the level of the lateral orbital tubercle (mini-cheek lift) can also be utilized for multiple functional as well as cosmetic applications of the lower eyelid and midface.

28.6 Teaching Points

- The eyelid's primary function is protection of the eyeball.
- Laxity of the lower eyelids and midface descent, in addition to being cosmetically unacceptable, also results in loss of the lower eyelid protection and results in worsening of dry eye symptoms as well as tearing due to inability of the lacrimal pump to pump tears medially to the nasolacrimal outflow system.
- Reattaching the lateral canthal tendon restores the normal functional and cosmetic appearance of the eyelid.
- Elevating the malar fat pad supports the lateral canthal tendon tightening and also provides a method of addressing malar festoons.

Acknowledgment

I would like to thank Aly McCanliss for the art and manuscript preparation.

Suggested Reading

[1] Mendelson BC, Hartley W, Scott M, McNab A, Granzow JW. Age-related changes of the orbit and midcheek and the implications for facial rejuvenation. Aesthetic Plast Surg. 2007; 31(5):419–423

[2] Lambros V. Observations on periorbital and midface aging. Plast Reconstr Surg. 2007; 120(5):1367–1376, discussion 1377

[3] Patipa M. Transblepharoplasty lower eyelid and midface rejuvenation: part I. Avoiding complications by utilizing lessons learned from the treatment of complications. Plast Reconstr Surg. 2004; 113(5):1459–1468, discussion 1475–1477

[4] Patipa M. Transblepharoplasty lower eyelid and midface rejuvenation: part II. Functional applications of midface elevation. Plast Reconstr Surg. 2004; 113(5):1469–1474, discussion 1475–1477

[5] Patipa M. The evaluation and management of lower eyelid retraction following cosmetic surgery. Plast Reconstr Surg. 2000; 106(2):438–453, discussion 454–459

29 Treatment of Vertical Lower Lid Restriction with Spacers

Dirk Richter and Nina Schwaiger

Summary

In this chapter, all types of vertical lower lid restrictions are described and related to anterior, mid, or posterior lamella scarring. We also demonstrate different kinds of spacers as well as the use of the subperiosteal midface elevation to recruit skin.

Keywords: lower lid retraction, spacer, midface lift, hard palate mucosal graft, scleral show

29.1 Vertical Restriction in All Lamellas

29.1.1 Patient History Leading to the Specific Problem

A 40-year-old patient presents with a history of previous lower lid blepharoplasty 1 year ago with fat distribution and transconjunctival revisional surgery to revise the scleral show of the first operation (▸ Fig. 29.1). He was a healthy nonsmoker with no significant medical issues.

29.1.2 Anatomic Description of the Patient's Current Status

The patient presents with the common problem of lower lid retraction after lower lid surgery. This can be due to overresection of skin or muscle denervation at the anterior lamellar, hematoma, or infection at the midlamellar or at the level of the posterior lamella with contraction of the conjunctiva or Müller's muscle after transpalpebral approach or Graves' disease. The lower lid malposition is often seen in negative vector patients with no lower lid support

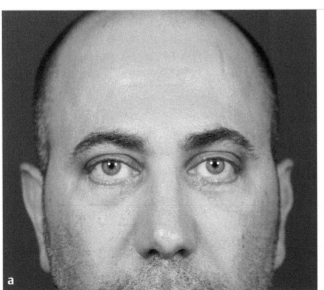
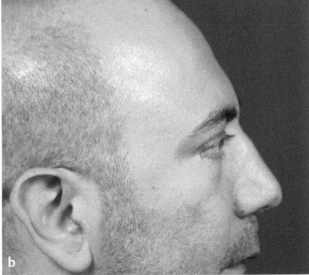

Fig. 29.1 (a,b) A 40-year-old patient with 3-mm scleral show after two previous operations. Vertical restriction in all lamella. Negative vector.

of soft tissue or bony structures. Care should be taken to analyze the patient's history and the anatomical situation according to the lamellas.

He provides a history of severe hematoma especially on the right side postoperatively with a long-lasting swelling, chemosis, and ectropion for several months, which was treated conservatively.

Analysis of the Problem

The patient shows moderate negative tilt on both eyes, vertical restriction of the midlamella with a horizontal lid lengthening of 6 mm left side and 8 mm right side, scleral show 3 mm right side and 2 mm left side, persisting tear trough deformity, and negative vector with Hertel value of 22 on the right side and 21 on the left. There is complete active lid closure but there is 2mm of lagophthalmos on passive closure of the eyelids. There is no conjunctival injection or chemosis. Blinking in all three orbicularis sections is normal with fishmouthing effect.

Diagnosis

This is a complex lower lid malposition with a small skin deficiency and midlamellar scarring, prominent eyes, horizontal lid lengthening, and aesthetic deformity of the arcus marginalis. There is mild posterior retraction with no conjunctival deficiency.

29.1.3 Recommended Solution to the Problem

- Convert the negative vector patient to a normal vector by a subperiosteal midface lift.
- Recruiting skin and releasing vertical restriction by the subperiosteal midface lift.
- Treatment of the horizontal lid laxity by a canthopexy with bony fixation on the left side and a tarsal strip procedure on the right side.
- Support and reconstruction of the midlamellar by acellular dermal matrix (ADM).

29.1.4 Technique

The revision procedure is started with the subperiosteal midface lift, as described by Hester et al, with an anterior skin incision. All attachments from the septum to the orbital rim and the periosteum down to the vestibulum oris are released to free the whole cheek. The periosteum is incised at a low level. Two 3–0 PDS sutures are used to lift the whole cheek up in order to recruit skin. Two drill holes are made at the level of the pupil and 1.5 cm laterally of the orbital rim to secure a stable fixation. Another two holes at the zygomaticotemporal suture for the canthopexy are drilled (▶ Fig. 29.2).

The ADM, 1 mm thick (Permacol), is sutured into the gap between tarsal plate and septum with 5–0 Vicryl, taking care not to suture it to the bone to prevent rendering the lid immobile (▶ Fig. 29.3).

The canthopexy with 4–0 Prolene is performed with the bridge-over-bone technique to slip into the orbit to prevent from lateral canthal displacement. A tarsal strip procedure is added to the right side to address the horizontal lid lengthening (▶ Fig. 29.4).

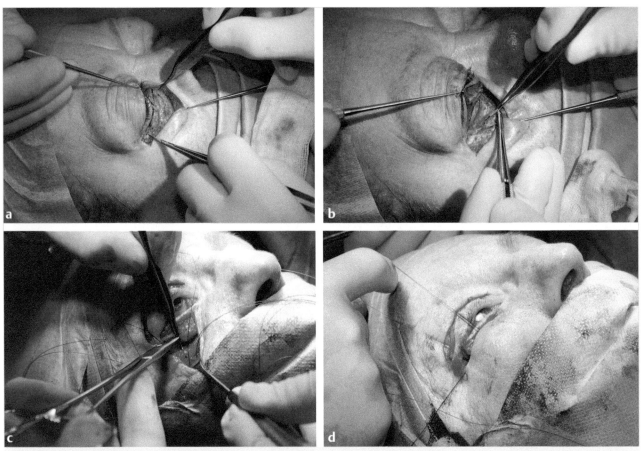

Fig. 29.2 **(a)** Anterior skin incision and approaching the posterior lamella; **(b)** splitting the retractors; **(c)** subperiosteal midface lift with drill holes at the level of the pupil and 1.5 cm laterally for two-point fixation; **(d)** vertical elevation with 3–0 nonresorbable stitches.

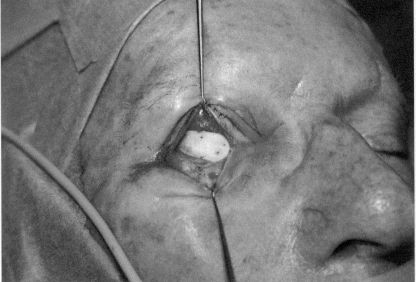

Fig. 29.3 Interpositioning of ADM (Permacol) and fixation with 5–0 resorbable stitches.

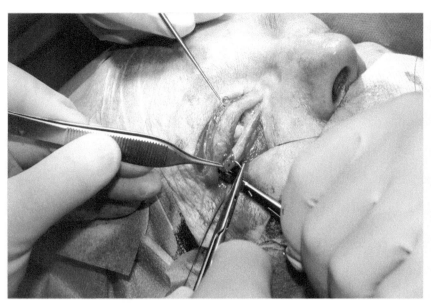

Fig. 29.4 Drill hole canthopexy with tarsal strip shortening.

29.1.5 Postoperative Photographs and Critical Evaluation of Results

▶ Fig. 29.5a shows the patient after 10 days, showing exact position of the lower lid margin touching the limbus and no more scleral show. Good support of the lower lid structures is achieved with a conversion into a normal vector. ▶ Fig. 29.5b,c shows complete lid closure after 1 year.

29.1.6 Teaching Points

- In order to avoid lower lid malposition, we must carefully analyze the individual anatomical situation regarding especially the lower lid tone and the vector.
- To treat complications such as vertical restrictions, it is mandatory to analyze which lamellae are involved. Especially in patients with a negative vector, we will need spacer grafts to support the lower lid structures and/or to change the negative vector into a normal or positive vector by a midface lift or implant.
- Stable bony fixations are key for a durable and reliable result.
- If there is horizontal lid lengthening more than 8 mm, a shortening procedure such as a tarsal strip needs to be performed.

29.2 Vertical Restriction in Mid- and Posterior Lamella

29.2.1 Patient History Leading to the Specific Problem

The patient is a 70-year-old man, who presented after complicated upper and lower blepharoplasty, with two corrections elsewhere (▶ Fig. 29.6). He does not want invasive surgery or midface lift. The patient only wants surgery on the right side and desires symmetry.

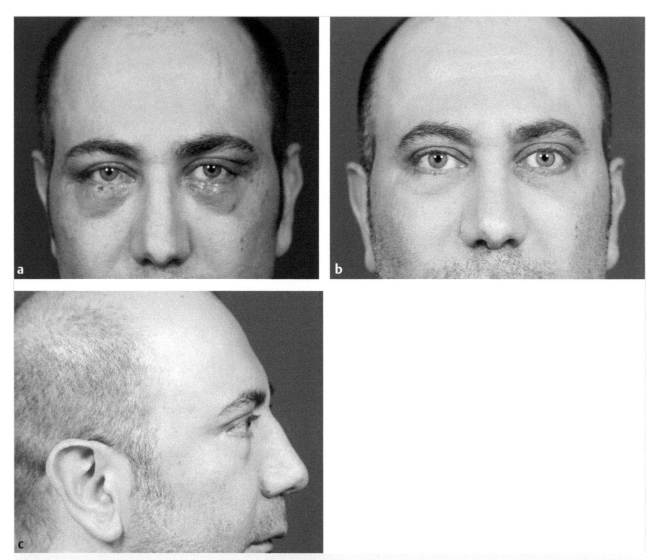

Fig. 29.5 **(a)** After 10 days and **(b, c)** after 1 year post-op.

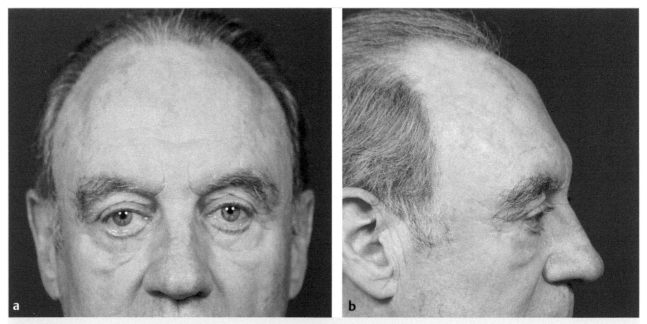

Fig. 29.6 **(a,b)** Vertical restriction in midlamella and posterior lamella. No skin deficiency, horizontal lid lengthening, negative vector, and scleral show 4 mm right eye.

29.2.2 Anatomic Description of the Patient's Current Status

He reports about a hematoma and mild infection on both sides after an upper and lower lid blepharoplasty treated conservatively with antibiotics. Two attempts with canthopexies were made with no results 2 years ago. He sleeps with a watch glass cover to treat the lack of closure with dry eyes and needs eye drops during the day.

Analysis of the Problem

Negative tilt on both eyes, vertical restriction of the midlamellar with a horizontal lid lengthening of 12 mm right side and 6 mm left side, scleral show 4 mm right side and 2 mm left side, negative vector with Hertel value of 20 on the right eye and 19 on the left eye, and hypoplasia of the zygoma were observed. There is also complete active lid closure and passive incomplete by 3 mm only on the right side. There were no symptoms on the left side. There was no conjunctival injection or chemosis. Blinking is reduced, and there was no fishmouthing on either side as a result from muscle denervation. The posterior lamella is free from cicatrix.

Diagnosis

This is a lower lid malposition with a midlamellar scarring, prominent eyes, horizontal lid lengthening, and malar mounds.

29.2.3 Recommended Solution to the Problem

- Treatment of the horizontal lid laxity by a tarsal strip procedure on the right side.
- Support and reconstruction of the midlamellar by hard palate mucosal graft.

29.2.4 Technique

According to the patient's desires, only the right side is operated. Incision is made with the Colorado needle just below the tarsal plate preserving the tarsal artery and splitting the retractors. We release the cicatrization of the septum and the fat arising from previous complicated surgery (▶ Fig. 29.7a).

We elevate a full-thickness hard palate graft, taking care about the palatine artery and leaving the periosteum intact (▶ Fig. 29.7b). The graft is trimmed and the mucosal glands are removed. We fit the graft into the gap and adjust the height to blend the limbus by the lid margin. The fixation is performed with 5–0 Vicryl stiches coming from outside to inside and going outside again to prevent chafing (▶ Fig. 29.7c).

A tarsal strip procedure is added to take care of the horizontal lid lengthening. The fixation is done by a double drill hole fixation at the lateral orbital rim and a 5–0 Prolene suture in a mild overcorrecting position.

29.2.5 Postoperative Photographs and Critical Evaluation of Results

▶ Fig. 29.8 shows the patient after 3 months with greatly improved position of the right lower lid margin. The patient was able to completely close the right eye. Note that the slight swelling on the right lower lid is due to the implant.

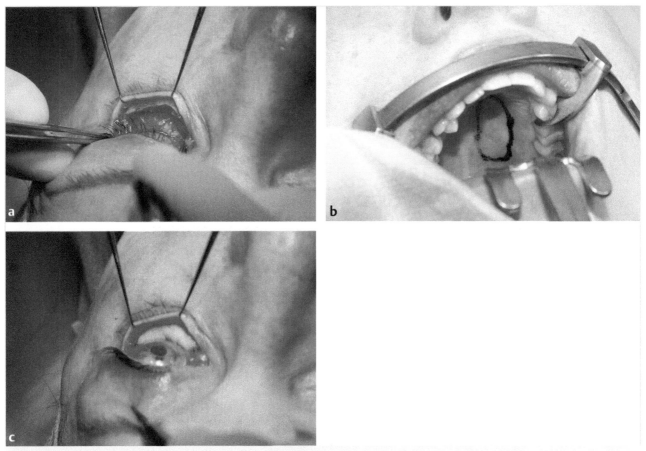

Fig. 29.7 **(a)** Transconjunctival approach and splitting retractors 2 mm below tarsal plate; **(b)** planning hard palate mucosal graft; **(c)** interpositioning of hard palate mucosal graft.

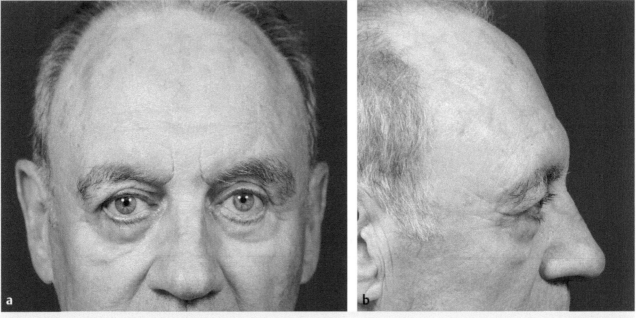

Fig. 29.8 **(a,b)** One year post-op.

29.2.6 Teaching Points

- A tarsal strip procedure alone would result in a bowstring phenomenon in patients with protruding eyes.
- Spacer grafts are essentially to support and unload the canthal fixation in negative vector patients.
- If there is a conjunctival deficiency in the posterior lamella, one needs to consider hard palate or ADMs as a spacer to replace the conjunctiva.

29.3 Vertical Restriction of the Posterior Lamella

29.3.1 Patient History Leading to the Specific Problem

A 57-year-old woman presented 1 year after transpalpebral orbital decompression by fat removal (Olivari technique) in Graves' disease. She had hypertension and Graves' disease, and smokes 10 cigarettes a day (▶ Fig. 29.9).

29.3.2 Anatomic Description of the Patient's Current Status

During her history of Graves' disease, she suffered from an upper and lower lid retraction and was unable to close the eyes during the night. After the orbital decompression with lengthening of the upper lid levator muscles, the Graves' symptoms improved but the lack of closure persisted.

Analysis of the Problem

The patient has preoperative severe Graves' disease with upper and lower lid retraction, protruding eyes (Hertel 30 both eyes), conjunctival injection, chemosis, lack of closure, and vertical restriction of the posterior lamella.

Postorbital decompression with Olivari technique and lengthening of the levators: negative tilt on both eyes, vertical restriction of the posterior lamella, no lid lengthening, scleral show 4 mm right and 3 mm left (Hertel 22 both eyes), no more conjunctival injection, no chemosis, and incomplete active and passive lid closure (2 mm). Regular orbicularis muscle function. No diplopia (▶ Fig. 29.10).

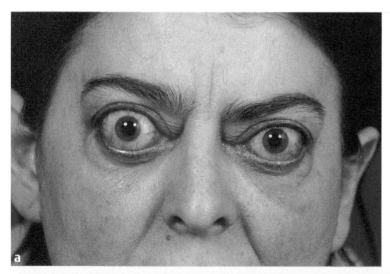
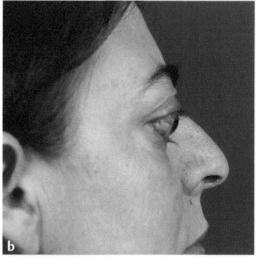

Fig. 29.9 (a,b) Patient with Graves' disease with upper and lower lid retraction (posterior lamella), protruding eyes, Hertel 30 right and 29 left, and scleral show 4 mm.

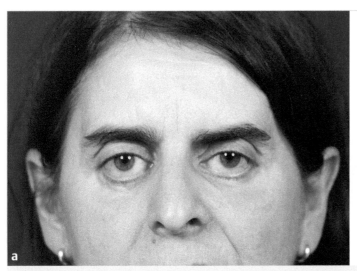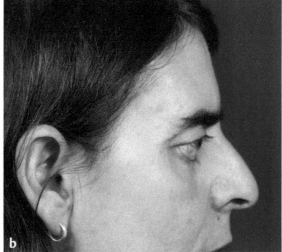

Fig. 29.10 (a,b) One year after transpalpebral orbital decompression by fat removal (Olivari technique), Hertel 22 bilateral, and scleral show 4 mm.

Diagnosis

Vertical restriction of the posterior lamella with no conjunctival deficiency.

29.3.3 Recommended Solution to the Problem

- Splitting and resecting the lower lid retractors.
- Support and reconstruction of the posterior lamellar with conchal cartilage.

29.3.4 Technique

Make a subciliary incision through the skin and orbicularis and separate them from the lower lid retractors down to the arcus marginalis. Separate the retractors from the inferior border of the tarsal plate and the underlying conjunctiva down to the inferior fornix. Take care to preserve the integrity of the conjunctiva. Now, completely resect the Muller muscle.

Harvest an appropriately sized piece of conchal cartilage and suture it into the gap between the inferior border of the tarsal plate and the cut end of the lower lid retractors. Also secure the lower edge of the cartilage graft to the inferior fornix to be certain that it slips into the orbit on downgaze. Additional lipofilling (9 mL/per side) is performed to blend the tear trough deformity and to augment the cheeks. Frost sutures are applied and only one eye is operated (▶Fig. 29.11).

29.3.5 Postoperative Photographs and Critical Evaluation of Results

▶Fig. 29.12 shows the patient 1 week after repair of the right side only with a good lower lid position, touching the limbus.

▶Fig. 29.13 shows the patient 1 year after repair of both sides with a good upper and lower lid position of both sides and complete lid closure. Note the stretched lid margin and a small step at the left eye due to the implant.

29.3.6 Teaching Points

- Concha cartilage is a very stable supporter of the lower lid margin.
- Complete splitting and resection of the retractors is key to success.
- Instead of concha cartilage, hard palate, ADMs, or Medpor implants may be used.

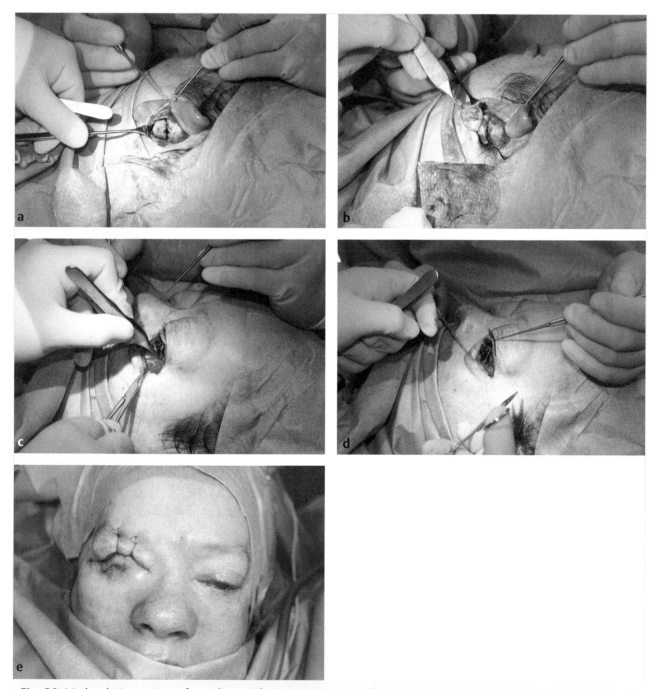

Fig. 29.11 (a-e) Harvesting of concha cartilage, suturing into the retractor gap.

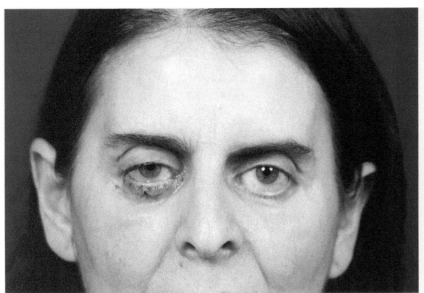

Fig. 29.12 One week after right side repair.

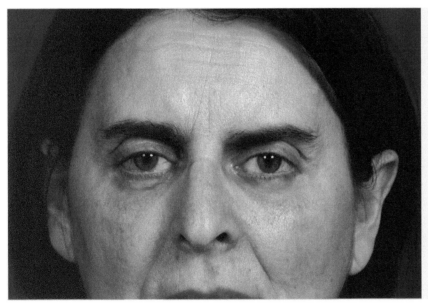

Fig. 29.13 One year after repair of both sides. Complete lid closure.

Suggested Reading

[1] Borrelli M, Unterlauft J, Kleinsasser N, Geerling G. Decellularized porcine derived membrane (Tarsys®) for correction of lower eyelid retraction. Orbit. 2012; 31(3):187–189

[2] Chang M, Ahn SE, Baek S. The effect and applications of acellular dermal allograft (AlloDerm) in ophthalmic plastic surgery. J Craniomaxillofac Surg. 2014; 42(5):695–699

[3] Hahn S, Desai SC. Lower lid malposition: causes and correction. Facial Plast Surg Clin North Am. 2016; 24(2):163–171

[4] Hester TR, Jr. Evolution of lower lid support following lower lid/midface rejuvenation: the pretarsal orbicularis lateral canthopexy. Clin Plast Surg. 2001; 28(4):639–652

[5] Jiaqi C, Zheng W, Jianjun G. Eyelid reconstruction with acellular human dermal allograft after chemical and thermal burns. Burns. 2006; 32(2):208–211

[6] Patel MP, Shapiro MD, Spinelli HM. Combined hard palate spacer graft, midface suspension, and lateral canthoplasty for lower eyelid retraction: a tripartite approach. Plast Reconstr Surg. 2005; 115(7):2105–2114, discussion –2115–2117

[7] Richter DF, Stoff A, Olivari N. Transpalpebral decompression of endocrine ophthalmopathy by intraorbital fat removal (Olivari technique): experience and progression after more than 3000 operations over 20 years. Plast Reconstr Surg. 2007; 120(1):109–123

[8] Taban MR. Lower eyelid retraction surgery without internal spacer graft. Aesthet Surg J. 2017; 37(2):133–136

[9] Tan J, Olver J, Wright M, Maini R, Neoh C, Dickinson AJ. The use of porous polyethylene (Medpor) lower eyelid spacers in lid heightening and stabilisation. Br J Ophthalmol. 2004; 88(9):1197–1200

[10] Wearne MJ, Sandy C, Rose GE, Pitts J, Collin JR. Autogenous hard palate mucosa: the ideal lower eyelid spacer? Br J Ophthalmol. 2001; 85(10):1183–1187

[11] Wong CH, Mendelson B. Midcheek lift using facial soft-tissue spaces of the midcheek. Plast Reconstr Surg. 2015; 136(6):1155–1165

30 Trauma-Related Lower Eyelid Retraction

Alison B. Callahan and Richard D. Lisman

Summary
Lower eyelid retraction is a well-known complication of orbital floor fracture repair, caused by violation of the eyelid's layered anatomy. Releasing the cicatrix and resuspending the canthus usually reveal a dead space that must be spanned and supported in order to maintain an elevated eyelid position. This chapter describes free fat transfer from the contralateral lower eyelid into this dead space in order to repair the lower eyelid retraction while simultaneously achieving a more symmetric result with improved aesthetics of *both* lower eyelids.

Keywords: retraction, lower eyelid, trauma, floor fracture, cicatrix, middle lamellar scar, symblepharon

30.1 Patient History Leading to the Specific Problem

This is a 46-year-old woman who sustained a right orbital blowout fracture that was repaired via transconjunctival approach (▶ Fig. 30.1). She presented to our care some years later with ocular surface irritation, redness, and tearing.

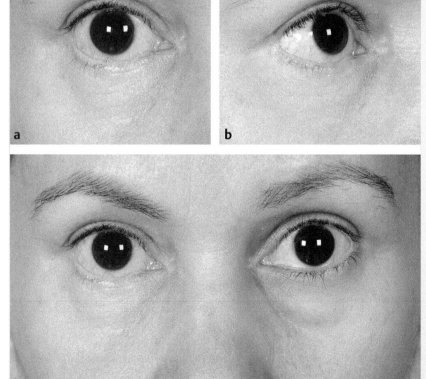

Fig. 30.1 Right lower eyelid retraction following transconjunctival orbital floor fracture repair. **(a)** Frontal plane, **(b)** lateral view demonstrating segmental entropion, and **(c)** contralateral comparison.

Cosmetically, she complained of more prominent lower eyelid bags under her uninjured eye. She was an otherwise healthy woman without other medical issues.

30.2 Anatomic Description of the Patient's Current Status

The patient demonstrates a retracted right lower eyelid with slightly irregular contour, presumably due to cicatrization of her wounds after surgical repair of her blowout fracture. The retraction is inducing approximately 2 mm of inferior scleral show as well as focal entropion with a few trichiatic lashes pressed against her inferior conjunctiva and limbus. The orbital fat is nonapparent in the right lower eyelid, thereby indirectly enhancing the prominence of the orbital fat pads in the contralateral uninjured lower eyelid. Her slit-lamp examination revealed moderate inferior superficial punctate keratopathy on the right side and a clear cornea on the left. These findings are the natural sequelae of combined inferior exposure due to her retracted eyelid with trichiatic lashes against the ocular surface.

30.2.1 Analysis of the Problem

The layered anatomy of the eyelid is complex and violation of its natural structure as in the case of penetrating or surgical trauma can lead to its dysfunction. Lower eyelid malposition including lower eyelid retraction is unfortunately a well-acknowledged complication following orbital floor fracture repair, and can occur following either transconjunctival or subciliary approach. Surgically correcting the eyelid malposition will undoubtedly require releasing the cicatrix, which can be accomplished by reopening the transconjunctival incision and releasing symblepharon (if apparent) as well as middle lamellar scar bands. Canthopexy, described elsewhere in this chapter, will also help elevate the eyelid to a more functional position with regard to the inferior limbus. However, one must anticipate that releasing the cicatrix and resuspending the canthus will reveal a dead space that will need to be spanned and supported in order to maintain the elevated eyelid position. While there are many ways to do so (spacer graft discussed elsewhere in the chapters, dermis fat graft, etc.), one possibility is to look to the contralateral inferior fat pads, which the patient herself noted to be relatively more prominent after her contralateral fracture. By harvesting a fat graft from the contralateral side, one can simultaneously fill and support the elevated right lower eyelid while reducing the prominence of the left inferior orbital fat pads. Thus, one borrows fat from the left side to place into the right, allowing for a more durable retraction repair on the right and a more symmetric result with improved overall aesthetic.

30.3 Recommended Solution to the Problem

Repair right lower eyelid retraction via the following:
- Transconjunctival incision.
- Release of conjunctival symblepharon and middle lamellar cicatrix.
- Right lateral canthopexy.
- Autologous fat graft from contralateral inferior orbital fat pads.
- Fat graft harvested from left inferior orbital fat pads via transconjunctival approach.

30.4 Technique

A transconjunctival approach to the right lower eyelid is taken. A skin hook placed under the tarsus may be used to slightly evert the right lower eyelid and give exposure of the palpebral conjunctiva. Any noted symblepharon should be lysed with Westcott scissors. The palpebral conjunctiva is then opened with cutting Bovie cautery. Grasping the conjunctiva and lower eyelid retractors in a toothed forceps, the Bovie is used to initiate the preseptal plane, which is then further carried to the inferior orbital rim with blunt, Q-tip dissection. Cicatricial bands encountered along the dissection should be lysed bluntly with Q-tips when possible or with Bovie cautery when sharp dissection is required. Once at the inferior orbital rim, a preperiosteal pocket is created by bluntly dissecting through the orbitomalar ligament with curved Steven's scissors (▶ Fig. 30.2). This pocket will receive the fat graft.

Attention is then directed toward harvesting the fat transfer from the contralateral lower eyelid. A similar transconjunctival approach is taken in a preseptal plane to the inferior orbital rim. The septum is then opened with Bovie cautery and fat carefully teased out and excised. The fat is directly posited into the previously created preperiosteal pocket in the right lower eyelid.

We recognize that there is variability in the closure (or lack thereof) of transconjunctival incisions. We prefer to minimize postoperative complications related to wound closure by leaving our wounds to heal primarily. Sparing use of ophthalmic ointment is advised to reduce the risk of ointment granulomas that can form in open inferior fornices.

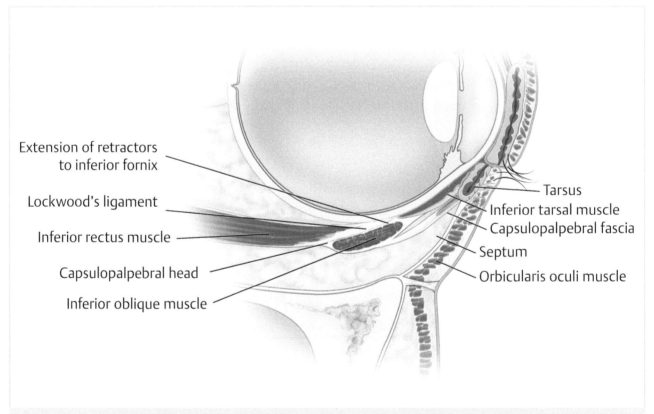

Fig. 30.2 Layered eyelid anatomy depicting location of preperiosteal pocket. (Reproduced with permission from Codner MA, McCord Jr CD. Eyelid & Periorbital Surgery. 2nd ed. New York, NY: Thieme; 2016.)

However, when placing a fat graft, we do recommend placing a modified Frost suture in the right lower eyelid to prevent the retractors from cicatrizing and to place tension on the preperiosteal pocket thereby restricting graft migration. This modified Frost suture is fashioned by placing each arm of a double-armed 6–0 silk suture through the inferior edge of the conjunctiva and retractors, then passing under the superior conjunctival edge, continuing through the eyelid to exit at the lower eyelid margin. Each arm is then passed into the superior eyelid margin exiting 3 mm above the margin and then finally passed to a bite transversing the brow. Two such sutures were passed dividing the stretched lower eyelid into approximately thirds (▶ Fig. 30.3).

30.5 Postoperative Photographs and Critical Evaluation of Results

The postoperative results are taken at 3 months (▶ Fig. 30.4). One can see an improved lid height with regard to the inferior limbus. Additionally, the inferior orbital fat pads have a more symmetric appearance.

The amount of benefit seen 3 months postoperatively is a relatively good estimate of the amount of fat that survived the transfer; however, a more conservative approach would wait until 6 months postoperatively to definitively evaluate the outcome. Still, these initial results seem to favorably demonstrate the impact of this procedure. Some may also question involving the unaffected side in the course of surgery. This is a valid concern and requires appropriate patient selection in, for example, a patient who notices and is bothered by fat herniation on the contralateral side. Effectively, you are repurposing a transconjunctival lower eyelid blepharoplasty to harvest a graft needed to assist in elevating and supporting the contralateral lower eyelid retraction repair. In the appropriately selected and counseled patient, we would argue that performing this type of bilateral surgery gives the surgeon more control to achieve a symmetric appearance and can result in an excellent functional and aesthetic outcome.

30.6 Teaching Points

- Correcting lower eyelid retraction that occurred in the setting of penetrating or surgical trauma can be surgically challenging and requires a good understanding of the layered eyelid anatomy and a multifaceted intervention.
- One should always consider the forces that created the initial problem and take care to avoid a similar complication. In this case, the modified Frost suture passing through the inferior conjunctival edge directly places it on stretch to avoid its retraction into the fornix and simultaneously helps stabilize the placement of the free fat transfer as the layers heal in place.
- Taking a broader perspective on the overall aesthetic of the patient and thinking creatively can enable you to achieve a more symmetric result, though patient counseling and selection are paramount to the success of such a bilateral procedure.

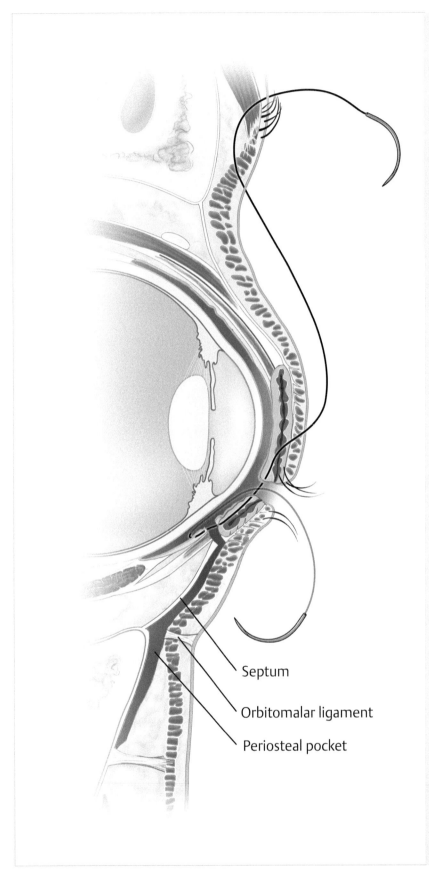

Septum

Orbitomalar ligament

Periosteal pocket

Fig. 30.3 Layered eyelid anatomy depicting modified Frost suture.

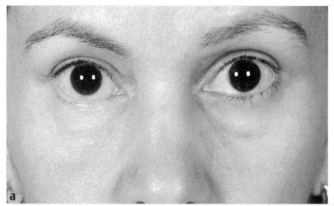 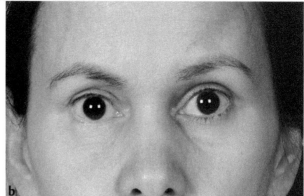

Fig. 30.4 (a,b) Preoperative and postoperative comparison.

Suggested Reading

[1] Belinsky I, Patel P, Charles NC, Lisman RD. Ointment granulomas following sutureless transconjunctival blepharoplasty: diagnosis and management Ophthal Plast Reconstr Surg. 2015; 31(4):282–286

[2] Gosau M, Schöneich M, Draenert FG, Ettl T, Driemel O, Reichert TE. Retrospective analysis of orbital floor fractures--complications, outcome, and review of literature. Clin Oral Investig. 2011; 15(3):305–313

[3] Patipa M, Patel BC, McLeish W, Anderson RL. Use of hard palate grafts for treatment of postsurgical lower eyelid retraction: a technical overview. J Craniomaxillofac Trauma. 1996; 2(3):18–28

[4] Raschke G, Rieger U, Bader RD, Schaefer O, Guentsch A, Schultze-Mosgau S. Outcomes analysis of eyelid deformities using photograph-assisted standardized anthropometry in 311 patients after orbital fracture treatment. J Trauma Acute Care Surg. 2012; 73(5):1319–1325

[5] Wray RC, Holtmann B, Ribaudo JM, Keiter J, Weeks PM. A comparison of conjunctival and subciliary incisions for orbital fractures. Br J Plast Surg. 1977; 30(2):142–145

31 Lower Lid Retraction

Sri Gore, Richard L. Scawn, and Naresh Joshi

Summary
Lower lid is a complex multilayered structure, which needs to be understood with regard to its anatomy, its interplay with the globe and surrounding facial structures, and its integrity in individual patients. Failure to appreciate these factors may lead to lower lid retraction, a common complication of eyelid surgery such as lower lid blepharoplasty. This chapter addresses anatomy and clinical evaluation of the lower lid in addition to providing illustrative examples of lower lid retraction and their surgical solutions.

Keywords: lower lid, retraction, scar, blepharoplasty, lamella, canthus, canthopexy, midface

31.1 Introduction

The normal lower lid position with the eye in primary gaze is at or slightly above the inferior corneal limbus. Lower lid retraction is an abnormally low position of the lower lid without eversion of the lid margin; retraction and canthal angle blunting are common complications of lower lid blepharoplasty, which not only result in an unaesthetic "sad," "tired" appearance but also may cause ocular irritation and epiphora due to an ineffective tear column–globe contact. Persistent long-term ectropion is a less common complication.

Understanding the complex interplay between the tissues and gravity, which "age" the lower lid, and addressing these appropriately decreases the possibility of lid malposition following blepharoplasty.

Careful preoperative evaluation and apt surgical planning and execution are paramount in avoidance of poor outcomes.

The lower lid must be evaluated anatomically, considering it in its three lamellae: anterior, middle, and posterior lamellae. Vertical shortening should be assessed in all three planes. Isolated posterior lamella deficiency tends to invert the lid. Middle lamellar shortening, which is sometimes difficult to judge, can be a cause of operative failure; the most common primary deficiency is that of the anterior lamellae, the restoration of which will be discussed in this chapter and elsewhere. The restoration of the lid to its normal position also requires the assessment of the horizontal plane, treating lid laxity where required, in conjunction with the anteroposterior plane, where the failure to consider the orbital vectors may result in unexpected poor results.

A three-dimensional and three-planar assessment is imperative before embarking on corrective surgery for lower lid retraction.

31.2 Evaluation

31.2.1 Horizontal Laxity and Lateral Canthal Tendon Laxity

The lateral canthal tendon is assessed by grasping the lid and pulling medially; the displacement of the lateral canthal angle is then observed. Up to 2 mm of movement is considered normal (►Fig. 31.1). The snap test is performed by pulling the central portion lid away from the globe and then allowing it

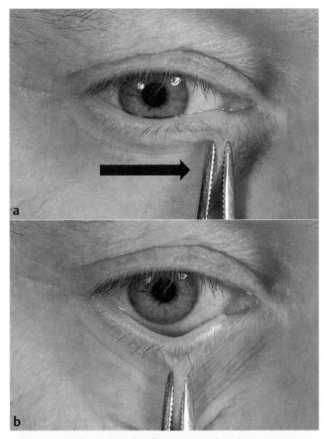

Fig. 31.1 Photographs illustrating the distraction tests of the lower lid; the use of forceps is for illustration only, and these tests should be performed in the outpatient setting with the clinician's finger. The patient's gaze should remain straight ahead (primary position). **(a)** The lid is distracted medially and the position and laxity of the lateral canthal is observed. **(b)** Vertical distraction of the lid downward can demonstrate the elasticity and laxity of the lower lid in its ability to "snap back" into position spontaneously or on blinking.

to snap back into position; upon release, a normal eyelid should snap back against the globe immediately without a blink. A severely lax eyelid may require one or more blinks to return to normal position. If the lower eyelid can be distracted more than 6 to 8 mm away from the globe, then horizontal laxity is present.

31.2.2 Orbital Vector Analysis

A patient's orbital vector is defined as the relationship between the globe (the corneal apex) and the malar eminence in the sagittal plane (▶ Fig. 31.2). The main purpose of assessing for the vector is to avoid complications that arise from lower lid surgery on negative vector patients, who have very little malar support.

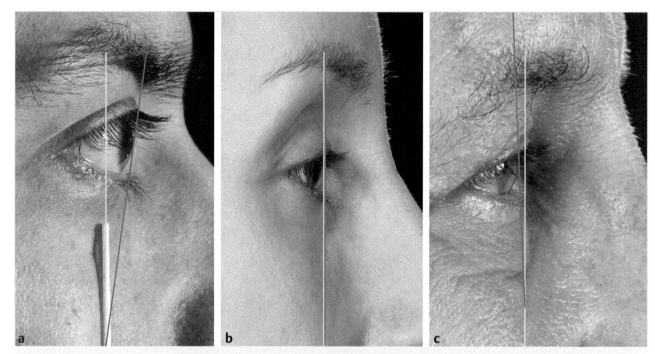

Fig. 31.2 Sagittal-plane photographs illustrating **(a)** negative, **(b)** neutral, and **(c)** positive orbital vectors. Red lines delineate the patient's orbital vector in relation to the green line, which represents the vertical plane of the malar eminence.

31.2.3 Evaluation of the Anterior Lamella: Skin and Orbicularis

The lower lid retraction may be exaggerated in up-gaze. It may be exaggerated further still by asking the patient to open their mouth while in up-gaze.

31.2.4 Evaluation of the Middle Lamella: Septum and Lower Lid Retractors

The middle lamella is evaluated by manual vertical distraction of the lower lid. While the patient is looking in the primary position, the lid is manually moved upward (opposite to that shown in ▶ Fig. 31.1b).

A patient with middle lamellar contracture will have lower lid tethering (▶ Fig. 31.3), and the lid cannot manually be moved upward over the surface of the globe. This is in contrast to the patient with lower lid retraction associated with an overresection of skin only.

31.2.5 Evaluation of the Posterior Lamella: Conjunctiva and Tarsal Plate

Direct visualization of the conjunctiva will reveal any scarring in the inferior fornix following transconjunctival techniques. Manually elevating the eyelid will result in the eyelid margin rolling inward toward the globe.

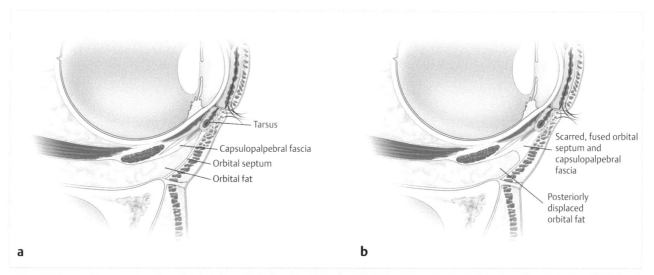

Fig. 31.3 **(a)** Normal lower eyelid anatomy showing the relationship of the lower lid retractors and the orbital septum. **(b)** Septum and retractor scarring and disruption. Note the contracted cicatrix shortening the middle lamellar.

31.3 Case 1. Postoperative Lower Lid Retraction Secondary to Anterior and Middle Lamella Complications

31.3.1 Patient History Leading to the Specific Problem

A 49-year-old lady had undergone bilateral lower lid blepharoplasties 6 months prior to presentation (▶Fig. 31.4). This surgery resulted in bilateral lower lid retraction and left lower lid diastasis from the globe. She then underwent a left lower lid canthoplasty elsewhere, but this failed to address the malposition. At presentation, she has bilateral lower lid retraction but the left was of particular concern due to the resultant corneal epithelial irregularity in her only-sighted eye; the other eye was affected by dense amblyopia. She was a nonsmoker and had no significant medical history.

Clinical photographs demonstrate postblepharoplasty syndrome with the eye in primary position and in up-gaze (▶Fig. 31.4). The purple skin markings illustrate the vector of retraction.

31.3.2 Anatomic Description of the Patient's Current Status

She demonstrates typical postblepharoplasty syndrome with rounding of the lateral canthal angles, bilateral lower lid retraction, and scleral show with a mild left lower lid ectropion. This patient demonstrated one of the

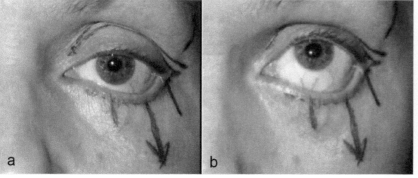

Fig. 31.4 Photographs of patient 1 illustrating retraction of the left eyelid with the patient's eye in **(a)** primary position and **(b)** up-gaze. Up-gaze visibly exacerbates the retraction. In both figures **(a)** and **(b)**, the purple arrow demonstrates the vector of maximal anterior lamella tethering.

commonest causes of postblepharoplasty complications, which was shortage of the anterior lamella due to overresection. In addition, the middle lamella of the lower lid was also scarred, leading to limited active and passive distraction of the lid on up-gaze. There was mild lid laxity present. It was decided to only operate on her left eyelids.

31.3.3 Recommended Solution to the Problem

- Middle lamella: cicatrix division and lower lid retractor recession.
- Lid support and soft tissue recruitment from the midface: transcanthal lateral canthopexy and midface support.
- Addition of anterior lamella: heteropalpebral flap (plus recruitment of skin from the midface area as a result of the midface lift).

Treatment Note

Treatment usually involves adding tissue, dissecting cicatrized tissue, and tightening or supporting the eyelid. We would like to stress that a combination of procedures may be necessary depending on the exact pathogenesis of iatrogenic lower lid retraction. If horizontal laxity is detected, it should be treated at the same time; a plethora of surgical procedures have been described to tackle this, including canthal tendon suspension and shortening. These techniques are described elsewhere in this book but we would like to highlight the need for vigilance for the negative orbital vector patient when planning to tighten an eyelid. Shortening the lateral canthal tendon in a negative orbital vector can lead to buckling of the eyelid underneath the globe and hence we suggest plication (▶Fig. 31.5).

31.3.4 Surgical Technique: Transcutaneous Approach for Midface Lift and Lower Lid Transcanthal Canthopexy

The scarring between the lower lid retractors and the orbital septum has to be divided and released and the retractors recessed to allow mobilization of the eyelid. The following surgical series has been divided into stages and demonstrated in different patients to aid understanding of each stage (▶Fig. 31.6). The surgical sequence demonstrates midface facelift via

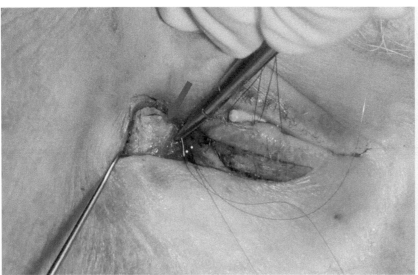

Fig. 31.5 Photograph demonstrating the plication of the right lateral canthal tendon. The yellow dots demonstrate the double passage of a 6–0 Prolene suture through an intact lateral canthal tendon. One needle (exiting at the green dot) is seen being passed through the periostium of the lateral orbital rim (purple arrow). Plication avoids the shortening affect that a lateral tarsal strip operation has.

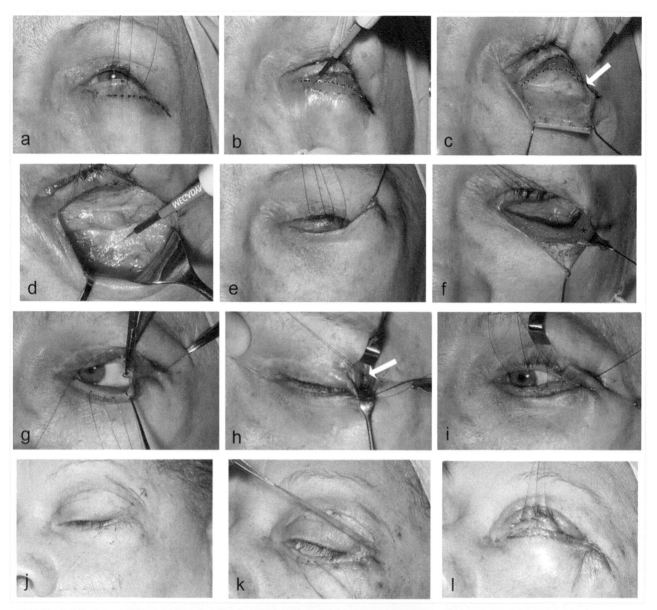

Fig. 31.6 The surgical sequence demonstrates midface lift via a subciliary incision, transcanthal canthopexy suture, and heteropalpebral flap from the upper lid into the lower lid. **(a)** A subciliary incision with lateral extension was made. **(b)** Pretarsal orbicularis is spared with this dissection; the dotted line delineates the preserved muscle. **(c)** A lateral skin and muscle composite was formed laterally. The white arrow shows the medial edge of this flap. **(d)** The orbicularis-retaining ligament was divided (demonstrated by the tip of the monopolar needle) and **(e)** the soft tissues midface mobilized to allow vertical lifting and recruitment of skin. **(f)** A lateral muscle–only flap (*) was created by dissection from the skin. Note that this skin is not excised. **(g)** This muscle flap is sutured to the lateral orbital rim just lateral to the canthopexy suture (different patient). A canthopexy suture was then passed through the canthal angle, via the inferior canthal tendon and tied at the level of the zygomaticofrontal **(h, i)** suture on the lateral orbital rim (white arrow). **(j)** Marking the heteropalpebral flap and dissection (different patient). **(k)** Mobilization of heteropalpebral flap. **(l)** Flap is positioned into the lower lid following the muscle flap suturing. The skin in the upper and lower lid is finally closed.

a subciliary incision, transcanthal canthopexy suture, and heteropalpebral flap from the upper lid into the lower lid. A subciliary incision with lateral extension was made (▶Fig. 31.6a). Pretarsal obicularis is spared with this dissection; the dotted line delineates the preserved muscle (▶Fig. 31.6b). A lateral skin and muscle composite was formed laterally (the white arrow shows the medial edge of this flap) (▶Fig. 31.6c). The orbicularis-retaining ligament was divided (▶Fig. 31.6d; demonstrated by the tip of the monopolar needle) and the soft tissues midface mobilized (▶Fig. 31.6e) to allow vertical lifting and recruitment of skin. A lateral muscle–only flap (*) was created by dissection from the skin (▶Fig. 31.6f). Note that this skin is not excised. This muscle flap is sutured to the lateral orbital rim just lateral to the canthopexy suture (▶Fig. 31.6g [different patient]). A canthopexy suture was then passed through the canthal angle, via the inferior canthal tendon and tied at the level of the zygomaticofrontal suture on the lateral orbital rim (white arrow) (▶Fig. 31.6h,i).

Surgical Technique: Heteropalpebral Flap

This technique was combined with that above for patient 1. For clearer photographic illustration purposes, a different patient's heteropalpebral flap is demonstrated here (▶Fig. 31.6j–l). The heteropalpebral flap was marked and dissected; the medial third is skin only and the final two-thirds are composed of skin and increasing thickness of orbicularis muscle (▶Fig. 31.6j). The flap was mobilized, hinged at the lateral canthal area (▶Fig. 31.6k), and sutured into the lower lid (▶Fig. 31.6l).

31.4 Postoperative Photographs and Critical Evaluation of Results

This patient's lower lid 1-week postcorrective operation is visibly higher in comparison to preoperatively (▶Fig. 31.7). The lateral canthal angle shape has also been restored. Six months postoperatively the lower lid is still in a reasonable position (at the level of the inferior limbus) but lower compared to the immediate postoperative photograph; patients must be counseled about this prior to the surgery.

31.5 Case 2. Complex Case of Postoperative Lower Lid Retraction in a Negative Orbital Vector Patient

31.5.1 Patient History Leading to the Specific Problem

This 69-year-old woman underwent bilateral upper and lower lid blepharoplasty at 30 years of age and, in the year prior to her presentation, she had this procedure repeated. Subsequently, she developed lower lid retraction and, thus, had bilateral lower lid tightening and bilateral heteropalpebral flaps as separate procedures at another institution to correct lower lid retraction. She was a nonsmoker and was in general good health. On presentation, she still had lower lid retraction with a mild left lower lid ectropion. She was unhappy with the lid positions but was also suffering symptoms of dry eye.

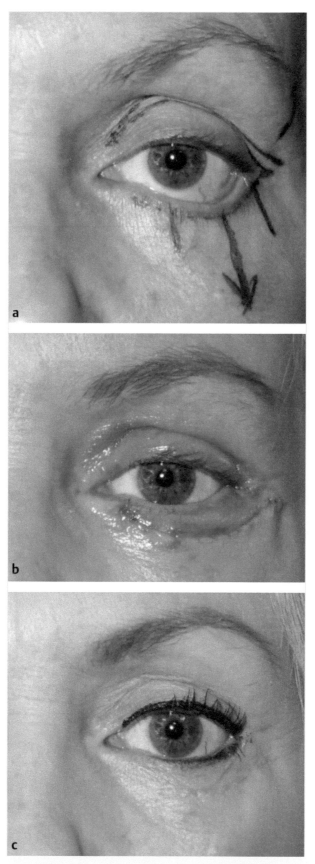

Fig. 31.7 Pre- and postoperative photos of the left eyelids. **(a)** Preoperative photo. **(b)** One-week postoperative photo. **(c)** Four-month postoperative photo.

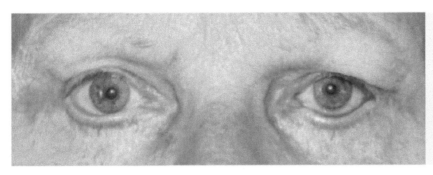

Fig. 31.8 Preoperative photo of patient 2 showing right lower lid retraction, left lower lid ectropion, and bilateral lateral canthal rounding. She has bilateral conjunctival infection as a sign of dry eye.

31.5.2 Anatomic Description of the Patient's Current Status

This patient demonstrated right lower lid retraction and left lower lid ectropion due to anterior lamellar shortage, middle lamella contracture, and lid laxity (▶ Fig. 31.8). She, unlike the previous case, had no redundancy of upper lid skin due to her previous lid surgeries. Notably, she did not want to have free skin grafts and had a negative orbital vector.

31.5.3 Recommended Solution to the Problem

- Osmotic expander insertion into the midface to increase the surface area of anterior lamella.
- Subperiosteal and supraperiosteal midface lift with endotine fixation to recruit this expanded tissue into the lower lid and provide vertical support.
- Lateral canthopexy to provide horizontal support.

Prior to surgery, she was counseled regarding the immediate and late postoperative complications including chemosis and overangulation of her lower lids.

Surgical Technique: Osmotic Expander Insertion into the Midface to Increase the Surface Area of Anterior Lamella

A mucosal incision was made 1 cm from the gingival margin (▶ Fig. 31.9a). The periostium of maxilla and periostium was dissected and elevated (▶ Fig. 31.9b,c). The osmotic expander was soaked in betadine prior to insertion high into this subperiosteal pocket (▶ Fig. 31.9d–f). A double-layer closure with absorbable suture was used. The appearance of the midface 1 day and 1 month postinsertion of bilateral osmotic expanders was demonstrated (▶ Fig. 31.9g,h). The osmotic expanders were left in situ for 1 month. At the second stage of the procedure, the osmotic expanders were removed and the additional tissue elevated with a midface lift via a subciliary incision into the eyelid area.

Surgical Technique: Subperiosteal and Supraperiosteal Midface Lift with Endotine Fixation to Recruit This Expanded Tissue into the Lower Lid and Provide Vertical Support

The authors no longer use endotines to provide fixation but, instead, apply the use of PDS sutures to the periostium and soft tissue flaps. In this surgical procedure (▶ Fig. 31.10), dissection along orbicularis–septal plane down to the orbital rim was made. The periostium was incised (▶ Fig. 31.10a) and a subperiosteal dissection performed (▶ Fig. 31.10b). An endotine fixation device was inserted (▶ Fig. 31.10c) and fixed to the orbital rim with titanium screws.

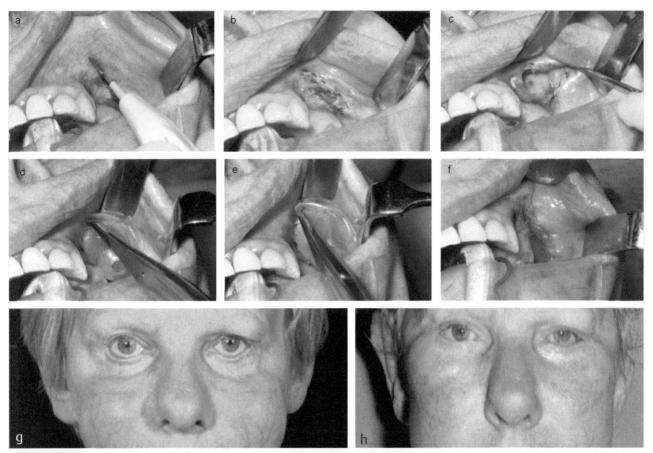

Fig. 31.9 **(a)** A mucosal incision was made 1 cm from the gingival margin. **(b,c)** The periostium of maxilla and periostium was dissected and elevated. **(d,e)** The osmotic expander was soaked in betadine prior to insertion high into this subperiosteal pocket. **(f)** A double-layer closure with absorbable suture was used. The appearance of the midface 1 day and 1 month postinsertion of bilateral osmotic expanders was demonstrated. **(g,h)** The osmotic expanders were left in situ for 1 month. At the second stage of the procedure, the osmotic expanders were removed and the additional tissue elevated with a midface lift via a subciliary incision into the eyelid area.

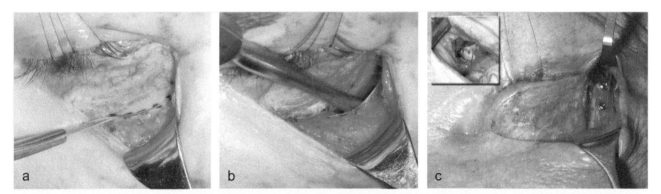

Fig. 31.10 In this surgical procedure, dissection along orbicularis–septal plane down to the orbital rim was made. The periostium was incised **(a)** and a subperiosteal dissection performed **(b)**. An endotine fixation device was inserted **(c)** and fixed to the orbital rim with titanium screws. The small insert-figure demonstrates the rakelike head of the midface endotine device, which grips the midface soft tissues.

The small image within ▶Fig. 31.10c demonstrates the rakelike head of the midface endotine device, which grips the midface soft tissues.

Lateral Canthopexy to Provide Horizontal Support

(▶Fig. 31.6h,i)

31.5.4 Postoperative Photographs and Critical Evaluation of Results

▶Fig. 31.11 illustrates preoperative and 4-month postoperative results of this patient. Both lower lid positions were elevated above the level of the limbus; her signs and symptoms of dry eye dramatically improved. The volume of cheek tissue elevated by the midface lift is also visible in the postoperative photograph. The patient was counseled about the overangulation of the lateral canthal area postoperatively but advised that this would settle with time. She failed to attend her 1-year follow-up but a telephone consultation revealed that she was very satisfied with her eyelid position, which had remained above the level of the limbus.

31.5.5 Teaching Points

- Revisional surgery of lower lid retraction requires the surgeon to meticulously assess and understand the dynamics of the lower lid. What we hope to have illustrated, through our cases, are the multifaceted aspects of corrective lower lid surgery and the importance of recognizing all the aspects of the pathology; these concepts are key in planning effective surgical treatment.
- Eyelid support, although covered in another chapter, cannot be overemphasized in corrective lower lid surgery.
- Supportive measures may range from a simple canthopexy to multilayer support with orbicularis muscle flaps, fascia lata slings, and bone-drilled canthoplasty; the choice depends on the surgical history and clinical needs of the patient.
- Medical devices, such as endotines and osmotic expanders, become "vogue" and then are rendered antiquated within a single generation of surgeons. Although we have used these devices in our cases as part of the surgical solutions, we wish to highlight their principles, namely tissue fixation and expansion, rather than promote the actual devices themselves.
- No doubt, the evolution of lower lid surgery, both primary and corrective, will continue to challenge and drive us.

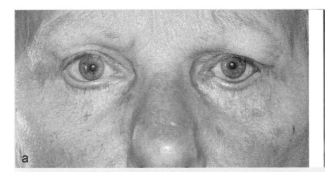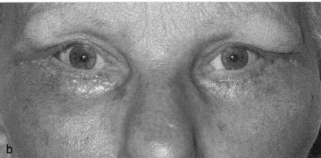

Fig. 31.11 Pre- and postoperative results. **(a)** Preoperative. **(b)** Four months postoperative.

Acknowledgments

Patient 2 was a joint-care patient with Mr. Simon Eccles, Craniofacial Consultant, Chelsea and Westminster Hospital, London.

Suggested Reading

[1] Jelks GW, Jelks EB. Preoperative evaluation of the blepharoplasty patient. Bypassing the pitfalls. Clin Plast Surg. 1993; 20(2):213–223, discussion 224

[2] McCord CD, Jr. The correction of lower lid malposition following lower lid blepharoplasty. Plast Reconstr Surg. 1999; 103(3):1036–1039, discussion 1040

[3] Morax S, Touitou V. Complications of blepharoplasty. Orbit. 2006; 25(4):303–318

[4] Patipa M. The evaluation and management of lower eyelid retraction following cosmetic surgery. Plast Reconstr Surg. 2000; 106(2):438–453, discussion 454–459

32 Recurrent Lower Eyelid Ectropion: Mastering the Sling Technique

Jose Rodríguez-Feliz and Mark A. Codner

Summary

Eyelid malposition is one of the most dreaded complications following elective lower eyelid blepharoplasty. Malposition of the lateral aspect presenting as either an eversion of the eyelid (ectropion) or retraction causing roundness of the lateral lower eyelid is commonly repaired with simpler techniques such as canthopexy or canthoplasty. It is important to understand that neither a canthoplasty nor a canthopexy will exert enough forces to reposition an ectropion of the medial lower eyelid. In this chapter, the authors describe in detail the use of tensor fascia lata allograft as a sling to correct a recurrent ectropion involving the medial and lateral aspects of the lower eyelid.

Keywords: ectropion, lower eyelid malposition, medial ectropion, blepharoplasty, lower blepharoplasty, complications, surgical technique, canthoplasty, canthopexy

32.1 Patient History Leading to the Specific Problem

The patient we present here is a 72-year-old woman with a complex surgical history, including multiple attempts by multiple surgeons at correcting her bilateral lower eyelid malposition. This problem developed secondary to one of the most common procedures performed today by plastic surgeons, an elective blepharoplasty.

Her first surgery was an elective upper and lower blepharoplasty approximately 30 years prior to presentation. The patient then developed severe bilateral lower eyelid ectropion with significant scleral show requiring correction with a porous polyethylene lower eyelid spacer (▶ Fig. 32.1). She then

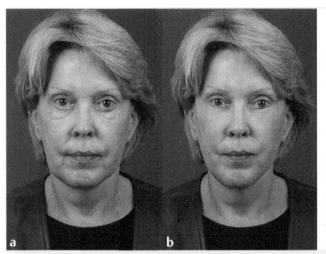
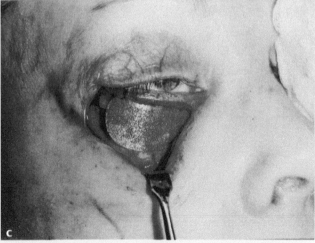

Fig. 32.1 **(a)** Patient is shown with bilateral lower eyelid retraction and significant scleral show after an elective upper and lower blepharoplasty. **(b)** Patient presented after initial correction with porous polyethylene implant used as a lower eyelid spacer. **(c)** Porous polyethylene implant used during the initial corrective surgery as a spacer via an anterior approach.

developed recurrent ectropion on the left lower eyelid (▶Fig. 32.2). Correction of this problem was performed with a canthoplasty and ear cartilage used as a spacer graft (▶Fig. 32.3). Months after, the patient presented with exposed ear cartilage, worsening left lower eyelid malposition, significant scleral show, lagophthalmos, persistent eye irritation, and epiphora (▶Fig. 32.4). The patient then underwent release of the anterior lamella scar, excision of the exposed ear cartilage, and a full-thickness skin graft to compensate for deficient skin in the anterior lamella.

After approximately 30 procedures (minor and major surgeries), the patient presented to us with persistent medial and lateral ectropion of the left lower eyelid (▶Fig. 32.5).

32.2 Anatomic Description of the Patient's Current Status

The left lower eyelid is the area of concern. The main anatomic problems are (1) recurrent left lower eyelid ectropion with an uncommon extension into the medial aspect of the eyelid, (2) inability to reposition the eyelid upward with the one-finger distraction test (▶Fig. 32.6), (3) deficient anterior lamella

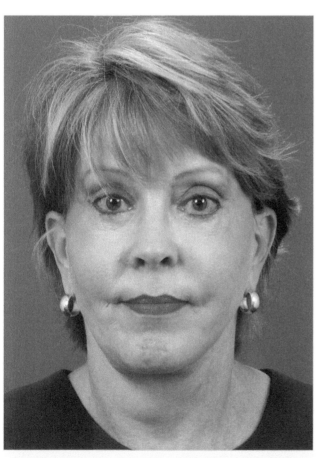

Fig. 32.2 Recurrence of lower lid retraction on the left lower eyelid.

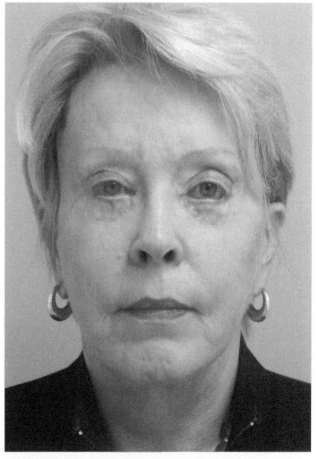

Fig. 32.3 Correction of left lower lid retraction with a canthoplasty and ear cartilage used as a spacer graft.

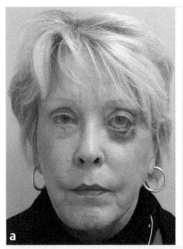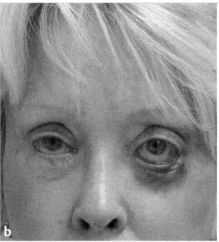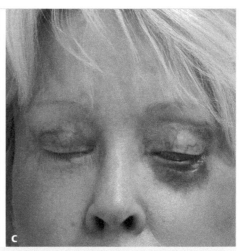

Fig. 32.4 (a–c) Patient developed extrusion of the spacer cartilage and worsening of ectropion with significant scleral show. The patient was unable to close the eye completely, which contributed to her eye irritation and constant lacrimation. This problem was addressed by trimming of the exposed graft and coverage with a full-thickness skin graft.

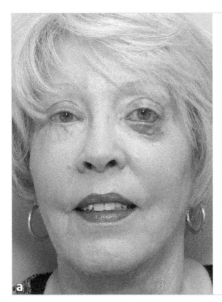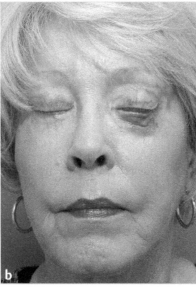

Fig. 32.5 (a,b) Due to lack of eyelid support and contraction from the anterior lamella skin graft during healing, the patient presented with recurrent ectropion of the medial and lateral lower eyelid.

skin with contracted skin graft, and (4) persistent scleral exposure causing constant eye irritation and excessive lacrimation.

32.3 Recommended Solution to the Problem

• Surgical release of the left lower eyelid with a lateral conthotomy and cantholysis via a lateral angled transcutaneous incision (▶ Fig. 32.7).
• Lower eyelid support with tensor fascia lata (TFL) allograft used as a lower eyelid sling in a pretarsal plane. Since repositioning of the left lower eyelid required a second finger support in the middle of the eyelid, additional support with a spacer graft was needed. Anterior and posterior approaches are both acceptable. In this case, we elected to use ear cartilage as a spacer graft via an anterior approach (▶ Fig. 32.8).

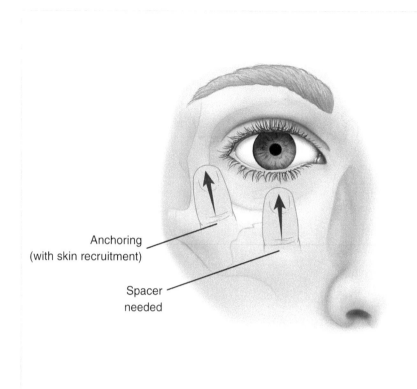

Anchoring
(with skin recruitment)

Spacer
needed

Fig. 32.6 One-finger distraction test. This test will evaluate the need for a spacer graft. If a second finger is needed at the midportion of the lower eyelid to correct the malposition, then a spacer graft should be considered as part of the surgical plan. (Reproduced with permission from Codner MA, McCord Jr CD. Eyelid and Periorbital Surgery. 2nd ed. New York, NY: Thieme; 2016.)

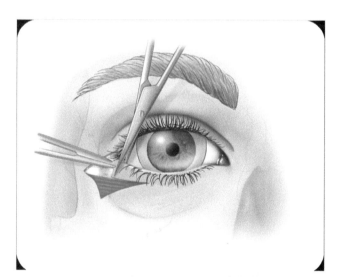

Fig. 32.7 Transcutaneous lateral angled incision used to perform lateral canthotomy and lower lateral canthal tendon lysis. (Reproduced with permission from Codner MA, McCord Jr CD. Eyelid and Periorbital Surgery. 2nd ed. New York, NY: Thieme; 2016.)

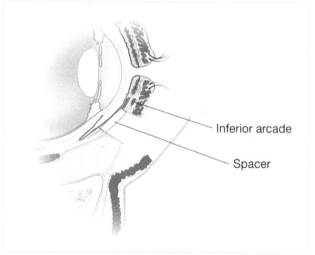

Inferior arcade

Spacer

Fig. 32.8 Placement of spacer graft to the lower eyelid. Anterior and posterior approaches are both acceptable. In this case, an anterior approach was used. (Reproduced with permission from Codner MA, McCord Jr CD. Eyelid and Periorbital Surgery. 2nd ed. New York, NY: Thieme; 2016.)

- Use of Mitek-anchoring devices (Mitek Products Inc., Westwood, MA) to support the TFL sling at the medial and lateral canthus, and resuspension of the skin-muscle (orbicularis oculi) flap at the lateral orbit rim considering the periosteum has been damaged from multiple prior surgeries.
- Recruitment of anterior lamella skin and release of lower eyelid pulling tension by performing a preperiosteal midcheek lift and resuspending the skin-muscle (orbicularis oculi) flap to the lateral orbit periosteum (▶ Fig. 32.9).
- Facelift was performed as an adjuvant technique to further release of pulling forces on the lower eyelids.

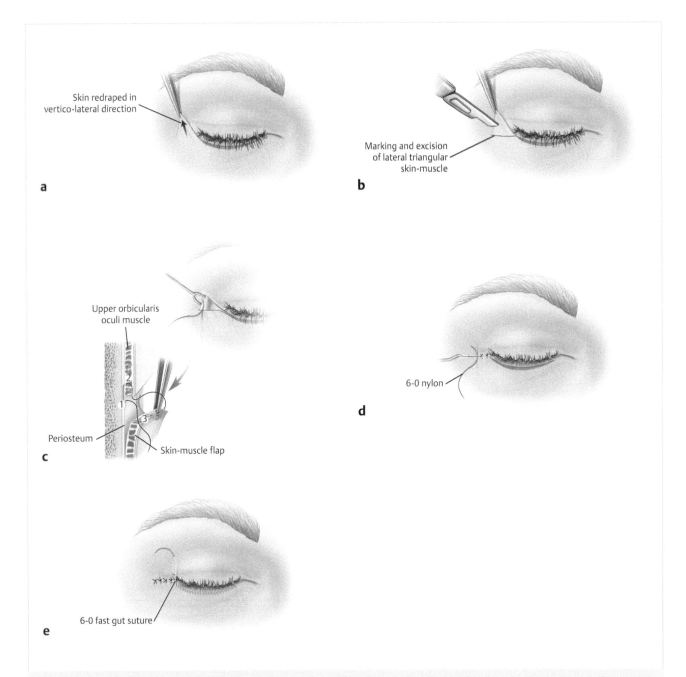

Fig. 32.9 (a–e) Lateral resuspension of skin–muscle (orbicularis oculi) flap will serve to recruit cheek skin into the lower eyelid and to relive pulling forces.

32.4 Technique

The medial canthal tendon is identified via a 1-cm vertical incision (▶Fig. 32.10). The TFL allograft sling is wrapped around the tendon and tied to itself with a 6–0 nonabsorbable monofilament suture.

A Mitek anchor device is placed into the lacrimal bone. The TFL allograft sling is then secured to the Mitek anchor for added medial support as the medial canthal tendon has been stretched (▶Fig. 32.11).

The TFL allograft sling is transferred to the lateral orbit in a pretarsal plane along the edge of the lower eyelid (▶Fig. 32.12).

A Mitek anchor is placed in the lateral orbit rim and used as an anchor point for the TFL allograft sling. This will provide added support now that the periosteum has been stripped away from previous surgeries (▶Fig. 32.13).

Immediate post-op picture is shown in ▶Fig. 32.14.

32.5 Postoperative Photographs and Critical Evaluation of Results

The patient is presented at 6 and 11 weeks postoperatively (▶Fig. 32.15). The left lower eyelid is now repositioned to its ideal location at the inferior corneal limbus. The medial and lateral scleral triangles are now smaller and more symmetrical in size when compared with the contralateral eye (right). This confirms adequate positioning of the lower eyelid and re-creates the visual symmetry of both eyes.

Despite adequate positioning of the lower eyelid, the patient continues to have lagophthalmos. Upon further evaluation, we noticed that the upper eyelid is now relatively longer after tightening of the lower lid with the TFL allograft sling. The problem is not the lower eyelid anymore, but less excursion of the upper eyelid as it is not tightly adhered to the lateral orbital rim. An upper eyelid canthoplasty will resolve this problem. In retrospect, this procedure could have been performed at the same time of the reconstruction with the TFL allograft sling. We understand the skin graft in the lower eyelid is not aesthetically pleasant and we discussed removing it during surgery, but due to multiple surgeries in the lower eyelid, the amount of available skin was limited. Complete excision of the skin graft in this case could increase the chances of recurrence despite recruitment of midcheek skin with resuspension of the skin–orbicularis oculi muscle flap at the lateral rim and a facelift.

32.6 Teaching Points

- Analysis of a complex reconstructive problem requires identification of the anatomic basis of each problem and an outlined plan to address each and every one of them.
- The ability to design a surgical plan different from what has already been done and the knowledge of a variety of surgical tools and skills will become useful to the plastic surgeon addressing a complex and recurrent problem.
- A lateral canthoplasty alone will not address laxity and eversion of the medial lower eyelid.
- TFL allograft (most commonly used for congenital upper eyelid ptosis) is a great option for support and repositioning of the lower eyelid when the laxity and eversion span the majority of the lower eyelid (medial and lateral ectropion).

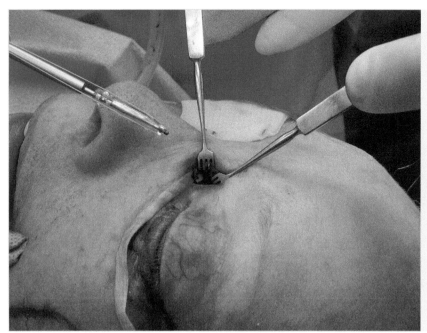

Fig. 32.10 The medial canthal tendon is identified via a 1-cm vertical incision. The TFL allograft sling is wrapped around the tendon and tied to itself with a 6–0 nonabsorbable monofilament suture.

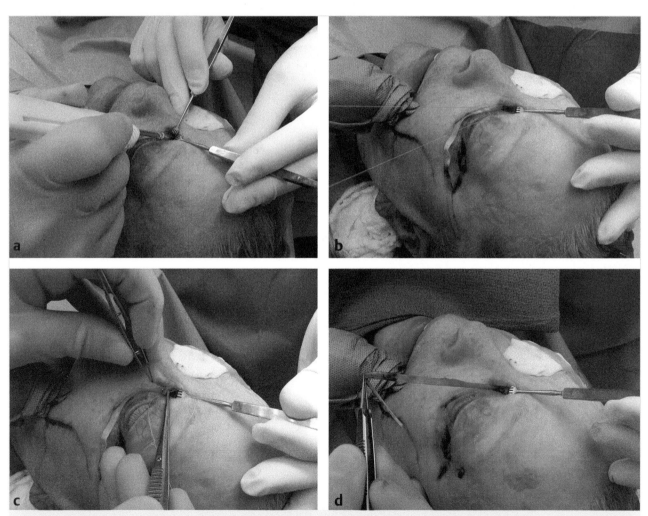

Fig. 32.11 (a–d) A Mitek anchor device is placed into the lacrimal bone. The TFL allograft sling is then secured to the Mitek anchor for added medial support as the medial canthal tendon has been stretched.

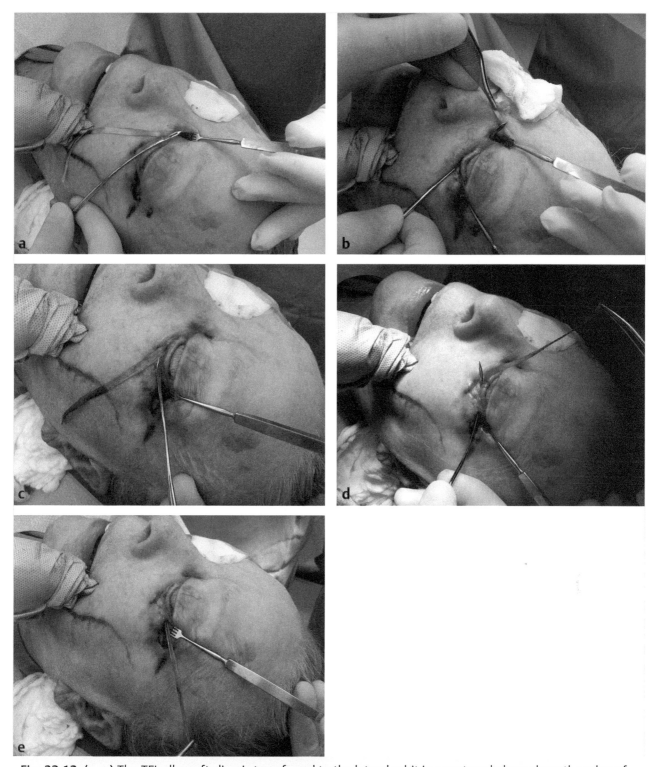

Fig. 32.12 (a–e) The TFL allograft sling is transferred to the lateral orbit in a pretarsal plane along the edge of the lower eyelid.

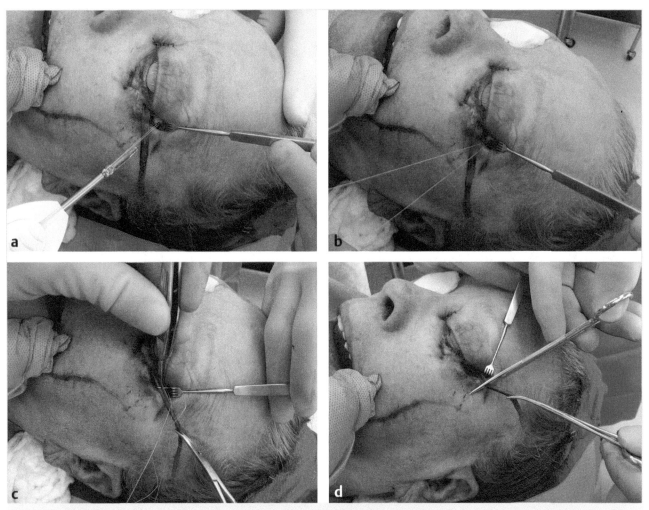

Fig. 32.13 (a–d) A Mitek anchor is placed in the lateral orbit rim and used as an anchor point for the TFL allograft sling. This will provide added support now that the periosteum has been stripped away from previous surgeries.

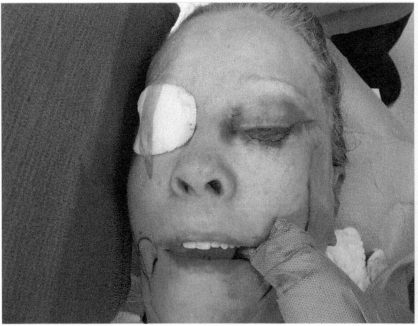

Fig. 32.14 Immediate post-op photo.

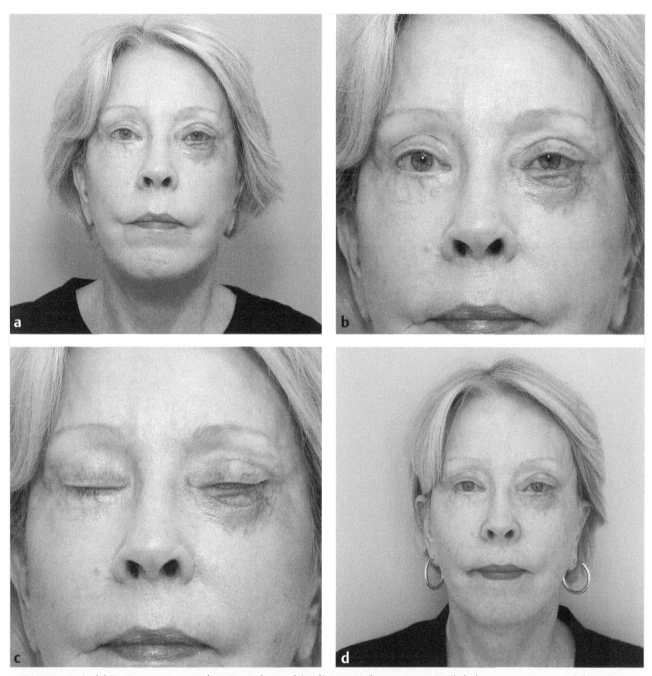

Fig. 32.15 (a,b) Patient presented at 6 weeks and **(c,d)** 11 weeks post-op. Eyelid closure is improved, but there is lagophthalmos present. The patient will benefit from upper eyelid canthoplasty to reduce the length of the upper eyelid and improved the mechanics of the upper eyelid.

- The one-finger distraction test (▶ Fig. 32.6) is a great method to select those patients who will benefit from additional support from a spacer graft in addition to a simple canthoplasty. If a second finger is needed in the midportion of the lower eyelid to achieve good positioning, then a spacer is included as part of the operative plan (as it was done in this case).
- Multiple operations in the periorbital area are a red flag. The surgeon must consider the periosteum to be damaged, which will prevent it from being used as an anchoring structure. In this case, we elected to use Mitek-anchoring devices to support the TFL sling and the skin–muscle (orbicularis oculi) flap to the facial bones.

- Tightening of the lower eyelid at the lateral canthus could result in a change in the mechanics of the upper eyelid, decreasing its excursion and preventing correction of lagophthalmos despite adequate repositioning of the lower eyelid. The surgeon performing these procedures should be also capable of performing an upper eyelid canthoplasty to shorten the upper eyelid. Drill hole canthoplasty should be considered if the periosteum is damaged.
- Preperiosteal midcheek lift with resuspension of the skin–muscle (orbicularis oculi) flap to the lateral orbital rim and/or a facelift are great adjuvant procedures to help recruit skin to the lower eyelid, also providing additional release of the pulling forces to the lower eyelid.

Suggested Reading

[1] Alfano C, Chiummariello S, Monarca C, Scuderi N, Scuderi G. Lateral canthoplasty by the Micro-Mitek Anchor System: 10-year review of 96 patients. J Oral Maxillofac Surg. 2011; 69(6):1745–1749
[2] Bartsich S, Swartz KA, Spinelli HM. Lateral canthoplasty using the Mitek anchor system. Aesthetic Plast Surg. 2012; 36(1):3–7
[3] McCord CD, Jr, Ellis DS. The correction of lower lid malposition following lower lid blepharoplasty. Plast Reconstr Surg. 1993; 92(6):1068–1072
[4] McCord CD Jr, Codner MC. Eyelid and Periorbital Surgery. St. Louis, MO: Quality Medical Publishing, Inc.; 2008
[5] Marshak H, Morrow DM, Dresner SC. Small incision preperiosteal midface lift for correction of lower eyelid retraction. Ophthal Plast Reconstr Surg. 2010; 26(3):176–181
[6] Jelks GW, Jelks EB. Repair of lower lid deformities. Clin Plast Surg. 1993; 20(2):417–425

33 Cicatricial Ectropion

Michelle Barbara Locke

Summary

This chapter reviews the surgical correction of cicatricial ectropion of the anterior lamella of the lower eyelid following resection of melanoma in situ and failed skin graft repair. Treatment involves excision of the scar, release of the remaining anterior lamella, and replacement with appropriate-sized full-thickness skin graft harvested from the ipsilateral upper eyelid. Repair is supported with a canthopexy suture.

Keywords: Cicatricial ectropion, ectropion, lower eye lid, scarring, anterior lamella, full-thickness skin graft, canthopexy

33.1 Patient History Leading to the Specific Problem

The patient is a 56-year-old European woman who underwent excision of melanoma in situ from her left lower eyelid and cheek on two occasions over the previous year. The first excision was performed by a surgeon at her regional hospital with a local flap repair. The second excision was performed by the dermatology service at a tertiary center due to incomplete excision of the lesion at the time of primary surgery. The second excision was reconstructed with a combination of a transposition flap from the left preauricular region together with a full-thickness skin graft placed at the superior aspect of the flap, harvested from the supraclavicular region. The recovery for the second surgery was complicated by infection and partial graft loss.

The patient was unhappy with the appearance of her right lower eyelid. She denied any symptoms of exposure. She presented to the Plastic Surgery department requesting treatment to obtain better symmetry. ▶ Fig. 33.1 shows frontal and oblique views of the patient on presentation.

She was also unhappy with the appearance of her donor site scar. ▶ Fig. 33.2 shows the undesirable scar from her previous supraclavicular skin harvest.

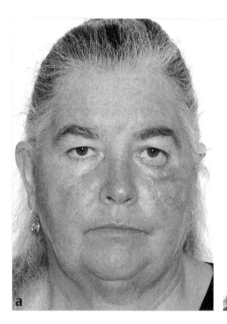
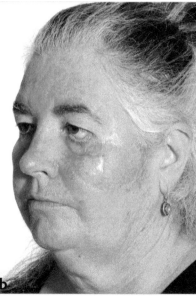

Fig. 33.1 (a) Frontal and **(b)** oblique views of the patient on presentation to the Department of Plastic Surgery.

233

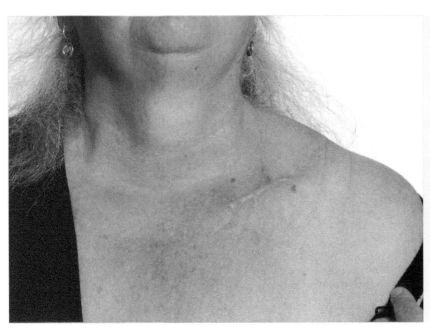

Fig. 33.2 Scar from her previous supraclavicular skin graft harvest.

She therefore requested that an alternative donor site be selected for future surgery.

33.2 Anatomic Description of the Patient's Current Status

The patient demonstrates significant left lower eyelid cicatricial ectropion. This is commonly due to shortening of the anterior lamella of the eyelid, which can be a result of tissue loss or scar contracture. Patients with ectropion commonly present with red or irritated eyes or a complaint of excessive tearing, especially if the punctum is pulled away from the globe.

In this case, review of the patient and the operative notes confirmed that previous resections had involved the anterior lamella only, with full-thickness skin and only partial orbicularis muscle resection. The likely cause of her ectropion was infection and subsequent graft loss from the lateral aspect of the left lower eyelid area. This region then healed by secondary intention and the subsequent scar contracture pulled the lower eyelid down and outward. Examination showed thick scar and a lower lid, which was unable to be manually repositioned into its anatomical position. The eye itself did not show any redness and the patient denied any symptoms of irritation or exposure. Surgical correction of the shortened anterior lamella was recommended. Due to the prior surgery, no local flap options from the cheek were available.

33.3 Recommended Solution to the Problem

- Excise the thickened scar and release remaining anterior lamella tissue.
- Measure the resulting defect and obtain appropriate full-thickness graft for reconstruction from upper eyelid(s).
- Stent graft with tie over dressing.
- Support the lower lid with horizontal tightening (canthopexy or canthoplasty as required).

33.4 Technique

The planned donor site is the ipsilateral upper eyelid. This donor site provides thin skin which is an excellent color and thickness match for the lower eyelid. It is also cosmetically favorable, with a well-hidden scar which potentially can provide the aesthetic benefit of an upper eyelid blepharoplasty. The upper eyelid crease is therefore marked preoperatively for future reference. A subciliary incision is planned at the superior aspect of the scarred area with a lateral extension to allow for canthal reset. ▶ Fig. 33.3 shows the extent of the incision planned preoperatively. Surgery is performed under general anesthesia, with local anesthetic infiltration. Flexible corneal protectors lubricated with eye ointment are placed to protect the globe. Following local anesthetic injection, incise with a blade through skin and orbicularis at the lateral aspect of the planned subciliary incision. With Westcott scissors, undermine medially in a subcutaneous plane along the planned subciliary incision and cut the skin as you progress. Extend your incision as far medially as required to reach normal, unscarred tissue.

With the orbicularis muscle exposed, dissection is performed inferiorly to allow release of the subcutaneous scarring (▶ Fig. 33.4). I prefer to use needlepoint monopolar diathermy ("Bovie") for this dissection. To assist with dissection, 4–0 silk sutures are placed through the ciliary margin and held superiorly to provide countertraction. Once the cutaneous release has been performed, any scarring or fibrotic attachments of the orbicularis muscles are also divided. After the complete release of all skin and muscle shortening, the maximum size of the defect under stretch is determined to facilitate appropriate donor skin harvest, as demonstrated in ▶ Fig. 33.5.

Prior to skin grafting, lateral canthal reset should be performed. Lateral canthopexy is performed in routine fashion with two core suture fixation from the lateral aspect of the lower eyelid to the medial aspect of the lateral orbital rim at an appropriate level to provide symmetry with the contralateral lower eyelid, as shown in ▶ Fig. 33.6. I prefer to use an absorbable, synthetic, braided suture such as 4–0 Vicryl, although permanent (nonabsorbable) sutures are also reasonable. Following canthopexy (▶ Fig. 33.7), lid position

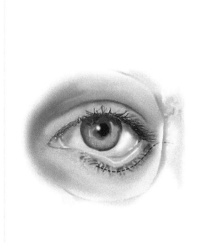
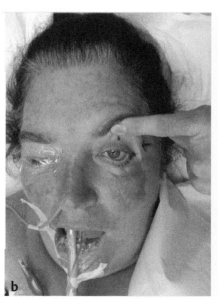

Fig. 33.3 (a) Extent of planned subciliary incision. (b) Intraoperative view with planned incision marked.

a

b

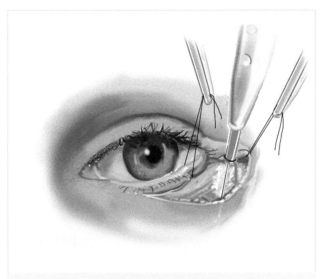

Fig. 33.4 With the orbicularis muscle exposed, dissection is performed inferiorly to allow release of the subcutaneous scarring.

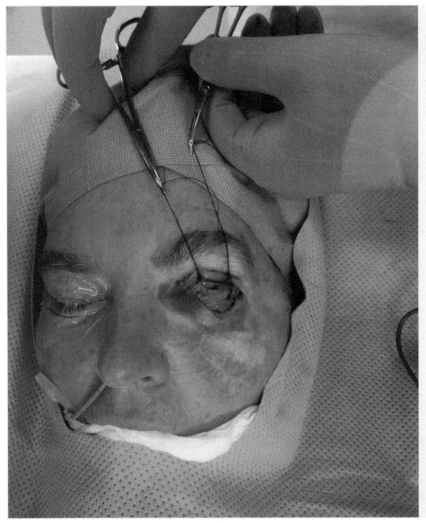

Fig. 33.5 After the complete release of all skin and muscle shortening, the maximum size of the defect under stretch is determined to facilitate appropriate donor skin harvest.

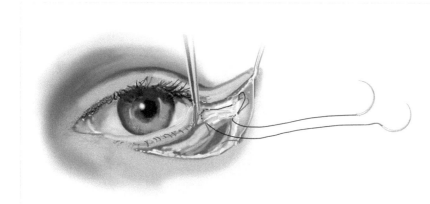

Fig. 33.6 Position of lateral canthopexy, performed with double-armed 4–0 suture. The first pass is through the lateral edge of the lower lid. Each arm in turn is then passed through the lateral orbital rim periosteum at the appropriate level. Figure shows passage of first arm of the suture through the orbital rim.

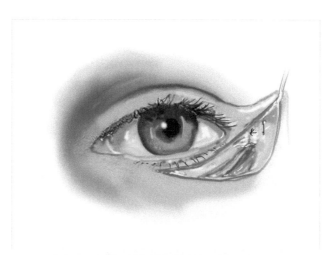

Fig. 33.7 Tying the lateral canthopexy suture repositions the lower lid appropriately.

and distraction are checked. In this case, lid distraction is less than 2 mm from the globe and the lateral canthal position was felt to be acceptable. However, if canthopexy did not provided an appropriately secure fixation, progression to formal canthoplasty would have been considered.

The maximum vertical height of the skin defect after canthopexy was measured at 13 mm. This height is then transposed onto the upper eyelid, measuring superiorly from the previously marked lid crease, with routine upper blepharoplasty planning. Nontoothed forceps are used to pinch the skin at the marks to estimate closure after skin removal. If it is felt that skin closure would be able to be performed without any tension or lagophthalmos, local anesthetic is infiltrated. Using a blade, incise through the skin of the upper eyelid as marked. With Westcott scissors, remove full-thickness upper eyelid skin and place it in a damp gauze sponge. ▶ Fig. 33.8 shows the upper eyelid skin after harvest. A thin strip of orbicularis oculi muscle can be excised from the donor site if necessary to facilitate closure. Following hemostasis, closure is performed with running 6–0 nonabsorbable monofilament suture.

While the 4–0 silk traction sutures maintain the cilial margin in a superior position, the full-thickness skin graft is secured in place with 6–0 absorbable sutures such as Vicryl Rapide or Fast Gut (▶ Fig. 33.9).

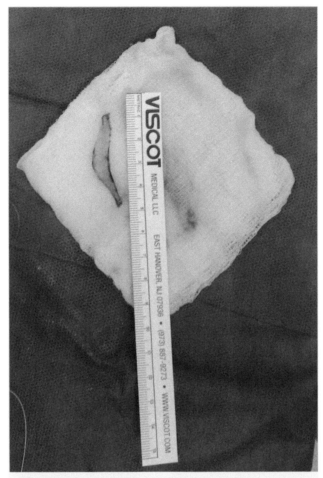

Fig. 33.8 Upper eyelid skin after harvest.

Paraffin gauze and paraffin-soaked cotton ball dressings are secured in place as a tie over dressing using 5–0 silk. The tie over dressing and upper lid sutures are removed 5 days postoperatively.

33.5 Postoperative Photographs and Critical Evaluation of Results

Postoperatively, the patient shows evidence of a well-healed skin graft at the lateral aspect of her left lower eyelid (▶ Fig. 33.10). The lower eyelid position is 1 to 2mm below the corneoscleral limbus on the left, which is symmetrical with her right lower eyelid position.

Harvesting of her left upper eyelid skin as donor for the lower eyelid graft has resulted in noticeable upper eyelid asymmetry. This would be most easily corrected by performing a right upper eyelid blepharoplasty under local anesthetic should the patient desire it.

33.6 Teaching Points

- Cicatricial ectropion can develop for a number of reasons, including poor planning (e.g., insufficient size of flap or graft), postoperative scar

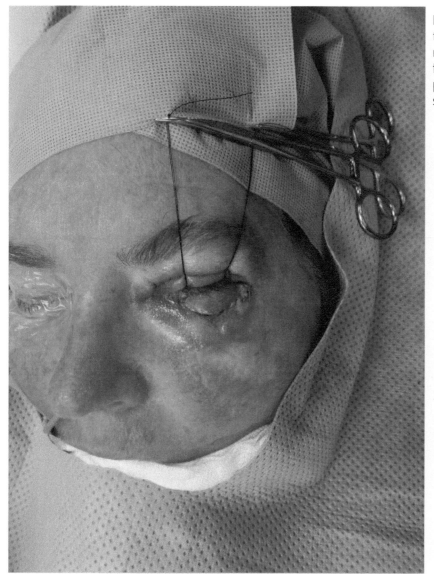

Fig. 33.9 While the 4–0 silk traction sutures maintain the cilial margin in a superior position, the full-thickness skin graft is secured in place with 6–0 absorbable sutures such as Vicryl Rapide or Fast Gut.

contracture, or postoperative complications (e.g., infection, delayed wound healing, graft or flap loss).

- Primary prevention is better than secondary correction.
- Appropriate repair requires recreation of the defect to allow analysis of the size and type of tissue deficiency.
- Recruitment of additional tissue to the anterior lamella can be in the form of a flap, a graft, or a combination of both. Each has advantages and disadvantages.
- Horizontal lid support in the form of canthopexy or canthoplasty is essential to reduce the risk of ectropion recurrence. However, horizontal lid support alone will not compensate for significant anterior lamella shortage.
- Active postoperative management with scar and lid massage can be helpful to prevent recurrence.

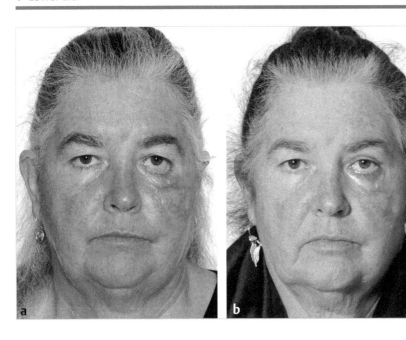

Fig. 33.10 (a,b) Postoperatively, the patient shows evidence of a well-healed skin graft and improved left lower eyelid position.

Suggested Reading

[1] Bedran EG, Pereira MV, Bernardes TF. Ectropion. Semin Ophthalmol. 2010; 25(3):59–65

[2] Fagien S. Algorithm for canthoplasty: the lateral retinacular suspension: a simplified suture canthopexy. Plast Reconstr Surg. 1999; 103(7):2042–2053, discussion 2054–2058

[3] Manku K, Leong JK, Ghabrial R. Cicatricial ectropion: repair with myocutaneous flaps and canthopexy. Clin Experiment Ophthalmol. 2006; 34(7):677–681

[4] McCord CD, Codner MA, eds. Eyelid and Periorbial Surgery. 1st ed. Boca Raton, FL: CRC Press; 2008

[5] Rathore DS, Chickadasarahilli S, Crossman R, Mehta P, Ahluwalia HS. Full thickness skin grafts in periocular reconstructions: long-term outcomes. Ophthal Plast Reconstr Surg. 2014; 30(6):517–520

[6] Spinelli HM. Eyelid malpositions. In: Spinelli HM, ed. Atlas of Aesthetic Eyelid and Periocular Surgery. New York, NY: Elsevier Inc; 2004:34–56

[7] Verity DH, Collin JR. Eyelid reconstruction: the state of the art. Curr Opin Otolaryngol Head Neck Surg. 2004; 12(4):344–348

34 The Spectrum of Postblepharoplasty Lower Eyelid Retraction (PBLER) Repair

Raymond Scott Douglas and Guy G. Massry

Summary

Postblepharoplasty lower eyelid retraction is a complicated and challenging problem to surgically address. Its etiology is multifactorial and can include eyelid scarring, eyelid laxity, volume deficit, orbicularis weakness, negative vector topography, and anterior lamellar deficit. Appropriate correction requires a detailed preoperative examination with identification of contributing factors to determine the best surgical plan. On occasion, nonsurgical intervention such as eyelid filler injection may suffice.

Keywords: lower eyelid retraction, postblepharoplasty lower eyelid retraction, eyelid vector, eyelid laxity, scleral show, Margin Reflex Distance 2, orbicularis strength, eyelid filler injection

34.1 Background

Postblepharoplasty lower eyelid retraction (PBLER) is a challenging and complicated eyelid malposition to address. Traditional teaching has been that it is caused by three principal factors: (1) unaddressed lower eyelid laxity, (2) anterior lamellar shortage, and (3) a "middle lamellar" or orbital septal scar. As such, the standard repair of these physical findings ("traditional surgery") has been a combination of (1) canthal suspension, (2) midface lifting to recruit skin, and (3) a posterior lamellar spacer graft. The authors have studied PBLER in depth and have found that this combination of procedures, applied universally, leads to patient satisfaction with surgery in only 40% of cases (surgeon satisfaction much higher at 80%); recurrence is not uncommon, and orbicularis deficit (innervational or biomechanical), a negative vector globe/midface morphology, and a volume-deficient lower eyelid/inferior orbit are also significant etiologic factors present (yet often unaddressed). Appropriate treatment for this complicated and multifactorial problem requires identifying (1) its primary component causes, (2) the degree of intervention patients are willing to undergo, and (3) patient expectations. Final treatment is then tailored accordingly. Examples of various presentations and treatment options are reviewed below.

34.2 Physical Examination

It is important to quantify the amount of PBLER to assess efficacy of surgery in an evidence-based manner. This can be standardized by measuring scleral show (the amount of sclera visible between inferior limbus and the lower lid margin) and the Margin Reflex Distance 2 (MRD2; distance of corneal light reflex to lower lid margin) (▶ Fig. 34.1). The authors prefer the MRD2 as an indicator of the degree of lower lid retraction. To best develop a plan to address PBLER, the authors have identified six critical factors that must be evaluated for each case. Assessing the presence and degree of each potential deficit directs treatment.

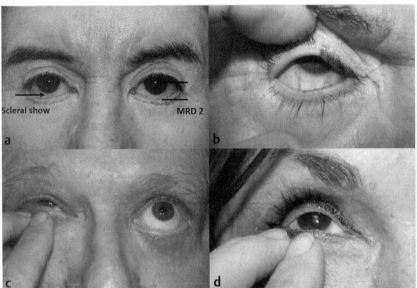

Fig. 34.1 (a) Scleral show and MRD2 are means of quantifying lower eyelid retraction. (b) Orbicularis strength is subjectively assessed by having the patient squeeze the eyelids closed while the examiner attempts to open the eyelids. With normal orbicularis function, the eyelids should not be pried open. The amount of deficit is graded (0: no strength; to 4: normal function). In this case, there is significant deficit. (c) A minimally positive FTT. (d) A significantly positive FTT.

These parameters and how they are evaluated are listed below.

- Orbicularis strength—lid squeezing (▶Fig. 34.1).
- Internal eyelid scar—forced traction test (FTT): limitation of free upward excursion of the eyelid (▶Fig. 34.1).
- Anterior lamellar shortage—patient looks up and opens mouth (▶Fig. 34.2).
- Eyelid/inferior orbit volume deficit—subjective grading by visual inspection (▶Fig. 34.2).
- Eyelid vector—subjective grading of globe/midface topography or slope (▶Fig. 34.2).
- Eyelid laxity—snap back and distraction test (▶Fig. 34.3).

34.3 Patient Examples

34.3.1 Case 1: Volume Deficit

A 36-year-old woman had transcutaneous (open approach) lower blepharoplasty 1.5 years ago. On examination, she primarily has volume-depleted lower lids, borderline anterior lamellar shortage, and no internal eyelid scar of significance. Her eyelid is not lax, there is good orbicularis function, and her eyelid vector is neutral. Her retraction was addressed well with lower lid filler treatment (▶Fig. 34.4).

Analysis

The predominant finding on this woman's examination is volume-deficient inferior orbits/lower eyelids, and she is not keen on invasive surgery. She was treated by stenting her lower lids with hyaluronic acid gel filler. This is best accomplished with a stiff (high G) and viscous product, which allows excellent three-dimensional tissue expansion. In her case, 1 cc of Restylane was given to both lower lids with a 25-G, 1.5 cannula. The authors have found the cannula technique leads to less bruising, and this length of cannula allows treatment of the entire eyelid with one skin penetration. The authors have also found that a malar entry (mideyelid location) versus an eyelid entry point, independent of the cannula device, leads to less bruising than direct eyelid injections. The gel is placed over the bone (using noninjecting finger to feel the location of the tip of

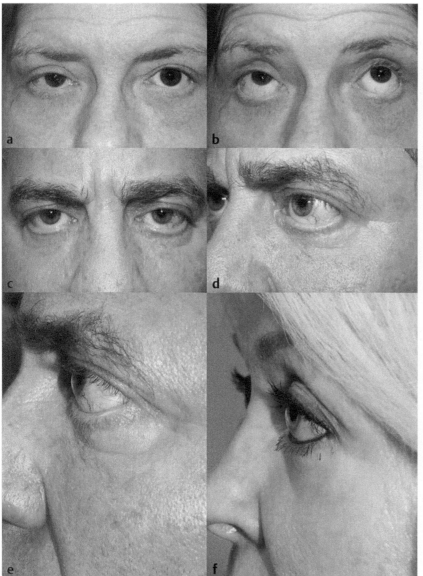

Fig. 34.2 **(a,b)** Anterior lamellar shortage is present with simultaneous supraduction (patient looks up) and mouth opening the lower lid retracts further. **(c,d)** Frontal and oblique view of inferior orbit/lower eyelid volume loss. **(e,f)** Two examples of negative vector globe/midface morphology (globe protrudes further than midface, thus lower lid must maintain position against a gradient).

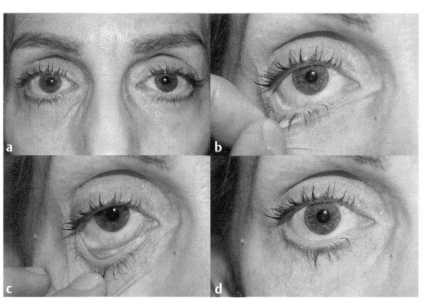

Fig. 34.3 **(a,b)** Eyelid distraction test. If the lower lid can be distracted more than 8 mm from the globe, eyelid laxity is present. **(c,d)** Eyelid snapback test. If the lower lid can be inferiorly displaced and not return to normal position without a blink, there is a positive test, which also signifies eyelid laxity.

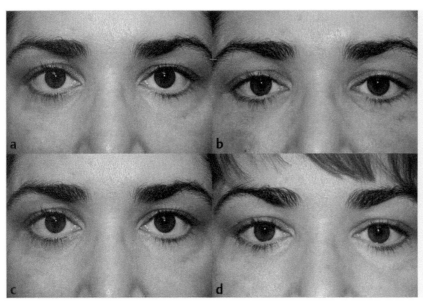

Fig. 34.4 **(a)** Before and **(b)** immediate after treatment with Restylane filler. The cannula entry site (red cheeks) is noted from the procedure. Note lower lid elevation with volumization of inferior periorbita. **(c)** Before and **(d)** after treatment at 4 months.

the cannula) of the inferior orbital rim in 0.1- to 0.2-mL deposits (after aspiration on plunger and retrograde injection), and is massaged on bone in a superior direction. The bone acts as a backstop for massage. Tissue expansion leads to lower lid elevation (▶Fig. 34.5). Original descriptions of this technique used a needle, and injections were given from the orbital rim to the lash line (▶Fig. 34.6). The authors prefer not to use needles in potentially scarred planes, as the scar may fix vessels in place and increase the likelihood of vascular complications. The authors also prefer to avoid injecting into the eyelid proper as they have found this leads to contour issues, significant bruising, and less predictable results. This procedure is less powerful when upward eyelid excursion is limited by severe scar or skin shortage. If there is significant negative vector present, the midface must be augmented simultaneously.

34.3.2 Case 2: Orbicularis Deficit

This 70-year-old woman had open approach lower blepharoplasty 10 years ago with resultant PBLER. The main findings on her examination are a degree of lower eyelid laxity, anterior lamellar shortage, volume deficit, and 2+ orbicularis deficit. She underwent minimally invasive retractor recession and closed canthal suspension (MIOS, minimally invasive, orbicularis-sparing lower lid recession) with an appropriate surgical outcome which met her expectations (▶Fig. 34.7).

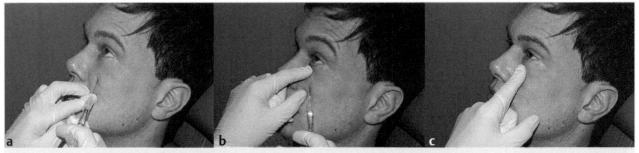

Fig. 34.5 **(a)** Malar entry with cannula. **(b)** Bimanual technique of identifying cannula location. **(c)** Massage on orbital rim.

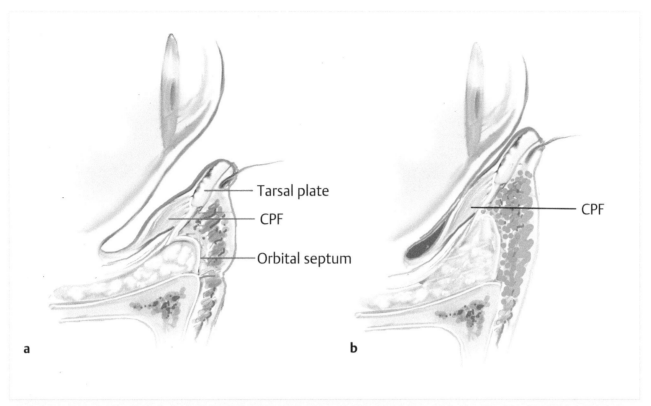

Fig. 34.6 Lower eyelid retraction **(a)** prior to filler placement and **(b)** after filler in green injected throughout eyelid (lashes to orbital rim). While this technique has shown to be effective, it is not the authors' preference.

Analysis

The patient was averse to placement of foreign materials (fillers) and "any significant surgery." As her orbicularis function was reduced, surgery was aimed at recessing the lower lid while preserving orbicularis integrity. She underwent an MIOS lower lid recession. In this procedure, the lower eyelid retractors are recessed transconjunctivally (▶ Fig. 34.8) and a closed canthal suspension via an upper lid crease is performed (dissection to canthal tendon

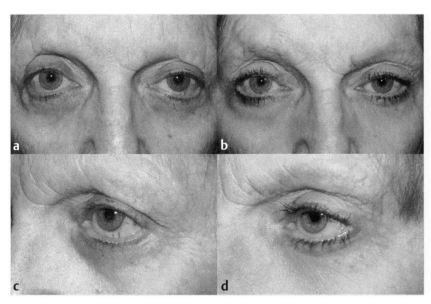

Fig. 34.7 **(a)** Before and **(b)** after frontal view of bilateral MIOS (orbicularis sparing) lower lid recession. **(c,d)** Oblique's views of same. While not a total correction, it is a significant improvement attained with minimal surgery.

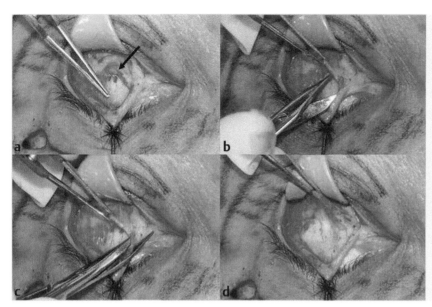

Fig. 34.8 Surgical series of lower lid retractor recession. **(a)** Initial release of retractors *(black arrow)* from conjunctiva, **(b)** retractor undermining. **(c)** Cutting retractors, **(d)** retractors recessed.

is suborbicularis and preperiosteal) (▶ Fig. 34.9). The access points in an MIOS procedure leaves the lower orbicularis relatively "untouched" (upper crease for canthal suspension and transconjunctival to recess the lower lid retractors). The closed canthal suspension combined with the retractor recession allows a degree of lift to the lower lid as long as there is minimal eyelid scar and the vector gradient is not too steep. Please refer to Yoo DB, Griffin GR, Azizzadeh BA, and Massry GG for a detailed description of the procedure.[14]

34.3.3 Case 3: Anterior Lamellar Shortage

This 56-year-old woman had previous transcutaneous lower blepharoplasty 1 year ago. She developed PBLER on the left primarily related to anterior lamellar shortage with mild internal eyelid scar (slightly reduced FTT). She underwent skin grafting for repair with 5FU supplementation to modulate scarring. She was very happy with her outcome (▶ Fig. 34.10).

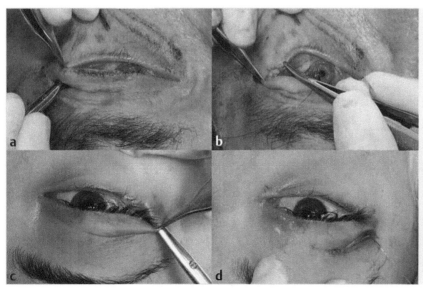

Fig. 34.9 (a,c) Upper lid crease access to release of the lateral canthal tendon (internal cantholysis). As a canthotomy has not been performed, this is considered a closed procedure. **(b)** Double-armed 5–0 PDS suture on RB-2 needle passed through commissure (both arms through same hole). **(d)** Pulling on suture after fixation to lateral orbital rim. Note natural canthal position with undisturbed canthal angle.

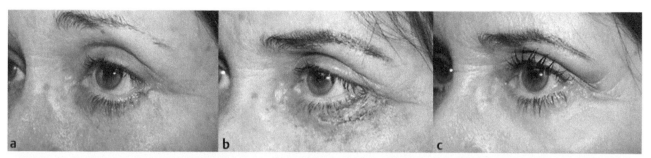

Fig. 34.10 **(a)** Lower lid retraction left after previous transcutaneous lower blepharoplasty. **(b)** Two weeks after skin grafting with a supraclavicular skin graft. **(c)** Nine month after surgery with makeup on. The scars are not noticeable. She underwent five separate injections of 5-FU per protocol.

Analysis

This patient was averse to the invasiveness of midface lifting and less concerned with a possible scar from skin grafting. The authors have found that skin grafting with meticulous technique, avoiding the thicker and less sun-exposed retroauricular skin as a donor site, and postoperative wound modulation with 5-FU have led to appropriate results by 3 to 4 months after surgery (refer to Yoo DB, Azizzadeh B, and Massry GG. for injection technique and timing), especially with makeup on.[15] In general, skin grafting has lost favor as a means of addressing PBLER, but, as stated, patient satisfaction with traditional midface lifting surgery is not high and lid malposition often recurs. This is a simpler procedure than skin recruitment via midface lifting, but patient selection is critical. The authors suggest trying skin grafting with wound modulation on reconstructive cases first to gain confidence.

34.3.4 Case 4: Internal Eyelid Scarring

This 40-year-old woman has PBLER after transcutaneous lower blepharoplasty 2 years ago. She has both anterior and middle lamellar deficits (skin shortage and an internal eyelid scar). She underwent traditional midface lifting with posterior lamellar spacer graft (hard palate) and canthoplasty. While long-term results of this procedure can be unpredictable, she attained an appropriate result (▶ Fig. 34.11; ▶ Fig. 34.12; ▶ Fig. 34.13; ▶ Fig. 34.14).

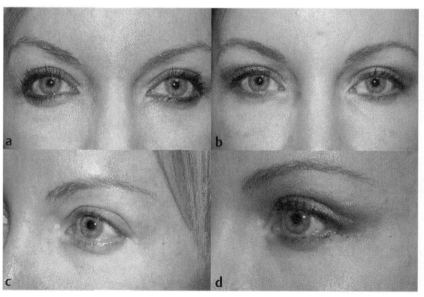

Fig. 34.11 **(a)** Before and **(b)** after (2 years) frontal view of patient with PBLER. **(c,d)** Oblique views of same.

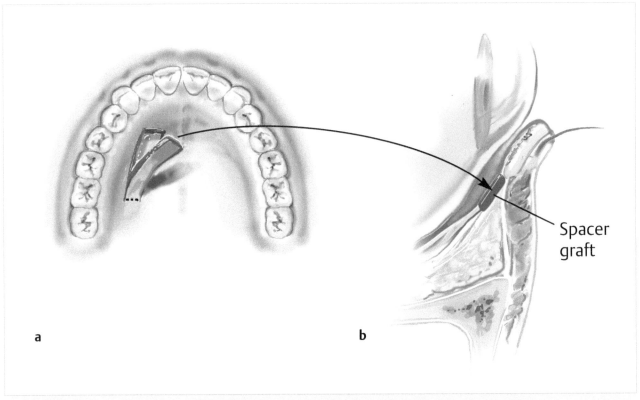

Fig. 34.12 (a) Removal of graft. (b) Sagittal view of placement of the graft as an eyelid spacer.

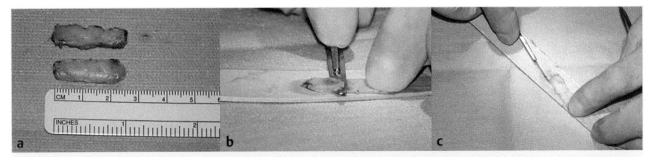

Fig. 34.13 (a) Harvested palate grafts measuring 25 mm in length. (b) Thinning of grafts. (c) Sizing of graft.

Analysis

This woman is a good candidate for traditional surgery as her deficits are not severe (patients do better in this scenario). She underwent open canthoplasty, placement of a posterior lamellar hard palate graft, and supraperiosteal transeyelid midface lifting. There are many nuances to this procedure and the authors have developed certain preferences including the following:

- The transconjunctival supraperiosteal approach (transconjunctival preseptal eyelid dissection, release of tear trough, and orbitomalar ligament), in the author's view, is more predictable especially when the midface glides freely over periosteum/bone. Elevating the midface subperiosteally in this scenario does not stabilize the midface soft tissue as predictably.
- Securing midface tissue for lift should be meticulous and lead to no or minimal skin pucker.

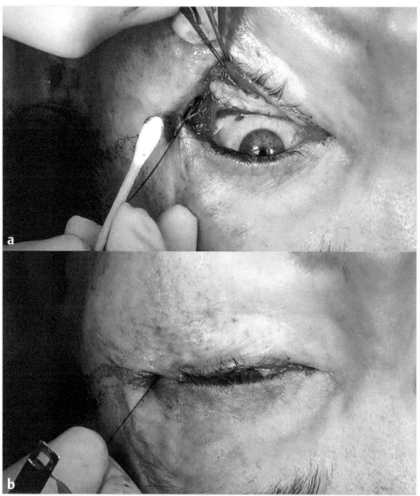

Fig. 34.14 (a) Palate graft interposed between the conjunctiva/lower lid retractors and the tarsus (inferior edge of tarsus just below forceps). This effectively recesses the retractors. The blue 4–0 Prolene suture which previously engaged the suborbicularis oculi (SOOF) fat for midface lift is seen exiting the eyelid at the lateral canthus. **(b)** Midface lifted as Prolene suture is elevated in the appropriate superolateral vector. This suture will be secured to the lateral orbital rim periosteum or deep temporalis fascia.

- Canthal suspension can be open or closed. When the midface is secured appropriately, there should be no tension on the canthus.
- Autologous spacer grafts are biocompatible and lead to less inflammation and shrinkage. Hard palate works well with few complications in experienced hands.

Clinical Pearl

Remember to select wisely in these cases. As stated, long-term patient satisfaction is not high even when the surgeon feels a good result was obtained.

34.4 Teaching Points

- PBLER is a complicated eyelid malposition whose correction must be planned based on physical findings and patient expectations.
- These cases are often unfixable to patient desires because the tissue biology has been critically altered from previous surgery and patient psyche is permanently negatively impacted.
- A "home run" result is a happy patient, not a happy surgeon (critical point).

- To improve surgical outcomes, more contemporary thought regarding the etiology of this problem should be considered. This includes the presence of orbicularis weakness, volume status, and eyelid vector.
- In this vein, consideration should be given to avoid the traditional approach to surgery in every patient, and to consider other options, when appropriate, as described in this chapter.

Suggested Reading

[1] Cotofana S, Schenck TL, Trevidic P, et al. Midface: clinical anatomy and regional approaches with injectable fillers. Plast Reconstr Surg. 2015; 136(5, Suppl):219S–234S

[2] DeLorenzi C. Complications of injectable fillers, part 2: vascular complications. Aesthet Surg J. 2014; 34(4):584–600

[3] Edgerton MT, Jr. Causes and prevention of lower lid ectropion following blepharoplasty. Plast Reconstr Surg. 1972; 49(4):367–373

[4] Ferri M, Oestreicher JH. Treatment of post-blepharoplasty lower lid retraction by free tarsoconjunctival grafting. Orbit. 2002; 21(4):281–288

[5] Goldberg RA, Lee S, Jayasundera T, Tsirbas A, Douglas RS, McCann JD. Treatment of lower eyelid retraction by expansion of the lower eyelid with hyaluronic acid gel. Ophthal Plast Reconstr Surg. 2007; 23(5):343–348

[6] Griffin G, Azizzadeh B, Massry GG. New insights into physical findings associated with postblepharoplasty lower eyelid retraction. Aesthet Surg J. 2014; 34(7):995–1004

[7] Korn BS, Kikkawa DO, Cohen SR, Hartstein M, Annunziata CC. Treatment of lower eyelid malposition with dermis fat grafting. Ophthalmology. 2008; 115(4):744–751.e2

[8] Marshak H, Morrow DM, Dresner SC. Small incision preperiosteal midface lift for correction of lower eyelid retraction. Ophthal Plast Reconstr Surg. 2010; 26(3):176–181

[9] Massry GG. A comparison of patient and surgeon satisfaction in revisional aesthetic eyelid and periorbital surgery. Presented at the: 44th annual fall meeting of the American Society of Ophthalmic Plastic and Reconstructive Surgery; New Orleans, LA; November 8, 2013

[10] Massry G. An argument for "closed canthal suspension" in aesthetic lower blepharoplasty. Ophthal Plast Reconstr Surg. 2012; 28(6):474–475

[11] Patipa M. The evaluation and management of lower eyelid retraction following cosmetic surgery. Plast Reconstr Surg. 2000; 106(2):438–453, discussion 454–459

[12] Patel BCK, Patipa M, Anderson RL, McLeish W. Management of postblepharoplasty lower eyelid retraction with hard palate grafts and lateral tarsal strip. Plast Reconstr Surg. 1997; 99(5):1251–1260

[13] Sundaram H, Cassuto D. Biophysical characteristics of hyaluronic acid soft-tissue fillers and their relevance to aesthetic applications. Plast Reconstr Surg. 2013; 132(4, Suppl 2):5S–21S

[14] Yoo DB, Griffin GR, Azizzadeh BA, Massry GG. The minimally invasive orbicularis sparing "MIOS" lower eyelid recession procedure for mild to moderate lower Lid retraction with reduced orbicularis strength. JAMA Facial Plast Surg. 2014; 16:140–146

[15] Yoo DB, Azizzadeh B, Massry GG. Injectable 5-FU with or without added steroid in periorbital skin grafting: initial observations. Ophthal Plast Reconstr Surg. 2015; 31(2):122–126

35 Filler Problems: Clinical Overview

Foad Nahai

Fillers and neuromodulators, known as the injectables, have had such a dramatic and disruptive effect that facial and periorbital rejuvenation are no longer solely in the surgical domain. Although injectables, particularly fillers, continue to evolve, they have already proven to be popular, safe, and efficacious. With minimal to no downtime and affordability, injectables continue to grow at a meteoric rate outpacing surgical procedure.

Although adverse events have been few, devastating complications including vision loss, soft tissue loss, and intracranial catastrophes have been reported with fillers. Fat grafting is also an option for volume replacement, as an isolated procedure or more commonly in conjunction with surgical rejuvenation of the face and the periorbital area. Fat too has proven to be safe and effective, though survival of grafted fat remains unpredictable.

Fillers and fat differ in many ways, and it can be argued that fat grafting is a surgical and not a cosmetic treatment; there are some similarities in terms of complications and adverse effects. ▶Box 35.1 lists complications common to fat and fillers, ▶Box 35.2 lists additional complications of fat only, and ▶Box 35.3 lists additional complications of fillers only.

While the most popular fillers, the hyaluronic acids, are readily reversible with administration of hyaluronidase, the other major categories of fillers are not. This makes dealing with complications such as infection, granuloma, overinjection, and misplaced injection very challenging. Similarly, overinjection or misplaced injection of fat is difficult to reverse and may require surgical excision.

Box 35.1 Complications Common to Fat and Fillers

- Loss of sight
- Loss of soft tissue
- Intracranial catastrophe
- Overinjection
- Underinjection
- Infection
- Misplaced injection

Box 35.2 Additional Complications of Fat Only

- Oil cysts.
- Fibrosis.
- Fat necrosis.
- Calcifications.
- Unpredictable survival.

Box 35.3 Additional Complications of Fillers Only

- Granuloma.

The volume of injected fat that takes or survives remains unpredictable, so we all overcorrect to some degree or other. This is not the case with fillers and is one of the advantages of fillers over fat. Unlike fillers, the volume of fat that takes is permanent.

The most devastating complications of fillers and fat are consequences of intravascular injections. A thorough knowledge of the vascular anatomy of the face and periorbital vasculature is essential. Injection technique is equally important. Injecting only while withdrawing the cannula or needle and avoiding excessive pressure on injection will minimize the chances of intravascular injection. Needles and cannulas both have a role in delivering fillers and fat into the tissues. Cannulas are felt to be safer in certain areas with less risk of vascular penetration.

Complications and adverse events are significantly reduced through experience and familiarity with the type of materials injected, how and where they are injected, and of course by whom these materials are injected.

Disastrous consequences of intravascular injections may be minimized or even avoided through early recognition and immediate aggressive treatment.

Suggested Reading

[1] Bailey SH, Cohen JL, Kenkel JM. Etiology, prevention, and treatment of dermal filler complications. Aesthet Surg J. 2011; 31(1):110–121

[2] Cavallini M, Gazzola R, Metalla M, Vaienti L. The role of hyaluronidase in the treatment of complications from hyaluronic acid dermal fillers. Aesthet Surg J. 2013; 33(8):1167–1174

[3] Cohen JL, Biesman BS, Dayan SH, et al. Treatment of hyaluronic acid filler-induced impending necrosis with hyaluronidase: consensus recommendations. Aesthet Surg J. 2015; 35(7):844–849

[4] Cosmetic Surgery National Data Bank Statistics. Aesthet Surg J. 2017;37(suppl_2):1–29

[5] DeLorenzi C. Complications of injectable fillers, part I. Aesthet Surg J. 2013; 33(4):561–575

[6] DeLorenzi C. Complications of injectable fillers, part 2: vascular complications. Aesthet Surg J. 2014; 34(4):584–600

[7] DeLorenzi C. New high dose pulsed hyaluronidase protocol for hyaluronic acid filler vascular adverse events. Aesthet Surg J. 2017; 37(7):814–825

[8] Kadouch JA, Tutein Nolthenius CJ, Kadouch DJ, van der Woude HJ, Karim RB, Hoekzema R. Complications after facial injections with permanent fillers: important limitations and considerations of MRI evaluation. Aesthet Surg J. 2014; 34(6):913–923

[9] Khan TT, Colon-Acevedo B, Mettu P, DeLorenzi C, Woodward JA. An anatomical analysis of the supratrochlear artery: considerations in facial filler injections and preventing vision loss. Aesthet Surg J. 2017; 37(2):203–208

[10] Ozturk CN, Li Y, Tung R, Parker L, Piliang MP, Zins JE. Complications following injection of soft-tissue fillers. Aesthet Surg J. 2013; 33(6):862–877

36 Complications of Periocular Injection: Nodules and Edema

Carisa K. Petris, Joseph A. Eviatar, and Richard D. Lisman

Summary

Periocular filler injection can result in various undesirable outcomes including nodules, overvolumization, bluish discoloration, and edema. This chapter provides a guide to addressing these challenging problems. Techniques for hyaluronidase injection, 5-fluorouracil injection, and surgical excision are described.

Keywords: filler, eyelid edema, festoons, periocular nodules, periocular overvolumization, filler granuloma, hyaluronidase

36.1 Patient History Leading to the Specific Filler Problem

36.1.1 Case 1

A 39-year-old man presented for persistent swelling of the lower eyelids, which began approximately 2 years ago (►Fig. 36.1). He had a history of Restylane and Perlane injections from 2002 to 2007 every 6 months. The patient reported that 6 months prior to the swelling, he was involved in a car accident without significant facial fractures. He also reported a sinus infection that resolved without complication 3 months prior to the onset of the lower eyelid fullness. One year ago, he had Botox injections.

36.1.2 Case 2

A 52-year-old woman presented with a 1-year history of lower eyelid fullness (►Fig. 36.2). She received Radiesse to the lower eyelid approximately 1 year before the lower eyelid swelling began. She was treated with hyaluronidase injection and antibiotics without benefit. An MRI of the orbits found no masses. She had a history of bilateral upper and lower eyelid blepharoplasty at

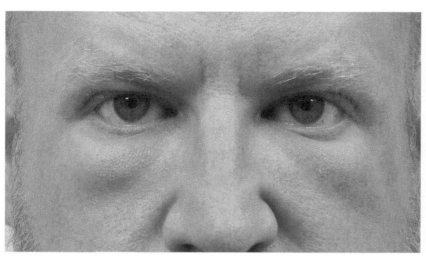

Fig. 36.1 Photograph of patient in case 1 demonstrating overvolumization of the lower eyelids.

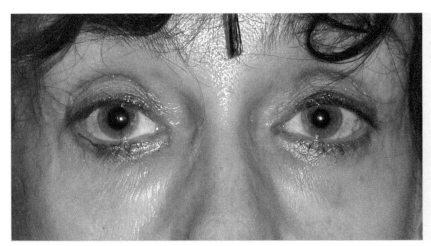

Fig. 36.2 Photograph of patient in case 2 showing bilateral lower eyelid swelling.

age 27 and no other surgeries. She had prior treatments of Botox to the glabella and lateral canthal region.

36.1.3 Case 3

A 57-year-old woman presented with a history of an unknown filler injection to the lower eyelids in Paris 3 years ago (▶Fig. 36.3). She reported that a physician attempted hyaluronidase to the lower eyelid 1 year ago without much effect.

36.2 Anatomic Description of the Patients' Current Status

Each patient experienced a suboptimal result from filler injectables for different reasons.

36.2.1 Case 1

This patient was injected multiple times and over time developed overvolumization of the lower eyelid. This may have become more obvious with time

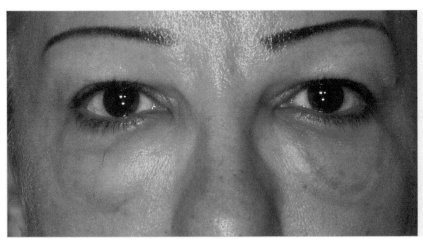

Fig. 36.3 Photograph of patient in case 3 showing prominent edema and nodules affecting bilateral lower eyelids.

as the orbicularis muscle became "stretched" and weakened from the mass effect of the filler.

There was no Tyndall's effect noted; therefore, the level of injection was likely suborbicularis and potentially retroseptal rather than subcutaneous.

36.2.2 Case 2

This patient received an irreversible filler to the lower eyelids, which resulted in palpable masses at the inferior orbital rims and festoon formation.

Injecting fillers in the lower eyelid and cheek (i.e., tear trough or nasojugal region) can be challenging. Complications often arise from poor placement, overinjection, and the tendency for swelling in this location. Retroseptal injection can result in a pronounced "bag" under the eye, while injection anterior to the infraorbital rim or anterior to the orbitomalar ligament often results in edema just inferior to the orbital rim, often referred to as festoons or malar bags. Injection of neuromodulator affecting the orbicularis in the area can exacerbate fluid collection.

Edema and festoons may result from filler injection due to the hydrophilic nature of the hyaluronic acid material. In addition to the ability of the material to imbibe water, we have also found profoundly decreased lymphatic drainage in one patient (case not presented) who had previously received Perlane and Restylane injections to the lower eyelids. This patient underwent lymphedema studies with Tc-99m injected into the central lower eyelid and lateral canthus. After 24 hours, there was virtually no lymphatic drainage noted on lymphoscintigraphy. Intralesional injection of hyaluronidase into reversible fillers may also correct edema as a result of removal of product, and result in improved lymphatic outflow as a result.

36.2.3 Case 3

This patient had a more complicated course. There was overinjection of an "unknown" filler material into the preseptal and premalar region of the lower eyelids and resultant edema and firm nodules. There was also significant lower eyelid laxity of both lower eyelids, which resulted in significant ectropion and lower eyelid retraction after removal of the filler.

36.3 Recommended Solution to the Problem

36.3.1 Case 1

- Hyaluronidase injection, about 200 IU to each lower eyelid (▶ Fig. 36.4).
- One week later, about 50 IU hyaluronidase injection was repeated to each lower eyelid.

36.3.2 Case 2

- Discuss direct excision of the palpable Radiesse nodules at the orbital rims via a transconjunctival approach.
- Lasix 40 mg plus KCl 20 mg taken daily as needed.
- Dexamethasone injection, given as 1-mL dexamethasone (4 mg/mL) distributed as three total injections to treat the entire body of the festoon to each eyelid.

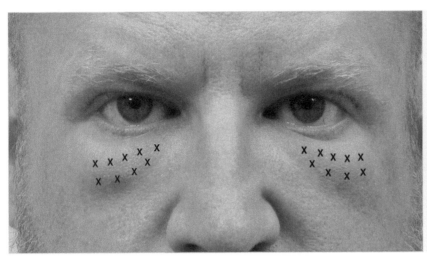

Fig. 36.4 Hyaluronidase injection technique in case 1. x = ~0.15 mL, Hylenex 22.5 IU.

36.3.3 Case 3

- Hyaluronidase 50 IU to bilateral lower eyelids.
- Surgical excision of filler material with intraoperative use of hyaluronidase.
- Ectropion repair.

36.4 Technique

36.4.1 Case 1

Hyaluronidase is the mainstay of treatment for overinjection and edema secondary to reversible fillers. When a reduction or contouring of a reversible filler is desired, we recommend starting with small doses of hyaluronidase (Hylenex 150 IU/mL). Starting with small doses can allow careful contouring without overcorrection or tissue atrophy. Treatment with hyaluronidase can be repeated weekly until the desired effect is achieved. This patient received small aliquots of hyaluronidase directly into the body of the lower eyelid in the location of the filler until the area was evenly treated (▶ Fig. 36.4).

He was seen 1 week later with much improvement. Additional injections were given and 1 week later he had excellent resolution of the lower eyelid fullness. He then elected to have treatment of his glabellar furrows with Dysport and improvement of volume loss of his cheeks with Radiesse. IPL was recommended for improved skin tone and texture.

Injecting fillers in the region of the lower eyelid and cheek junction (i.e., tear trough or nasojugal region) can be problematic. Complications often arise from poor placement, overinjection, and the tendency for swelling in this location. Retroseptal injection can result in a pronounced "bag" under the eye. Injection anterior to the infraorbital rim or anterior to the orbitomalar ligament can result in edema just inferior to the orbital rim, often referred to as a festoon or malar bag. Injections to the lower eyelid in the area should be performed using a conservative amount of filler placed deep to the orbicularis oculi and anterior to the orbital septum. In the area below the orbital rim, filler should be injected deep to the orbitomalar ligament and care should be taken as inadvertent retroseptal injection may occur for patients who have a lower lying orbital septum. Less biphasic material is preferred in this location.

For those without significant experience injecting irreversible fillers, reversible agents should be first line of treatment. Physicians should consider the anatomic deformity and the cause in order to provide an appropriate correction. For example, in an older patient with bone resorption, injection of a more robust filler to support the midface and cheek needs to be performed before periorbital treatment can be initiated. The structure should be first set with supraperiosteal injections below the orbital rim, if needed, followed by treatment of periorbital volume deficits using submuscular injection with a hyaluronic (HA) product with good spread (less cohesivity). Fillers can be customized for the patient by the addition of lidocaine to thin a high G prime filler in this delicate area. Finally, one can treat subcutaneously for fine lines and more superficial volume loss with a very fine filler in tiny aliquots with a technique of subcision and spread (▶ Fig. 36.5).

Of note, all the periocular injections discussed are off-label use of the various products discussed.

36.4.2 Case 2

Various options for treating eyelid edema exist but the treatment of festoons can be very challenging. In patients with suboptimal response to hyaluronidase injection with prior reversible filler or for patients with edema following irreversible filler injections, one can consider a trial of diuretics for temporary improvement. In this case, the patient deferred surgical excision and elected treatment with Lasix 40 mg plus KCl 20 mg taken daily as needed. She appreciated a 50% improvement when taking the diuretic. Later, she elected for dexamethasone injection, given as 1-mL dexamethasone (4 mg/mL) distributed as three total injections to treat the entire body of the festoon to each eyelid.

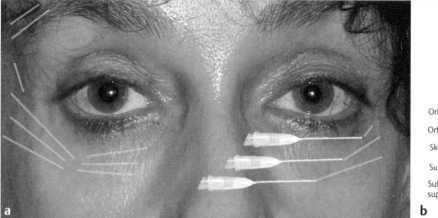
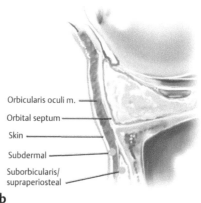

Orbicularis oculi m.
Orbital septum
Skin
Subdermal
Suborbicularis/
supraperiosteal

Fig. 36.5 (a) Left side of the image shows a linear threading technique for filler injection. The right side shows gentle injection of filler material upon withdrawal of the needle or cannula. (b) The preferred level of filler injection. Deeper injections for structural loss are performed in a supraperiosteal plane. Periorbital volumization can be addressed with submuscular injections. Lastly, fine lines may be addressed with subcutaneous injections with the use of alternating subcision and injection with very small aliquots. If a patient has festoons, care should be taken to avoid injection near that location.

For treatment of nodules from products such as Radiesse or Sculptra, a shift from treatment with steroid injections to 5-fluorouracil (5-FU) has gained support. Direct injection to break up nodules with saline or lidocaine plus sodium bicarbonate mixed with 5-FU avoids the adverse events of steroid injection, including depigmentation of the dermis and dermal thinning, and is the treatment of choice by many.

The appearance of festoons can be improved by lifting and supporting them with deep injections under the muscle with nonhydrophilic products (i.e., Radiesse, Sulptra, Voluma) and then treated directly if further treatment is required. Radiofrequency devices are increasingly being used for treatment in these cases as well as tetracycline injections to create an adhesion of skin to muscle in this potential space.

36.4.3 Case 3

Lumps and nodules usually occur as a result of too much filler being injected into a small area. Records could not be obtained to ascertain the type of filler material previously used in this; therefore, hyaluronidase 50 IU were injected to bilateral lower eyelids to assess response to possible hyaluronic acid–based material. In this case, there was no appreciable response to hyaluronidase. Next, pockets of filler were opened with a 22-gauge needle through which the gelatinous material was manually expressed. Residual nodules and granulomas were excised via a subciliary approach. A skin and muscle flap was created to the infraorbital rim and nodules deep and superficial to this plane were directly accessed and excised. Hyaluronidase was also injected as needed. Pathology revealed fibroadipose tissue with abundant interstitial exogenous material and noncaseating granulomas.

Later, a canthopexy was required for cicatricial ectropion on the right. Surgery on these patients can be challenging because the filler is often integrated within multiple tissue layers so the use of injections to mechanically break up the fillers and transdermal devices such as Ulthera or radiofrequency can be offered with varying results. The exception is a discrete nodule which can be easily identified and excised.

When the nature of lower eyelid swelling is uncertain, imaging may be utilized to rule out masses, inflammatory, or infectious etiologies, among others.

36.5 Postoperative Photographs and Critical Evaluation of Results

36.5.1 Case 1

Resolution of lower eyelid swelling following hyaluronidase injection (►Fig. 36.6).

36.5.2 Case 2

Improved lower eyelid masses over the inferior orbital rim and associated festoons/edema following dexamethasone injection (►Fig. 36.7).

36.5.3 Case 3

Improvement of lower eyelid edema, nodules, and granulomas. Residual ectropion of the right lower eyelid (►Fig. 36.8).

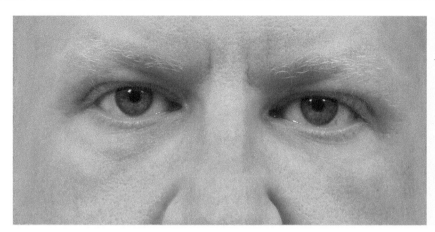

Fig. 36.6 Patient in case 1 shows resolution of lower eyelid swelling following hyaluronidase injection.

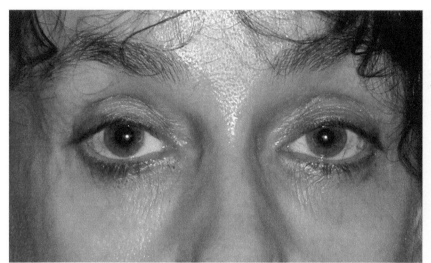

Fig. 36.7 Patient in case 2 with improved lower eyelid masses over the inferior orbital rim and associated festoons/edema following dexamethasone injection.

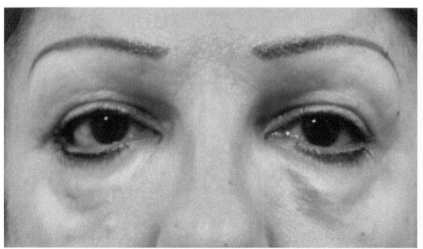

Fig. 36.8 Patient in case 3 with improvement of lower eyelid edema, nodules, and granulomas. Residual ectropion of the right lower eyelid.

36.6 Teaching Points

- While more serious complications, such as infection, vascular compromise, and even stroke, are rare (see Chapter 31 on vascular compromise related to fillers), other complications, including overinjection, lumpiness, granuloma formation, and edema, are more common and usually amenable to treatment. Key to prevention of these devastating complications is good knowledge of the anatomy, meticulous slow implantation of the material using a retrograde injection technique, the use of sterile technique, and treating conservatively in the periocular area. Adding 0.2 mL of lidocaine to an HA product, for example, and treating to full correction is one technique employed to allow for good spread and helps to prevent overcorrection. Highly cross-linked HA products (i.e., Juvederm) may be less preferable in this area because of their tendency to remain cohesive compared with less cross-linked products such as Restylane or Belotero. In the case of overinjection, the product can be treated through the same needle tract or with a new entry point with a larger bore needle if needed.

- Records may not always be available and the patients may not recall the type of injectable filler they have received. In the event that records cannot be obtained, hyaluronidase is a safe first step in treating lower eyelid edema, nodules, or overinjection. Always ask patients if they received fillers to the periorbital region even many years after implantation; often, patients assume that these fillers have already been resorbed by the body.

- Other causes of lower eyelid edema should always be ruled out afterward if clinically suspected (i.e., thyroid eye disease, allergy, orbital inflammation/masses, medication-induced edema, lymphoproliferative disease, etc.). I have seen countless patients who have been referred after extensive workup because they had not thought to disclose or had forgotten that they had received filler injections many years prior. Lastly, we commonly perform filler injections on patients who have had blepharoplasty surgery years before and in these patients the tissue planes may be altered and more care and smaller aliquots of filler are recommended over several treatment sessions for optimal correction. This is especially true when adding volume to the upper eyelid or superior sulcus.

- Of note, all periocular injections discussed are an off-label use of the various products.

Suggested Reading

[1] DeLorenzi C. Complications of injectable fillers, part I. Aesthet Surg J. 2013; 33(4):561–575

[2] Goldberg RA, Fiaschetti D. Filling the periorbital hollows with hyaluronic acid gel: initial experience with 244 injections. Ophthal Plast Reconstr Surg. 2006; 22(5):335–341, discussion 341–343

[3] Lowe NJ, Maxwell CA, Patnaik R. Adverse reactions to dermal fillers: review. Dermatol Surg. 2005; 31(11, Pt 2):1616–1625

[4] Sharad J. Dermal fillers for the treatment of tear trough deformity: a review of anatomy, treatment techniques, and their outcomes. J Cutan Aesthet Surg. 2012; 5(4):229–238

[5] Perry JD, Mehta VJ, Costin BR. Intralesional tetracycline injection for treatment of lower eyelid festoons: a preliminary report. Ophthal Plast Reconstr Surg. 2015; 31(1):50–52

37 Filler Problems

Hema Sundaram, Mark R. Magnusson, and Tim Papadopoulos

Summary

This chapter provides case-based discussions with photographic and video illustrations of nodular complications from injection of soft tissue fillers in the periorbital region, and the appropriate strategies to remediate them, based on integrative clinical and anatomical analysis. A case discussion of a complication with injectable botulinum toxin is also included because it provides insight into the sequelae of volume loss in the periorbital region. The authors emphasize a diagnostic, evidence-based approach to injectables complications.

Keywords: soft tissue augmentation, fillers, botulinum toxin, filler complications, toxin complications, injectables complications, hyaluronidase, biofilm, laser complications, periorbital

Key Points

- Most specialists who inject fillers will encounter patients with complications during the course of their careers, whether from their own treatments or in consultation following treatment by other injectors. In our opinion, it is the ability to diagnose and appropriately treat complications that distinguishes those who are appropriately qualified to inject fillers.
- A number of authors have expressed the concern that complications are more frequent when injectable procedures are performed by physicians and nonphysicians who lack the requisite understanding of facial anatomy and appropriate injection technique.
- There are different ways in which to classify injectables complications, including the following:
  - By onset and time course: acute versus subacute or chronic.
  - By nature of the complication, e.g., vascular versus infectious versus reactive.
  - By the type of filler, e.g., reversible versus irreversible.
- Some problems can occur after injection of either irreversible or reversible fillers. Some are specific to the type of filler. Some are exacerbated or more difficult to resolve when they occur with certain types of filler. Some are more common in certain regions of the face or body, due to the anatomical and functional characteristics of these regions.
- This chapter is classified according to the onset and time course of the complication. This is a useful classification because it allows an etiology-driven, patient-tailored parsing of the complication and its remedy. This classification also permits evidence-based analysis of the roles played by the type of filler and regional characteristics in development of the complication.
- Physicians who treat patients with filler complications may encounter significant challenges. These include poor patient compliance with recommendations and follow-up, and considerable patient anxiety and distress at sequelae of treatment for the complication, even when temporary, such as ecchymosis. In addition, patients may attribute blame to the physician treating the complication, for problems related to the original filler injection that cannot be fully resolved. These challenges are understandable in the light of the embarrassment, fear, and even anger that patients feel when they develop a problem from a filler injection procedure that they anticipated to be quick, uneventful, and with little or no recovery time. Establishment of good

physician–patient rapport and realistic patient expectations are essential prior to embarking on treatment of a filler complication.

- For the reader's general reference when reviewing the cases in this chapter, a series of anatomical drawings has been provided (▶Fig. 37.1; ▶Fig. 37.2; ▶Fig. 37.3; ▶Fig. 37.4; ▶Fig. 37.5)

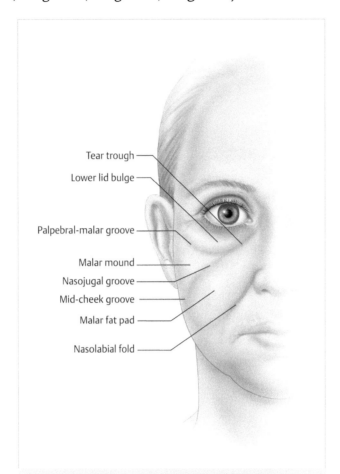

Tear trough
Lower lid bulge
Palpebral-malar groove
Malar mound
Nasojugal groove
Mid-cheek groove
Malar fat pad
Nasolabial fold

Fig. 37.1 Surface anatomy of the aging lower lid and midface. Facial aging is characterized by facial volume loss, loss of bony support, and soft tissue descent due to gravity. Collectively, these changes unveil the underlying bony and ligamentous anatomy, creating the typical grooves and expansions of the aged face. The tear trough deformity, palpebral-malar groove, nasojugal groove, midcheek groove, and nasolabial fold develop at the sites of relative fixation associated with underlying ligaments and fascial adhesions. In contrast, the lower lid bulge, malar bag, and malar fat pad form protuberances in the relatively mobile areas between these more stable, fixed points. For nonsurgical rejuvenation of the lower lid, it is important to note the tear trough deformity; this is the medial extension of the palpebral-malar groove at the lid–cheek junction, arising at the site of the tear trough ligament, which is the only direct bony attachment of the orbicularis oculi muscle.

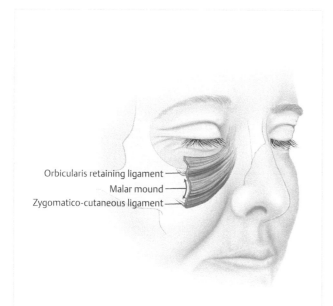

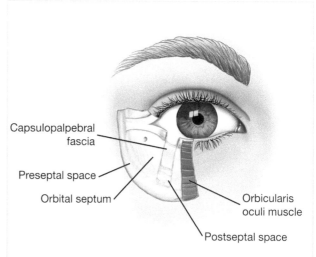

Fig. 37.2 Anatomical relationship of the orbicularis retaining ligament and zygomaticocutaneous ligament in the aging lower lid and midface. Age-related changes in the periorbital region may have different patterns. The positions of the fixed and immobile areas of the orbicularis retaining ligament and zygomatic cutaneous ligament remain stable and contribute to these age-related patterns. Soft tissue laxity, attenuation of the orbital septum, and changes to bony support can lead to soft tissue bulging and fat herniation. This may manifest as the lower lid bulge and malar mound, which are distinct from each other.

Fig. 37.3 Layered anatomical structures of the lower lid and lid–cheek junction. Note that there is no fat between the tarsal and preseptal parts of the orbicularis oculi muscle and the overlying skin. In the region of the preseptal space, there is a 5–8 mm vertical bony rim where inadvertent placement of filler may produce nodules, contour irregularities, or prolonged soft tissue swelling. Since these layered anatomical structures are in intimate apposition, placement of filler in an unintended location can occur quite easily unless there is a sound understanding of anatomy.

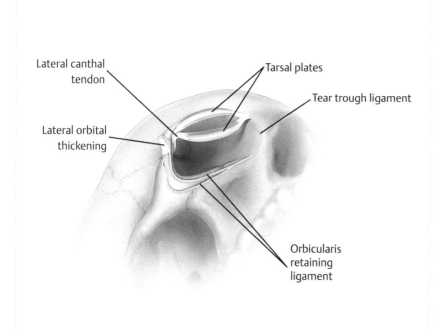

Fig. 37.4 Position of key attachments to the inferior bony orbit including the orbital retaining ligament. The term "tear trough deformity" should be applied to the medial periorbital hollow extending obliquely from the medial canthus to the mid-pupillary line. The tear trough deformity associated with aging has been attributed to gravitational descent, including laxity of the supporting ligaments and descent of the mid-face. The orbicularis retaining ligament creates a V-shaped deformity that correlates with the lid-cheek junction. The tear trough is often related to the underlying bony changes particularly associated with age-related maxillary hypoplasia. Lower eyelid skin progressively loses its elasticity and thickness with aging. Hyperpigmentation and actinic changes may also play a role.

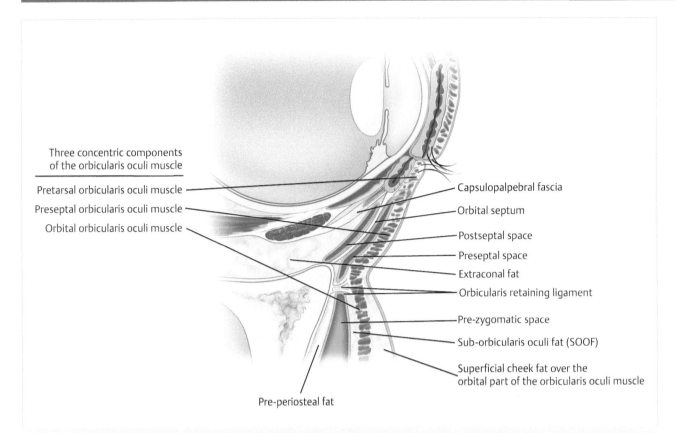

Three concentric components
of the orbicularis oculi muscle

Pretarsal orbicularis oculi muscle

Preseptal orbicularis oculi muscle

Orbital orbicularis oculi muscle

Capsulopalpebral fascia

Orbital septum

Postseptal space

Preseptal space

Extraconal fat

Orbicularis retaining ligament

Pre-zygomatic space

Sub-orbicularis oculi fat (SOOF)

Superficial cheek fat over the
orbital part of the orbicularis oculi muscle

Pre-periosteal fat

Fig. 37.5 Cross-sectional anatomy of the lower lid and midface, including the suborbicularis oculi fat (SOOF), the orbital septum with associated preseptal and postseptal spaces, and the orbicularis retaining ligament. The relationship of these structures and spaces in this compact area is illustrated in a sagittal plane. As noted in Fig. 37.3, there is no fat between the muscle of the tarsal and preseptal parts of the orbicularis oculi and the overlying skin. Beyond the orbicularis retaining ligament in the area known as the orbital part of orbicularis oculi, the normal subcutaneous fat layer separates skin and muscle. It is demonstrated that a combination of anatomical elements contributes to the tear trough deformity and palpebral-malar groove—the tear trough ligament medially and the orbicularis retaining ligament laterally, in combination with the cheek fat overlying the orbital part of orbicularis but not the preseptal part.

37.1 Case 1: Acute-Onset Periocular Swelling following Injection of Filler, Presumed to be Hyaluronic Acid

37.1.1 Patient History Leading to the Specific Problem

This 52-year-old Middle Eastern woman reported injection of cross-linked hyaluronic acid (HA) filler for correction of infraorbital hollows, with immediate onset of postprocedural swelling. She reported that the filler was injected overseas in a group setting, with several patients in one examination room and the physician moving quickly from injection of one patient to the next. One milliliter of filler was injected to each side. The onset of swelling was within 24 hours of injection. It worsened over the ensuing week. The treating physician advised the patient that the swelling would resolve spontaneously. At the time of consultation, the swelling had persisted for 3 months. The patient reported that it was often more pronounced in the mornings.

37.1.2 Anatomic Description of the Patient's Current Status

On visual inspection and palpation, the patient presented with bilateral, diffuse, soft, compressible infraorbital swelling. The swelling was more pronounced on the left than the right side. There were no symptoms or signs of inflammation, such as erythema, pain, tenderness, or warmth of the swollen regions. The patient had mild limitation of lower eyelid movement due to the swelling. She reported no paresthesia (▶ Fig. 37.6).

37.1.3 Diagnosis

Inappropriate placement of HA filler.

37.1.4 Recommended Solution to the Problem

- The acute-onset, persistence, and noninflammatory nature of the swelling were consistent with inappropriate placement of the filler and/or overfilling, causing lymphatic outflow obstruction. The increased swelling in the mornings was also consistent with lymphatic outflow

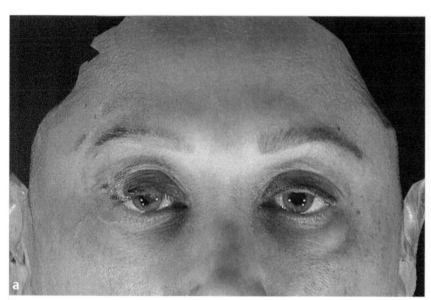
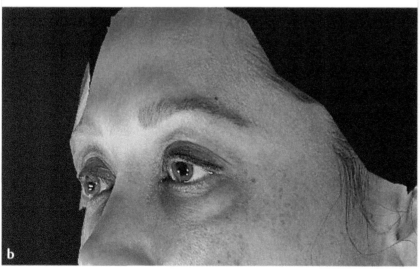

Fig. 37.6 Patient at first consultation, presenting with acute-onset, persistent, bilateral, noninflammatory swelling of the infraorbital regions. **(a)** Front view and **(b)** oblique view.

obstruction, since fluid will accumulate after several hours lying down.

- Diagnostic ultrasonographic imaging would be optimal prior to intervention, to determine the precise location of the filler and to provide evidence confirming it as HA. The patient declined this investigation.
- Hyaluronidase will enzymatically break down unwanted HA filler. It may also be considered for the tissue surrounding non-HA filler deposits, to aid in their dispersion (this is discussed further in case 3 below). The Lambros method entails dilution of the hyaluronidase with lidocaine to decrease discomfort during and after injection, plus epinephrine with the objective of localizing the hyaluronidase, to maximize its efficacy and limit its dispersion to areas where it is not indicated.
- After careful analysis of the risks versus the benefits of empiric treatment with hyaluronidase, this was performed as described in the following.

37.1.5 Technique

Ovine hyaluronidase (Vitrase, 200 USP Units/mL, Bausch & Lomb) was diluted 1:4 with 1% lidocaine (10 mg/mL) plus epinephrine (1:100,000) suspension. Using sterile technique, 0.6 mL of this diluted hyaluronidase was injected intralesionally and in the adjacent, surrounding subcutaneous tissue, via serial 0.1-mL boluses with a 32-G needle. Mild tissue pressure and molding were applied after injection, with the aim of dispersing the hyaluronidase throughout the areas of swelling.

37.1.6 Postoperative Photographs and Critical Evaluation of Results

At follow-up, 12 days after hyaluronidase injection, the infraorbital swelling was significantly improved. There was mild residual bilateral swelling. The patient was advised that further hyaluronidase injection could achieve further improvement. The patient was noncompliant with recommended follow-up 2 to 3 weeks later, stating that she wished to return for further treatment after overseas travel (▶ Fig. 37.7).

37.1.7 Teaching Points

- Acute-onset swelling or nodules may be defined as those that occur within 48 hours of filler implantation. If they are noninflammatory on the basis of history, visual inspection, and palpation, they may be a result of filler misplacement or overfilling. Postinjection displacement of filler may also occur, especially in highly mobile regions or when the filler has been implanted into muscle.
- The periocular region is vulnerable to swelling and nodules because of its anatomically unforgiving nature, its thin skin which makes underlying contour abnormalities more visible, and its propensity for lymphatic outflow obstruction.
- Different fillers have different propensities to absorb water. Highly hygroscopic HA fillers are not ideally suited to the periorbital area, and especially not to the region of the lower lid–cheek junction. Physiological hydration of an inappropriate product may exacerbate preexisting edema or create it.
- A common cause of acute swelling following periocular filler injection is inadvertent, misplaced implantation, resulting in lymphatic outflow

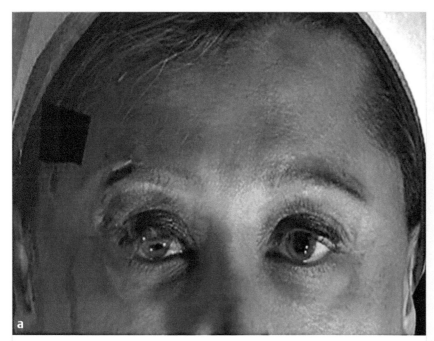
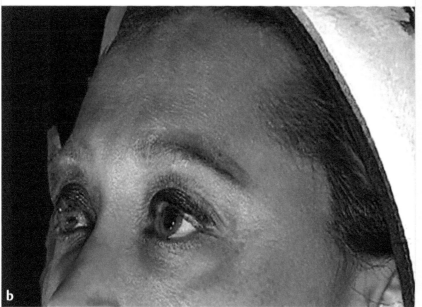

Fig. 37.7 Patient 12 days after the first session of hyaluronidase injection to the areas of acute-onset, persistent, noninflammatory infraorbital swelling. (a) Front view and (b) oblique view.

obstruction. The aging eyelid may have an increased susceptibility to this, due to deflation and descent of its supporting fat compartments. Anatomical study of the lower eyelid by Shoukath et al, and correlation with postoperative chemosis and edema, has provided insights into the principal points within the lymphatic system at which obstruction is likely to occur. The deep lymphatic system of the eyelid commences at the conjunctiva, pierces the tarsal plate, and descends deep to the orbicularis oculi. This connects through the muscle with a superficial lymphatic system. Lymphatic vessels then travel through the orbicularis retaining ligament, to run within the suborbicularis oculi fat (SOOF), in the roof of the prezygomatic space. At the zygomaticocutaneous ligament, the vessels descend to preperiosteal fat and then follow branches of the facial nerve to lymph nodes within the parotid gland. The superficial lymphatic system drains the eyelid skin, passing superficial to the orbicularis oculi muscle, with connections through the muscle to the deep system. Laterally, it reaches preauricular lymph nodes, while, medially, it parallels the path of the facial vein and drains into mandibular and submandibular lymph nodes. The key regions at which obstruction of the lateral deep lymphatic system is most likely are at the orbicularis retaining ligament and the zygomaticocutaneous ligament.

- Preexisting malar or lower lid edema may be considered a contraindication to infraorbital filler injection, since it confers an increased risk for prolonged, postprocedural swelling. The incidence of malar or lower lid edema is relatively high. In a series of 114 randomly selected patients, Goldberg et al found that 32% had some degree of it, and 13% had malar mounds (i.e., triangular areas of fullness inferior and lateral to the orbital rim [▶ Fig. 37.1]).

- HA fillers are strongly recommended for the periocular region, since their reversibility with hyaluronidase confers maximal safety and allows misplaced or excessive filler to be removed noninvasively.

- Slight undercorrection of the infraorbital region is recommended to avoid aesthetically undesirable convexity, with no more than 0.5 mL of filler implanted per side during each session. An interval of at least 3 to 4 weeks is recommended before further injections are performed.

- In general, as in all branches of medicine and surgery, filler problems are best diagnosed definitively and a treatment plan formulated based on this diagnosis. However, it is not uncommon for patients with filler problems to refuse diagnostic investigations. This is primarily due to a desire for prompt treatment with rapid resolution of the problem. It is the responsibility of the treating physician to determine what is in the patient's best interests, considering the risks versus the benefits of empiric treatment. In situations where the risks outweigh the benefits, patients should be counseled that diagnostic investigations must be undertaken prior to treatment, to assure safe and effective management.

- Since intracutaneous and subcutaneous injection of exogenous hyaluronidase has a favorable safety profile, its empiric use is justified when risk–benefit analysis indicates this to be appropriate. Besides the specific preparation of ovine hyaluronidase used for treatment of this patient, other hyaluronidase preparations are available on a geographic basis. Another preparation of ovine hyaluronidase (Hyalase, 1500 IU as a freeze dried powder 1 mL ampule, Sanofi-Aventis Australia Pty Ltd) can be diluted with saline to 50 IU per mL for treatment of aesthetic complications (compared with 150 IU per mL or greater for vascular indications). Recombinant human hyaluronidase (Hylenex, 150 USP units/mL, Halozyme Therapeutics, San Diego, CA) can be diluted in a similar manner to ovine hyaluronidase (Vitrase).

- Patients should be advised as part of the informed consent process for hyaluronidase that temporary bruising and swelling are expected after injection. Multiple sessions of hyaluronidase injection are often required, particularly with HA fillers of high longevity. An interval of at least 1 week is recommended between sessions. Infraorbital hollows are likely to reappear after hyaluronidase. Their correction will require injection of filler with appropriate technique.

- Patients should also be warned that the extent of improvement with hyaluronidase cannot be predicted and may be incomplete. In the anecdotal experience of one of the authors (H. S.), some patients who experience an episode of swelling after suboptimal periocular filler injection are prone to swelling after the filler is removed and even if filler is reimplanted subsequently with appropriate technique.

- Hyaluronidase has also been advocated as a rescue treatment in cases of inadvertent intra-arterial injection of HA filler and consequent filler embolization. In a real-time, fresh, frozen cadaver model, Magnusson and Papadopoulos demonstrated that HA filler implanted into facial arteries can be degraded transarterially by exogenous hyaluronidase injected into the surrounding soft tissue. DeLorenzi has described transarterial degradation of HA filler within closed cadaveric arterial segments immersed in hyaluronidase at therapeutic doses. Zhu et al prospectively evaluated the efficacy of retrobulbar hyaluronidase injection in four patients whose vision loss was due, respectively, to branch retinal artery occlusion, posterior ischemic optic neuropathy (PION), ophthalmic artery occlusion, and both branch retinal artery occlusion and PION. None of the patients achieved substantial retinal artery recanalization or improvement in visual acuity following one or two retrobulbar injections of high-dose (1,500 or 3,000 units) ovine testicular hyaluronidase (Shanghai First Biochemical Pharmaceutical Corporation) at least 4 hours after the onset of vision loss. In support of this finding, the authors recently reported failure of hyaluronidase to pass transarterially in a pilot, real-time, in vivo model, suggesting that permeability of the living arterial wall differs significantly from permeability in the cadaver.

37.2 Case 2: Subacute-Onset Periocular Nodules following Injection of Permanent Filler

37.2.1 Patient History Leading to the Specific Problem

This 48-year-old Caucasian man in good health received injections of a non–U.S. FDA approved permanent filler to his face over a period of 1 year in Canada, where this product was approved for aesthetic use. The filler was an HA–acrylic hydrogel. Fourteen months after the last injections, the patient developed multiple red nodules on his cheeks and under his eyes. Over the ensuing 6 years, he was treated empirically with multiple sessions of intralesional steroid injections to the nodules. The patient experienced what he described as "rebound inflammation" within 4 weeks of each intralesional steroid session. He was treated over the subsequent 2 years with oral corticosteroids, allopurinol, cyclosporine, and antibiotics; higher doses of intralesional steroids; and topical imiquimod. He experienced recurrent, worsening episodes of nodules, some of which occurred after dental cleanings. He developed renal insufficiency as a result of the cyclosporine.

37.2.2 Anatomic Description of the Patient's Current Status

At the time of his first consultation, the patient was taking oral cyclosporine 100 mg twice daily. His last intralesional steroid injections were over a year previously. He had bilateral, moderately erythematous nodules of the midface, lid–cheek junctions, and infraorbital regions, with no apparent exudate or discharge. Palpation indicated that the nodules were located subcutaneously. They were mildly tender and nonfluctuant. The patient was afebrile and had no palpable face or neck lymphadenopathy (▸ Fig. 37.8).

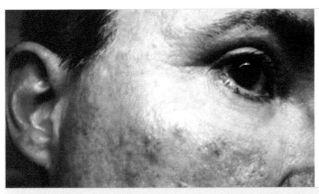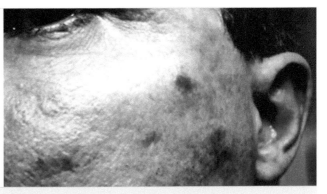

Fig. 37.8 Patient at first consultation, presenting with bilateral, multiple inflammatory subcutaneous nodules of the malar regions, lid–cheek junctions, and infraorbital regions. **(a)** Right side view and **(b)** left side view.

37.2.3 Diagnosis

Inflammatory nodules following injection of permanent filler.

37.2.4 Recommended Solution to the Problem

- These symptoms and signs are consistent with inflammatory nodules.
- Diagnostic ultrasonographic imaging would be helpful for further evaluation. The patient declined this investigation.
- The subacute onset and presentation of these inflammatory nodules is consistent with microbial contamination, most likely at the time of filler injection. Therefore, antibiotics are indicated. Immunosuppression with corticosteroids or cyclosporine is contraindicated, since this would exacerbate the infection.
- Antibiotic treatment to address microbial contamination of an implanted foreign body (filler material) should be more aggressive and for a longer duration than the short antibiotic courses that are typically prescribed for minor, self-limiting infections.
- A macrolide antibiotic, such as azithromycin or clarithromycin, is an appropriate choice. In addition to the broad-spectrum antimicrobial activity of macrolides, their polymodal immunomodulatory activity confers anti-inflammatory benefits without immunosuppression, as discussed by Kanoh and Rubin.

37.2.5 Technique

- Cyclosporine was discontinued.
- Oral clarithromycin at a dosage of 500 mg twice daily was started. The patient was advised to take adjunctive probiotic capsules.
- The patient was advised that continuous treatment for several months would be required, with follow-up appointments as appropriate to evaluate his status. He was also advised that removal of the permanent filler was desirable after the infection was controlled, to maximize the probability of complete and permanent resolution of the nodules.

37.2.6 Postoperative Photographs and Critical Evaluation

(▶ Fig. 37.9)

- At follow-up 5 weeks later, the nodules had decreased in number, size, elevation, and erythema. Induration was still present at the sites of the nodules.
- To date, the patient has continued oral clarithromycin for 6 months. He reports that the episodes of nodules have diminished in frequency and severity.
- To date, the patient has declined interventions to remove the filler.

37.2.7 Teaching Points

- The evidence for infection as a primary cause of filler nodules of sub-acute or late onset that persist or recur is compelling enough to justify empiric, broad-spectrum antibiotic therapy.
- In many case reports of nodules following filler injection, a presumptive diagnosis of granuloma or cutaneous hypersensitivity reaction to

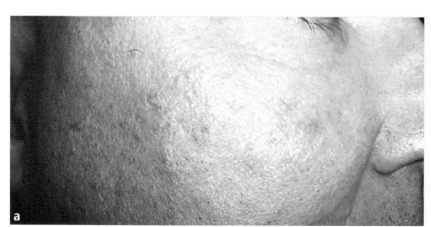
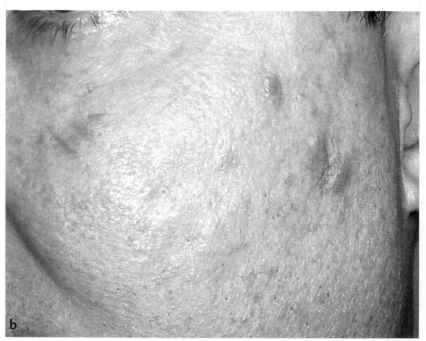

Fig. 37.9 Patient, 5 weeks after initiation of oral clarithromycin and discontinuation of oral cyclosporine. **(a)** Right side view and **(b)** left side view.

the filler has been made, based on signs and symptoms of inflammation. However, these signs and symptoms, including tenderness, erythema, swelling, and induration, also occur in the presence of infection.

- Infection itself can result in secondary granulomas or hypersensitivity.
- Since infection is the most likely cause of persistent nodules, until proven otherwise, corticosteroids and other immunosuppressive therapies should not be prescribed empirically. They are only appropriate after infection has been absolutely ruled out.
- The empiric use of treatments without a rationale, such as furosemide and other diuretics, should be avoided.
- A macrolide antibiotic is an appropriate empiric, first-line treatment due to its broad-spectrum antimicrobial and polymodal immunomodulatory activities.
- Addition of a fluoroquinolone antibiotic such as levofloxacin or moxifloxacin may also be considered. As discussed by Lewis, this genre of antibiotic readily equilibrates across biofilms and is therefore somewhat effective in impeding their growth.
- Lack of improvement after a few days of antibiotic treatment or negative cultures should raise the suspicion of resistant microbes, mycobacteria, or biofilm.
- Infection can occur with reversible or irreversible fillers. Removal of the contaminated filler is always the treatment of choice. When the filler is irreversible, removal is more difficult, and hence treatment is more challenging.
- Negative cultures from a filler nodule do not exclude the diagnosis of bacterial or fungal infection. Rimmer and colleagues have described the classic presentation of mycobacterial infection in breast implants as "sterile" nodules or abscesses. Rodriguez et al recently associated cutaneous inflammation at the site of HA filler implantation with *Mycobacterium chelonae* infection. Through fluorescence in situ hybridization, Bjarnsholt and colleagues demonstrated bacteria in seven of eight biopsy specimens taken from culture-negative nodules arising after implantation of polyacrylamide gel filler.
- A skin procedure or a procedure room can be clean but is never completely sterile. Several factors heighten the risk of bacterial contamination during a filler injection entailing the repeated piercing of nonsterile skin in a nonsterile environment. These include passage of the injection needle through a sebaceous gland containing bacteria; incidental bacteremia at the time of the procedure resulting from tooth brushing, dental flossing, sinusitis, and other everyday activities; and physiologic fluctuations in the skin's inherent immune surveillance.
- Furthermore, several pathogenic bacteria possess the ability to use HA as a nutrient source. These include *Staphylococcus* and *Streptococcus* species, which synthesize the enzymes that are necessary to break glycosidic bonds and grow well on HA-supplemented culture media. Costagliola et al and Lee et al have both reported that the in vitro growth of mycobacteria is enhanced by the presence of HA. The possibility of infection should always be considered when persistent or recurrent filler nodules occur with subacute or late onset. When any type of infection is suspected, this should obviate the use of systemic or intralesional immunosuppressants such as corticosteroids before a diagnosis has been made.

- It is important that the recent focus on biofilms does not prompt clinicians to label all cases of persistent filler nodules as biofilms. The hallmarks of a biofilm distinguish it clearly from other subacute or chronic infections. Biofilm reactions manifest little or no antibody response, are frequently culture-negative, are resistant to antibiotic treatment, and tend to present as low-grade rather than fulminant inflammation. To date, the strongest evidence for biofilm formation after soft tissue filler implantation has been with permanent fillers. Saththianathan et al recently published a combined laboratory study and clinical review, in which they discussed the role of bacterial biofilm in adverse reactions to soft tissue fillers. They found that all studied fillers (HA, polyacrylamide gel, and poly-L-lactic acid) supported the growth of bacterial biofilm in vitro, and suggested a high correlation between chronic granulomatous inflammation and biofilm in the clinical cases that they reviewed.

37.3 Case 3: Early-Onset Persistent Periocular Nodules following Injection of Unknown Filler

37.3.1 Patient History Leading to the Specific Problem

This 56-year-old woman presented with persistent right lower eyelid nodules, following injection of unknown fillers over 15 years prior to her consultation. She stated that the nodules had appeared soon after the filler injection, and that they had remained unchanged since then. The patient reported severe distress and social embarrassment from this problem. She had been told previously that it could not be improved without surgical excision, which she declined. During the consultation, she stated that she could not tolerate treatment that carried even a small risk of bruising, as it would worsen her distress and embarrassment. The patient declined ultrasonographic or other evaluation of the nodules.

37.3.2 Anatomic Description of the Patient's Current Status

At the time of first consultation, the patient had bilateral, firm, non-erythematous nodules of the infraorbital regions, with no exudate or discharge. The nodules were nontender and nonfluctuant, with no overlying warmth. Palpation indicated that the nodules were located subcutaneously, including supraperiosteally. The patient was afebrile and had no palpable face or neck lymphadenopathy (▶ Fig. 37.10).

37.3.3 Diagnosis

Noninflammatory nodules following injection of unknown filler.

37.3.4 Recommended Solution to the Problem

- The longevity of the nodules suggests that they were derived from a permanent or semi-permanent filler rather than HA.
- The absence of signs and symptoms of inflammation from the time of injection until the time of presentation suggests "cold nodules" without evidence of acute or subacute infection.

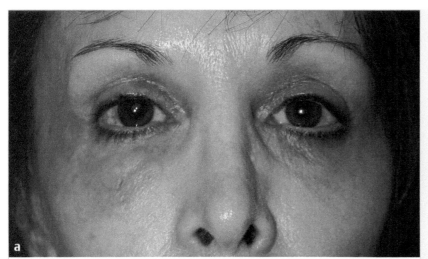

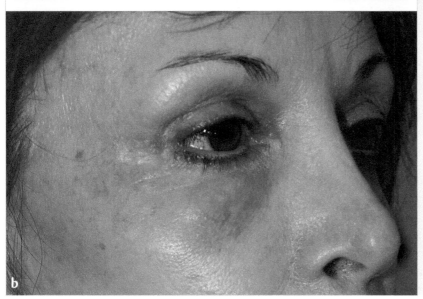

Fig. 37.10 Patient prior to treatment of early-onset, persistent, noninflammatory nodules of the infraorbital region. **(a)** Front view and **(b)** right oblique view.

- However, biofilm or another chronic infection cannot be conclusively ruled out on the basis of clinical evaluation alone. Therefore, it would be wise to initiate prophylactic antibiotic coverage prior to any attempted manipulation of the nodules.
- Voigts and colleagues have reported the dispersion and elimination of calcium hydroxylapatite filler nodules with a sharp needle, preceded by injection of lidocaine suspension to minimize patient discomfort.
- Injection of hyaluronidase has been advocated even when filler nodules are not composed of HA, to help break up surrounding tissue and improve access of the subcision instrument to the nodules.
- Since this patient stated that she could not tolerate any ecchymosis from attempts to remove the nodules, the decision was made to use a blunt-tipped microcannula.

37.3.5 Technique

- Oral clarithromycin, at a dosage of 500 mg twice daily with food, was commenced 1 week prior to the first session of treatment for the nodules. This was to minimize the risk of disseminating any bacterial infection or biofilm during manipulation of these long-standing nodules.
- A 27-G, 38-mm blunt-tipped microcannula was selected for treatment, with the objective of purposefully penetrating the nodules. In contrast, the treating author (H. S.) prefers a 22- or 23-G, 50-mm microcannula for filler injection itself, in order to minimize the risk of tissue trauma and penetration of vascular, neurological, or other vital structures.
- The microcannula was inserted via a single entry point on the right supramedial midface, and passed gently back and forth subcutaneously to subcise and gently break up the nodules. During this procedure, a total of 1 mL of ovine hyaluronidase, diluted 1:5 with lidocaine 1% plus epinephrine, was injected with retrograde threading technique.
- This technique had not been reported previously.
- The microcannula procedure was repeated 4 weeks later, with injection again of 1 mL of ovine hyaluronidase, diluted 1:5 with lidocaine 1% plus epinephrine.

37.3.6 Postoperative Photographs and Critical Evaluation of Results

(▶Fig. 37.11; ▶Fig. 37.12)

The patient reported no bruising after the first session of treatment, and started to see improvement after 1 week. On re-evaluation 4 weeks after the first treatment session, the nodules had decreased in diameter and elevation. The second session of treatment was performed at this time with further improvement apparent on re-evaluation 6 weeks later. No nodules were visible or palpable, and the right lower eyelid had no contour irregularities. The patient reported that she was very satisfied with the results.

37.3.7 Teaching Points

- This case history presents a novel treatment paradigm that may be of value for chronic nodules without signs or symptoms of inflammation following filler implantation.
- The nodules were dispersed by a blunt microcannula with simultaneous injection of hyaluronidase, under prophylactic macrolide antibiotic coverage.
- The aim of using the microcannula for subcision and break-up of the nodules was to provide nontraumatic, mechanical dispersal, and also to increase the surface area of contact between the nodule's constituents and the injected hyaluronidase.
- From an evidence-based perspective, the diagnosis and management of filler nodules are greatly facilitated by ultrasonographic imaging, performed and interpreted by an ultrasonographer with expertise in facial anatomy. This can reveal the presence of unreported, previously implanted materials that could form a nidus of infection; help to determine the nature of these materials; and indicate their precise location and whether they encroach on vital structures.

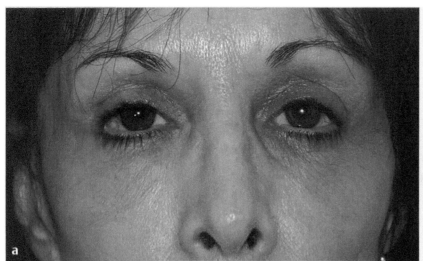

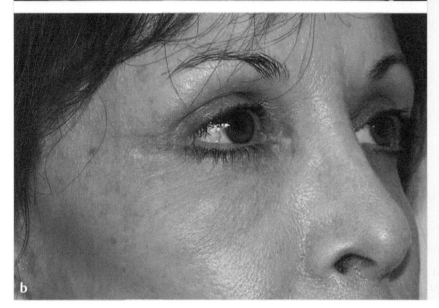

Fig. 37.11 Patient 4 weeks after first treatment session. **(a)** Front view and **(b)** left oblique view. Subcision and gentle break-up of nodules was performed with a 27-G, 38-mm blunt-tipped microcannula via a single entry point on supramedial midface, while injecting ovine hyaluronidase diluted 1:5 with lidocaine 1% plus epinephrine. Total injected volume was 1mL.

- Lesional biopsy has been recommended previously to aid in the diagnosis of nodules following filler implantation. The advantages of ultrasonographic imaging over lesional biopsy are that it is noninvasive and does not create scarring and that the risk of sampling error is significantly diminished or eliminated.

- It is important to appreciate that a histopathological diagnosis of granuloma does not rule out infection, and hence obviate the need for antibiotic therapy. Infection may exist concomitantly with granulomas. In addition, as noted in case 2, mycobacterial and other infections can lead to granuloma formation.

- The best course of action for this patient would have been to perform diagnostic ultrasonographic imaging prior to attempting any intervention to address the nodules. However, she declined this. In light of the complete absence of signs or symptoms of inflammation or infection for over 15 years, the decision was made in this particular patient to perform empiric treatment under prophylactic antibiotic coverage.

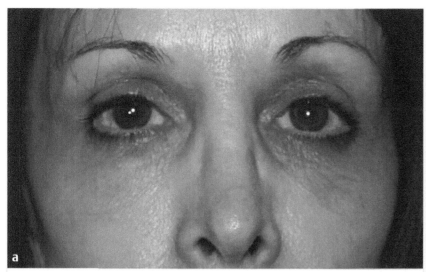

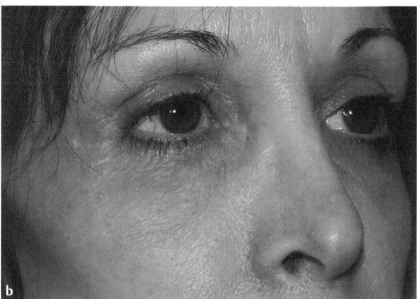

Fig. 37.12 The patient 10 weeks after first treatment session and 6 weeks after second treatment session. **(a)** Front view and **(b)** left oblique view. The same protocol of filler nodule subcision and dispersion with a microcannula was used. A total of 1 mL of ovine hyaluronidase diluted with 1% lidocaine plus epinephrine was injected via a 25-G, 38-mm blunt-tipped microcannula.

37.4 Case 4: Subacute Onset of Inflammatory Nodules following Same-Day Microdermabrasion and Filler Injection

37.4.1 Patient History Leading to the Specific Problem

This 52-year-old Caucasian woman reported onset of redness and swelling of her left lower eyelid and adjacent cheek, 7 days after receiving crystal-free microdermabrasion of her face including her lower eyelids, and injections of HA filler to her lower eyelids, during the same session. At the time of first consultation, the redness and swelling had persisted for 10 days without change. The patient reported no pain, malaise, or fever.

37.4.2 Anatomic Description of the Patient's Current Status

At the time of first consultation, the patient had soft, erythematous nodular swelling of the left infraorbital region, with satellite inflammation of the left malar region. There was mild overlying warmth of the inflamed regions, and no exudate or discharge. The swelling was nontender and nonfluctuant. Palpation indicated that the swelling was located subcutaneously, including supraperiosteally. The patient was afebrile and had no palpable face or neck lymphadenopathy (▶ Fig. 37.13).

37.4.3 Diagnosis

Inflammatory nodules following same-day microdermabrasion and injection of HA filler.

37.4.4 Recommended Solution to the Problem

- The subacute onset of persistent, inflammatory swelling (48 hours to 2 weeks after filler implantation) was consistent with microbial contamination of the filler.

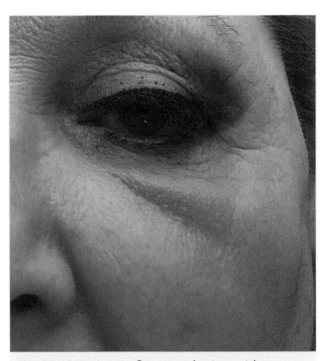

Fig. 37.13 Patient at first consultation, with subacute-onset inflammatory nodules of the left infraorbital and cheek region. Onset was 7 days after receiving same-day treatment with crystal-free microdermabrasion of the face including the lower eyelids, followed by injection of hyaluronic acid filler to the lower eyelids. Patient presented 10 days after onset, i.e., 17 days after microdermabrasion and filler injection.

- The recommended solution to the problem was to remove the HA filler enzymatically from the inflamed areas, by infiltration of hyaluronidase. The Lambros method for hyaluronidase was selected. As described above for case 1, this entails dilution of the hyaluronidase with lidocaine to decrease discomfort during and after injection, with the addition of epinephrine to localize the hyaluronidase, hence maximizing its efficacy and limiting its spread to areas where it is not indicated.
- Given the presumptive diagnosis of microbial contamination, prophylactic antibiotic coverage would be advisable prior to mechanical manipulation of the inflamed area while injecting hyaluronidase.
- A macrolide antibiotic, azithromycin, was selected for its broad-spectrum antimicrobial activity and also for its anti-inflammatory effects without immunosuppression, due to polymodal immunomodulatory activity.

37.4.5 Technique

- Oral azithromycin, at a dosage of 500 mg once daily with food, was commenced.
- One week later, the left lower eyelid and malar region were infiltrated with a total of 1.5-mL ovine hyaluronidase, diluted 1:5 with lidocaine 1% plus epinephrine (0.3-mL hyaluronidase plus 1.2-mL lidocaine 1% plus epinephrine). Injection was performed into the dermis and superficial subcutis with a 30-G needle and retrograde threading technique.

37.4.6 Postoperative Photographs and Critical Evaluation of Results

At follow-up, 2 weeks after hyaluronidase injection, the erythema and swelling had resolved completely. Reinjection of HA filler was performed 6 weeks later without sequelae.

37.4.7 Teaching Points

- The presumptive clinical diagnosis for this patient was secondary microbial contamination of the HA implant, most likely on the day of filler injection following microdermabrasion.
- In a recent consensus of plastic surgeons and dermatologists, Sundaram et al recommended that "any procedures that de-epithelialize the skin or cause tissue edema, such as laser resurfacing, should be avoided on the same day as filler or botulinum toxin procedures."
- Same-day microdermabrasion may have increased the risk of contamination of the HA implant, by causing subclinical trauma to the epidermis, and hence providing a portal of entry for microbes into the skin.
- The skin of the eyelids is especially susceptible to trauma, because it is thinner and more friable than the skin in nonperiocular regions of the face.
- As discussed above for case 2, no procedure that breaches the skin can ever be completely sterile. The skin itself is a repository of bacteria, and contamination can also occur from environmental microbes. Therefore, if inflammation occurs after filler implantation, the presumptive diagnosis should be infection until proven otherwise.
- As in all cases of infection due to a contaminated implant, the first line of treatment is to remove the implant. This is relatively easy with an HA

filler, since it can be enzymatically targeted with hyaluronidase. Patients should be advised that more than one session of hyaluronidase treatment may be required to completely remove the filler.

• Prophylactic antibiotic coverage helps to reduce the risk of spreading infection during infiltration of contaminated areas with hyaluronidase.

37.5 Case 5: Decompensation of Partially Compensated Upper Eyelid Ptosis following Injection of Botulinum Toxin

37.5.1 Patient History Leading to the Specific Problem

A 62-year-old woman complained that her right eyebrow had dropped following facial surgery and injectable procedures in Asia, including botulinum toxin injection to the forehead for improvement of wrinkles. She requested elevation of her right eyebrow to match the height of the left.

37.5.2 Anatomic Description of the Patient's Current Status

At the time of first consultation, the patient had asymmetry of the position of her eyebrows, with the peak of her left eyebrow approximately 1 cm above the peak of her right eyebrow. She had mild bilateral upper eyelid ptosis, which was more pronounced on the right side. She had transverse horizontal rhytids of moderate severity on the left side of her forehead. Rhytids were barely visible on the right side of her forehead. The patient's brow depressor activity was intact, as evinced by her ability to frown (▶ Fig. 37.14).

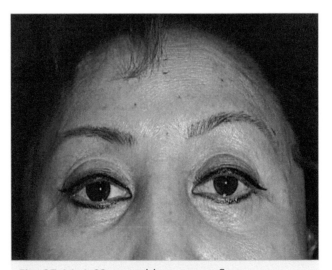

Fig. 37.14 A 62-year-old woman at first consultation. She complained of dropped eyebrow on the right side, following facial surgery and injectable procedures in Asia, including botulinum toxin. Patient requested re-elevation of the right eyebrow. She declined treatment strategies to lower the left eyebrow to the same height as the right.

37.5.3 Diagnosis

Eyebrow and eyelid ptosis following injection of botulinum toxin.

37.5.4 Recommended Solution to the Problem

- This patient's history and presentation were consistent with preexisting bilateral upper eyelid ptosis, with partial compensation through over-contraction of the frontalis muscle. This had become decompensated on the right side by her prior procedures—most likely the botulinum toxin injection and consequent weakening of frontalis muscle activity. The result was to lower the right eyebrow and to unmask preexisting right eyelid ptosis.
- The patient had loss of bone and soft tissues from her forehead and temples. Volume replacement would improve tissue support, hence restoring a more aesthetically appropriate eyebrow position bilaterally and improving eyebrow projection.
- Improved tissue support could also have reduced the need for frontalis to compensate by overcontracting, thereby ameliorating the forehead rhytids.
- Based on this understanding, botulinum toxin would be avoided, as it would weaken frontalis contraction and unmask eyelid ptosis. Injection of filler would be considered the preferred treatment.
- Although the right eyebrow was at a more natural-looking height from an aesthetic perspective, the patient declined lowering of the left eyebrow to match the height of the right. Since activity of the brow depressor muscles was intact, injection of botulinum toxin to weaken them would elevate the right eyebrow, as the patient requested, by allowing relatively unopposed activity of the frontalis muscle.
- Despite the aesthetic shortcomings of elevating the right eyebrow with botulinum toxin, this could be justified from a functional perspective if it ameliorated the right upper eyelid ptosis, which had become more pronounced than on the left following postprocedural decompensation.

37.5.5 Technique

- Botulinum toxin type A was injected to the medial and lateral brow depressors. The dosage was 4 units of onabotulinum toxin A to the procerus muscle, and 1 unit to the superolateral aspect of the right orbicularis oculi muscle.
- At follow-up, 3 weeks later, the patient agreed to injection of 1-mL HA filler supraperiosteally to the inferior aspects of both eyebrows. She continued to decline filler to the forehead and temples.

37.5.6 Postoperative Photographs and Critical Evaluation of Results

- At follow-up, 3 weeks after botulinum toxin treatment, the right eyebrow was elevated almost to the same height as the left eyebrow. Upper eyelid ptosis was diminished on the right side, and there was also some improvement on the left side.
- The small volume of filler that was injected subsequent to the botulinum toxin resulted in elevation of the right eyebrow to the same height as the left. This was the same pattern and degree of bilateral eyebrow elevation

that the patient reported prior to her procedures in Asia. The position of both eyebrows and the appearance of the frontalis muscle were consistent with bilateral partial compensation for eyelid ptosis. Upper eyelid ptosis was diminished on both the right and left sides.

- Although this treatment plan fulfilled the patient's request, it did not restore optimal brow position and projection, as could have been achieved by injection of a sufficient volume of filler to the forehead and temples (▶ Fig. 37.15)

37.5.7 Teaching Points

- The frontalis and levator palpebrae muscles are integrally linked in a periorbital gestalt that maintains vision in response to dermatochalasis, lid ptosis, or brow ptosis. The patterns of muscular activity are frequently asymmetric to provide preferential support to the neurologically dominant eye. The presenting complication was caused by inappropriate injection of botulinum toxin to the frontalis muscle, in an attempt to improve rhytids on the forehead.
- This commonly encountered situation can be avoided by pretreatment analysis that considers the anatomy of facial muscles and their three-dimensional, mechanical relationships—including the specific understanding that frontalis is the sole elevator of the eyebrows.
- For the patient under discussion, this analysis would yield the understanding that the forehead rhytids were due to physiologically appropriate contraction of frontalis, to compensate for upper eyelid ptosis. The optimal treatment, from an analytical perspective, would be to correct the primary cause of frontalis overcontraction.
- This case history illustrates a common situation when consulting with patients who desire cosmetic procedures—a discrepancy between what the patient requests and what is medically appropriate. After an extensive discussion with this patient, it was elected to follow her request, because the outcome she desired did not pose any medical dangers, even though it was aesthetically inappropriate.

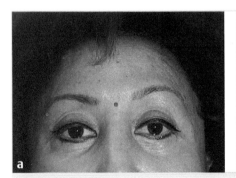 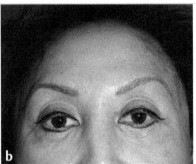 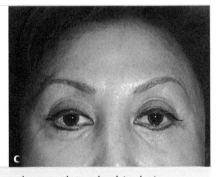

Fig. 37.15 **(a)** Points of injection of botulinum toxin type A to the procerus and superolateral orbicularis oculi muscles. Four units of onabotulinum toxin A were injected to the procerus, and 1 unit was injected to the superolateral aspect of the right orbicularis oculi. **(b)** The patient before and 3 weeks after injection of botulinum toxin type A to the procerus and superolateral orbicularis oculi muscles. Elevation of the right eyebrow is seen. This is due to weakening of the injected brow depressors, allowing less opposition of brow elevator activity by the frontalis muscle. Slight improvement of eyelid ptosis is also seen. **(c)** 3 weeks after injection of hyaluronic acid filler supraperiosteally to the lateral tail of the eyebrows. The patient declined injection of filler to the forehead and temples.

- The levator muscles of each eyelid obey Hering's law of equal innervation, in that they are innervated symmetrically, resulting in equal central neural output. Therefore, in cases of bilateral asymmetric ptosis, the less affected eyelid may maintain a normal level of elevation due to excessive innervational stimulation determined by the more ptotic eyelid. This condition can be detected prior to procedures by manual elevation of the more ptotic eyelid. An immediate fall of the contralateral eyelid confirms the presence of bilateral, asymmetrical ptosis, masked by levator "overaction."

Suggested Reading

[1] Arron ST, Neuhaus IM. Persistent delayed-type hypersensitivity reaction to injectable non-animal-stabilized hyaluronic acid. J Cosmet Dermatol. 2007; 6(3):167–171

[2] Bjarnsholt T, Tolker-Nielsen T, Givskov M, Janssen M, Christensen LH. Detection of bacteria by fluorescence in situ hybridization in culture-negative soft tissue filler lesions. Dermatol Surg. 2009; 35(Suppl 2):1620–1624

[3] Christensen L. Normal and pathologic tissue reactions to soft tissue gel fillers. Dermatol Surg. 2007; 33(Suppl 2):S168–S175

[4] Cassuto D, Pignatti M, Pacchioni L, Boscaini G, Spaggiari A, De Santis G. Management of complications caused by permanent fillers in the face: a treatment algorithm. Plast Reconstr Surg. 2016; 138(2):215e–227e

[5] Cassuto D, Sundaram H. A problem-oriented approach to nodular complications from hyaluronic acid and calcium hydroxylapatite fillers: classification and recommendations for treatment. Plast Reconstr Surg. 2013; 132(4, Suppl 2):48S–58S

[6] Chabra I, Obagi S. Severe site reaction after injection hyaluronic acid-based soft tissue filler. Cosmet Dermatol. 2011; 24:14–21

[7] Costagliola C, Del Prete A, Winkler NR, et al. The ability of bacteria to use Na-hyaluronate as a nutrient. Acta Ophthalmol Scand. 1996; 74(6):566–568

[8] DeLorenzi C. Complications of injectable fillers, part I. Aesthet Surg J. 2013; 33(4):561–575

[9] DeLorenzi C. Complications of injectable fillers, part 2: vascular complications. Aesthet Surg J. 2014; 34(4):584–600

[10] DeLorenzi C. Transarterial degradation of hyaluronic acid filler by hyaluronidase. Dermatol Surg. 2014; 40(8):832–841

[11] Friedman PM, Mafong EA, Kauvar AN, Geronemus RG. Safety data of injectable nonanimal stabilized hyaluronic acid gel for soft tissue augmentation. Dermatol Surg. 2002; 28(6):491–494

[12] Glashofer MD, Cohen JL. Complications from soft tissue augmentation to the face: a guide to understanding, avoiding, and managing periprocedural issues. In: Jones DJ, ed. Injectable Fillers: Principles and Practice. Oxford: Wiley-Blackwell; 2010:121–139

[13] Glashofer MD, Flynn TC. Complications of temporary fillers. In: Carruthers J, Carruthers A, Dover JS, Alam M, eds. Procedures in Cosmetic Dermatology: Soft Tissue Augmentation. 3rd ed. London: Elsevier Saunders; 2013:179–187

[14] Goldberg RA, McCann JD, Fiaschetti D, Ben Simon GJ. What causes eyelid bags? Analysis of 114 consecutive patients. Plast Reconstr Surg. 2005; 115(5):1395–1402, discussion 1403–1404

[15] Hering E. The Theory of Binocular Vision. New York, NY: Plenum Press; 1977

[16] Kanoh S, Rubin BK. Mechanisms of action and clinical application of macrolides as immunomodulatory medications. Clin Microbiol Rev. 2010; 23(3):590–615

[17] Criollo-Lamilla G, DeLorenzi C, Karpova E, et al. Anatomy and Filler Complications. Paris: Medical Publishing; 2017

[18] Lambros V. The use of hyaluronidase to reverse the effects of hyaluronic acid filler. Plast Reconstr Surg. 2004; 114(1):277

[19] Lee YN, Kim JD, Lew J. Comparison of mycobacterial growth in Dubos medium, hyaluronate supplemented medium and umbilical cord extract based medium. Yonsei Med J. 1977; 18(2):130–135

[20] Lewis K. Riddle of biofilm resistance. Antimicrob Agents Chemother. 2001; 45(4):999–1007

[21] Lupton JR, Alster TS. Cutaneous hypersensitivity reaction to injectable hyaluronic acid gel. Dermatol Surg. 2000; 26(2):135–137

[22] Rimmer J, Hamilton S, Gault D. Recurrent mycobacterial breast abscesses complicating reconstruction. Br J Plast Surg. 2004; 57(7):676–678

[23] Rodriguez JM, Xie YL, Winthrop KL, et al. Mycobacterium chelonae facial infections following injection of dermal filler. Aesthet Surg J. 2013; 33(2):265–269

[24] Saththianathan M, Johani K, Taylor A, et al. The role of bacterial biofilm in adverse soft-tissue filler reactions: a combined laboratory and clinical study. Plast Reconstr Surg. 2017; 139(3):613–621

[25] Sclafani AP, Fagien S. Treatment of injectable soft tissue filler complications. Dermatol Surg. 2009; 35(Suppl 2):1672–1680

[26] Shoukath S, Taylor GI, Mendelson BC, et al. The lymphatic anatomy of the lower eyelid and conjunctiva and correlation with postoperative chemosis and edema. Plast Reconstr Surg. 2017; 139(3):628e–637e

[27] Signorini M, Liew S, Sundaram H, et al; Global Aesthetics Consensus Group. Global aesthetics consensus: avoidance and management of complications from hyaluronic acid fillers-evidence- and opinion-based review and consensus recommendations. Plast Reconstr Surg. 2016; 137(6):961e–971e

[28] Sundaram H, Kiripolsky M. Nonsurgical rejuvenation of the upper eyelid and brow. Clin Plast Surg. 2013; 40(1):55–76

[29] Sundaram H, Liew S, Signorini M, et al; Global Aesthetics Consensus Group. Global Aesthetics Consensus: hyaluronic acid fillers and botulinum toxin type A-recommendations for combined treatment and optimizing outcomes in diverse patient populations. Plast Reconstr Surg. 2016; 137(5):1410–1423

[30] Van Dyke S, Hays GP, Caglia AE, Caglia M. Severe acute local reactions to a hyaluronic acid-derived dermal filler. J Clin Aesthet Dermatol. 2010; 3(5):32–35

[31] Voigts R, DeVore P, Grazer J. Dispersion of calcium hydroxylapatite accumulations in the skin: animal studies and clinical practices. Dermatol Surg. 2010; 36:798–803

[32] Zhu GZ, Sun ZS, Liao WX, et al. Efficacy of retrobulbar hyaluronidase injection for vision loss resulting from hyaluronic acid filler embolization. Aesthet Surg J. 2017; 38(1):12–22

38 Filler Problems: Vascular Complications

Joseph A. Eviatar, Carisa K. Petris, and Richard D. Lisman

Summary

Vascular occlusion is the most feared complication of filler injection. This chapter provides two case presentations, their management, and outcomes. A treatment algorithm based on time since vascular occlusion is presented.

Keywords: filler, vascular occlusion, blindness, necrosis, hyaluronidase, hyperbaric oxygen therapy, central retinal artery occlusion

38.1 Patient History Leading to the Specific Filler Problem

38.1.1 Case 1

A 39-year-old man presented for a second opinion following Sculptra injection to the face for HIV lipoatrophy approximately 2 weeks prior. The patient was treated with oral antibiotics, ice, massage, and topical Mederma prior to his presentation. Despite these measures, the patient reported the "blood spot" under his eye was not improving. He had a history of HIV for 10 years with a CD4 count of 220 and viral load of 0. He had no previous injections (▶ Fig. 38.1).

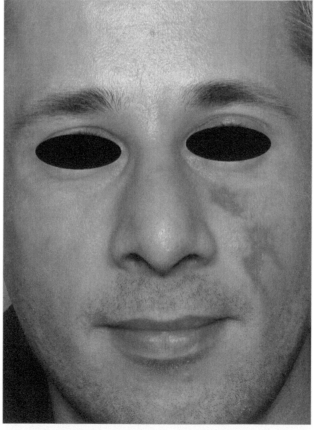

Fig. 38.1 Photograph of patient in case 1 demonstrating atrophy and erythema of the dermis of the left cheek in a reticulated pattern.

38.1.2 Case 2

A 48-year-old woman presented with redness of her glabella, nasal dorsum, and right nasal sidewall and right nasolabial region after Juvederm injections 2 days previously. She was reported having transgingival block prior to injections and began to notice immediate facial swelling. Juvederm was injected over the area of swelling. She returned to the doctor the following day due to pain and facial swelling and was given hyaluronidase and nitropaste. She was otherwise healthy without history of scarring or previous injections (▶ Fig. 38.2).

38.2 Anatomic Description of the Patient's Current Status

Both patients presented with one of the most feared complication of injectable fillers: vascular occlusion. **Case 1** presented in the late remodeling phase after vascular occlusion affecting the dermis of the left cheek, and **case 2** presented 2 days following vascular compromise of the branches of the facial artery and angular artery (i.e., superior labial artery, inferior alar artery, lateral nasal

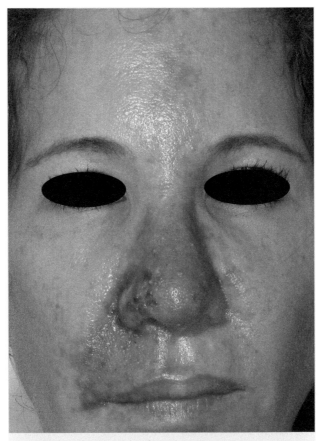

Fig. 38.2 Photograph of patient in case 2 demonstrating dusky, blue-red discoloration with blister formation involving the glabella, right nasal sidewall, nasal dorsum, right nasal ala, right superior labial region, and right nasolabial region.

artery, and dorsal nasal artery), involving the right nasolabial region, right superior labial region, right nasal ala, right nasal sidewall and dorsum, and the glabella region. There was a classic dusky, blue-red discoloration with blister formation, hyperemia, and necrosis.

Injectable fillers are increasing in popularity for use in facial volume augmentation and treatment of rhytides. The mechanism of tissue ischemia is likely a result of direct occlusion of small arteries and arterioles with the injectable particle rather than external pressure on the arterial supply. Intravenous injection is unlikely to cause significant side effects. Depending on the particle size of the particular filler, intra-arterial injection may occlude small arteries or arterioles. In cases 1 and 2, arterial occlusion likely occurred at the level of small arteries and arterioles supplied by the facial artery. The particle size of poly-L-lactic acid (PLLA; Sculptra, Valeant Aesthetics, Bridgewater, NJ) Sculptra (PLLA) is 40 to 63 μm. Small superficial arteries of the face may be around 1 mm, while arterioles are 17 to 22 μm.

The quantity and extrusion are more likely to account for vascular occlusion. Injection of 0.1 mL or less to any single area may minimize the risk of vascular occlusion. Dilution or reconstitution of the filler material in saline or lidocaine may help decrease the total filler delivered to any given location.

It is our practice to only inject filler slowly as the needle is being withdrawn to minimize the risk of intra-arterial injection. Additionally, the use of larger gauge needles or cannulas can lessen the risk of cannulating a facial artery during deep injections.

Blindness is also a known risk of intra-arterial filler injection. This is believed to be related to the pressure of the injection causing the injected filler to pass via bridging collateral arteries from the external carotid circulation to the internal carotid circulation (e.g., to the ophthalmic artery) before returning to normal anterograde flow. Therefore, gentle force should always be used when injecting fillers to minimize this risk.

38.3 Recommended Solution to the Problem

38.3.1 Case 1

- Topical hydrocortisone cream to the affected area.

38.3.2 Case 2

- Prompt infiltration of the affected area with hyaluronidase (150 IU).
- Nitropaste applied over the affected areas.
- Warm compresses.
- Doxycycline 100 mg twice daily.
- Initiation of hyperbaric oxygen therapy (HBOT) to promote healing in the ischemic areas.
- Medrol dose pack.
- Vicodin as needed for pain.
- After the area of necrosis was healed, she was treated with
  - Hydroquinone 2.5% cream twice daily to massage to the area for 3 weeks for hyperpigmentation.
  - Aquaphor as needed as a moisturizer.
- Later intense pulsed light (IPL) for residual redness.

38.4 Technique

38.4.1 Case 1

The patient was treated with topical steroid only. However, if deep dermal scarring were to occur, the use of Kenalog and/or 5-FU injections may be considered. We now prefer 5-FU (50 mg/mL) combined with saline or 2% lidocaine + sodium bicarbonate injection into the scar. If necessary, the scar is first treated with subcision with a needle and then infiltrated with a small amount of 5-FU solution. This can be repeated every 2 weeks, up to four injections as needed until the desired effect is achieved.

38.4.2 Case 2

When arterial occlusion is not transient, we recommend first infiltrating the areas affected by ischemia with hyaluronidase (150 IU/mL) for reversible fillers. More hyaluronidase will be needed for monophasic (i.e., Juvederm) than biphasic fillers (i.e., Restylane, Perlane). Biphasic fillers will have greater spread within the tissues and a greater surface area on which the hyaluronidase may act. This may be subcutaneous or supraperiosteal injection followed by massage. This can be effective even if the artery is not cannulated since diffusion of the hyaluronidase can occur through an intact vessel wall, leading to the resolution of the intra-arterial particles. In addition to massage start aspirin 81mg orally daily. We also recommend doxycycline for the antibacterial and matrix metalloproteinase inhibition effects on wound healing effects. Given her significant area and depth of necrosis, she received 3 cycles of HBOT.

The role of nitropaste has recently come into question, after a recent article by Hwang et al. This article has shown that vasodilation could propagate intra-arterial particles and potentially decrease the potential of collateral circulation worsening end point ischemia. We, therefore, do not advocate the use of nitropaste in the early postocclusion state (within minutes of the occlusion).

The use of prostaglandin E1, to promote vasodilation, has been reported to be effective in the treatment of acute retinal artery occlusion; however, the authors do not have experience with such complications or the use of this medication.

Ophthalmic artery or central retinal artery occlusion from a reversible filler may benefit from retrobulbar injection of hyaluronidase. Another consideration could be high-dose intravascular injection, as for myocardial infarction. The additional consideration of hyaluronidase for reversible filler products may be used in conjunction with standard treatment of a central retinal artery occlusion, including ocular massage, anterior chamber paracentesis, intraocular pressure reduction, and possible hyperventilation. HBOT can also be considered.

The algorithm given in ▶ Fig. 38.3 may be used as a guide for treatment depending on timing post–vascular occlusion.

38.5 Postoperative Photographs and Critical Evaluation of Results

38.5.1 Case 1

There was minimal scarring in the area of vascular occlusion. The patient was happy with his final outcome and elected to continue Sculptra approximately 6 months after he was completely healed (▶ Fig. 38.4).

If vascular compromise is recognized within minutes of vascular compromise from filler injection
o Immediate infiltration of the affected tissue with hyaluronidase (150 IU/ml) using multiple vials if needed. o Massage the area after hyaluronidase injection o Oral aspirin 81 mg o If reperfusion is achieved follow closely
If vascular re-perfusion is not achieved with the above measures in the first hour(s)
o Consider intra-arterial injection of hyaluronidase or additional hyaluronidase injection o Consider use of nitropaste or phosphodiesterase inhibitor o Consider starting HBOT o Start doxycycline 100 mg twice a day by mouth o Start aspirin 81 mg daily o Follow closely
If a patient presents days to weeks after vascular occlusion without optimal-perfusion
o Give additional hyaluronidase injections as needed o Aspirin o Nitropaste o Doxycycline 100 mg twice a day

Fig. 38.3 Treatment algorithm following filler associated vascular occlusion

38.5.2 Case 2

The patient healed very well with minimal scarring. She had IPL for treatment of residual erythema. She later elected to have Sculptra and Botox to elevate the brows. Focused ultrasound (Ultherapy) was also recommended for further brow elevation (▶ Fig. 38.5).

38.6 Teaching Points

- Early recognition and prompt treatment of vascular occlusion is imperative.
- The algorithm may be very helpful to guide treatment of vascular occlusion for filler depending on presentation and timing (▶ Fig. 38.3).

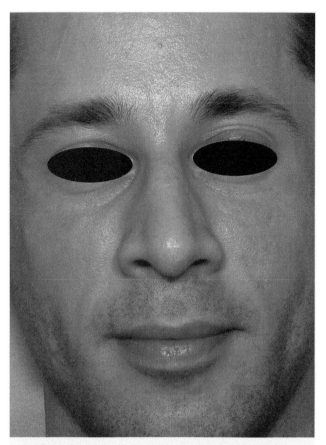

Fig. 38.4 Patient in case 1 showing mild atrophic scar in the area of the previous vascular occlusion of the left cheek.

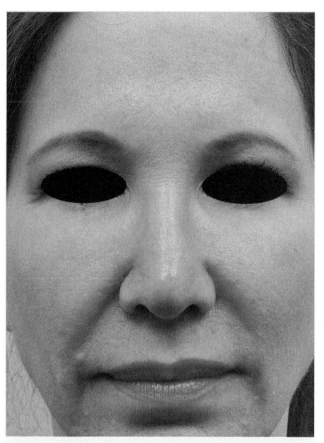

Fig. 38.5 Patient in case 2 showing minimal scarring in the right nasolabial region 5 months after vascular occlusion. Patient underwent IPL for residual redness which has also improved.

Suggested Reading

[1] DeLorenzi C. Complications of injectable fillers, part I. Aesthet Surg J. 2013; 33(4):561–575

[2] DeLorenzi C. Complications of injectable fillers, part 2: vascular complications. Aesthet Surg J. 2014; 34(4):584–600

[3] Hwang CJ, Morgan PV, Pimentel A, Sayre JW, Goldberg RA, Duckwiler G. Rethinking the role of nitroglycerin ointment in ischemic vascular filler complications: an animal model with ICG imaging. Ophthal Plast Reconstr Surg. 2016; 32(2):118–122

[4] Carruthers JD, Fagien S, Rohrich RJ, Weinkle S, Carruthers A. Blindness caused by cosmetic filler injection: a review of cause and therapy. Plast Reconstr Surg. 2014; 134(6):1197–1201

[5] Takai Y, Tanito M, Matsuoka Y, Hara K, Ohira A. Systemic prostaglandin E1 to treat acute central retinal artery occlusion. Invest Ophthalmol Vis Sci. 2013; 54(4):3065–3071

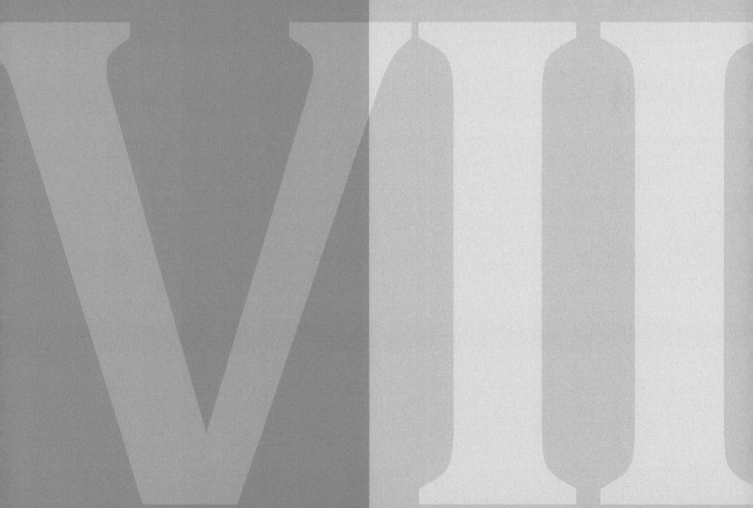

Part VII

Resurfacing Complications

39 Resurfacing Complications: Clinical Overview

Foad Nahai

Noninvasive and minimally invasive procedures including injectables and resurfacing continue their meteoric rise, by far outpacing the growth in surgical procedures. The "new normal" for us as surgeons means that periorbital rejuvenation is no longer solely surgical. For our patients, the noninvasive procedures offer convenience, faster recovery with less downtime, and, in general, less morbidity. At least the complications are perceived to be less in severity. The reality is that all operations and procedures, whether surgical or not, do carry risk of serious complications, including those threatening life and eyesight. Periorbital resurfacing is no exception. Whether the laser or peels, injudicious application or less-than-thorough pretreatment evaluation may lead to serious consequences, including skin burns, contractures, and lid retraction.

Prior to any resurfacing procedure, a thorough history and eyelid evaluation is essential, noting any history of previous eyelid procedures, dry eyes, or other conditions, which may affect the outcome of the procedure. Evaluation of lid position and lid tone, including the distraction and snap tests, must be undertaken. Preexisting malposition or poor lid tone will only be worsened by the resurfacing and should be concomitantly dealt with.

As the eyelid skin is far thinner than the adjacent skin, especially that of the brow, laser settings and peel concentrations must be adjusted accordingly. All laser devices have recommended settings according to skin thickness and must be calibrated prior to each case. The energy levels, patterns, and number of passes must be adjusted for each patient based on the condition of the eyelid and the skin.

Peels, whether glycolic acid based, trichloroacetic acid (TCA), phenol, or croton oil, must be diluted sufficiently for eyelid application. Our preference is to only apply 20% TCA and 0.1% croton oil to the eyelids while limiting the number of "passes" based on skin quality, skin excess, and, of course, experience.

Combining surgery with peels requires special caution. Surgical procedures where middle lamellar modification and skin excision is undertaken and then followed by a peel or laser resurfacing are best combined with canthal anchoring to minimize the risk of lid retraction. Needless to add, the skin excision must be conservative if it is followed by resurfacing of any kind.

Suggested Reading

[1] Nahai F. The aesthetic surgeon's "new normal". Aesthet Surg J. 2015; 35(1):105–107

40 Laser Resurfacing Burn to the Lower Lid

Ryan Scot Burke and T. Roderick Hester Jr.

Summary

A 48-year-old woman underwent carbon dioxide laser resurfacing of the bilateral lower eyelids, resulting in full-thickness burns. The burn injury resulted in both lid retraction and unsatisfactory scar appearance. In addition to multiple canthoplasty procedures to maintain lid position, the patient underwent a subperiosteal midface lift to recruit healthy tissue and resect burn scar. This chapter outlines the technique of the subperiosteal midface lift and its utility to decrease the size or eliminate the need for a full-thickness skin graft of the lower eyelid when attempting to correct lid retraction.

Keywords: laser, burn, cheek lift, scar, lid retraction, lower eyelid

40.1 Patient History Leading to the Specific Problem

The patient is a 48-year-old woman who underwent carbon dioxide laser resurfacing of the bilateral lower lids and perioral area (wavelength of 10,600 nm, pulse energy of 0.5 J, and output power of 100 W). She returned 2 weeks following treatment complaining of delayed wound healing, persistent erythema, and fibrinous discharge (▶ Fig. 40.1). The patient denied vision changes and dry eye, and was otherwise healthy. Cultures (viral and bacterial) were obtained to rule out infection, and a trial of oral antibiotics was attempted with no improvement of symptoms. Area was determined to be a full-thickness burn injury to the subtarsal lower lid with surrounding partial-thickness burn to the pretarsal and malar skin in addition to perioral skin. Prior to our initial evaluation, patient developed bilateral ectropion and underwent bilateral tarsal sling and steroid injections in the burn scars in another state.

40.2 Anatomic Description of the Patient's Current Status

The patient presented to Paces Plastic Surgery, to Doctors Hester and McCord, 6 months following the laser resurfacing and two previous attempts to correct lid retraction. She had worsening lid retraction resulting in significant

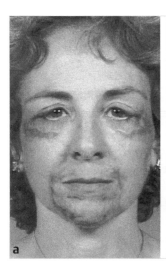
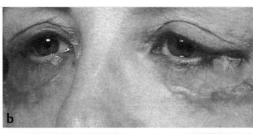
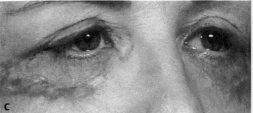

Fig. 40.1 (a–c) Patient photographs upon initial presentation to Paces Plastic Surgery. Significant burn scar is noted in the periorbital/cheek region as well as the perioral region. The patient recently had a canthoplasty temporarily correcting the lower eyelid position.

scleral show. The patient had developed hypertrophic scarring involving her pretarsal, subtarsal, and malar skin, resulting in lid malposition. Additionally, the patient has developed hypertrophic scarring of the perioral skin, particularly affecting the oral commissure.

The evaluation of the patient's problem begins with assessment of burn depth and affected structures. The area must initially be allowed to demarcate prior to any procedures to correct the aesthetic deformity, which will allow recovery of adjacent areas with partial-thickness injury and proper assessment of the necessity to replace them. Additionally, incompletely healed burn will continue to contract, thereby adversely affecting an already completed reconstruction.

Lid position is often assessed by evaluation of the lid margin's position relative to the limbus. A youthful eye is synonymous with a 0.5-mm overlap of these structures with no scleral show at rest. Assessment of the eye must include evaluation of upper lid excursion for complete eye closure and presence of Bell's phenomenon. Bell's phenomenon, which is present in 75% of the population, is an upward and outward movement of the eye upon closure. Incomplete eye closure, particularly in the absence of Bell's phenomenon, increases the risk of exposure keratopathy and damage to the cornea. Lid retraction is a result of shortening of both anterior and posterior lamella combined with tarsoligamentous laxity. This is of particular importance when attempting to correct the deformity as in the patient with a full-thickness injury, as both lamellae must be addressed.

Assessment of the lower lid laxity should always involve a "snap back" test or a more objective skin distraction test. The skin distraction test involves measuring the distance from the globe to the lid margin while traction is applied away from the globe. A distance of 2 mm or greater indicates lid laxity, which can be addressed with tightening of the tarsoligamentous sling, while a distance of 6 mm or greater requires skin resection in the horizontal plane. The "snap back" aspect of the examination refers to a firm return of the lower lid margin to the globe when released after distraction (▶Fig. 40.2). A delayed return would also indicate a requirement of tarsoligamentous sling tightening.

The approach to the anatomy of this region can be daunting, especially when the goal is resection of a significant surface area of skin to address a poorly aesthetic scar. Scar resection must be balanced with lid position as they are competing forces. This patient presents with a lid distraction test greater than 2 mm with delayed "snap back" indicating tarsoligamentous laxity. Additionally, the patient has scleral show, indicating there is a shortening of both the anterior lamellar skin/orbicularis and the posterior lamella tarsus/conjunctiva. She had persistently irritated eyes secondary to incomplete lid closure, which was addressed in the short term with eye drops.

40.3 Recommended Solution to the Problem

- Stabilize the lid position during scar maturation utilizing canthoplasty while augmenting scar development with judicious use of steroid injection.
- Close monitoring for dry eye, evidence of ectropion, retraction, and/or lagophthalmos, which requires canthoplasty.
- Evaluation of surrounding skin laxity and recruitment of adjacent tissue utilizing subperiosteal cheek lift.

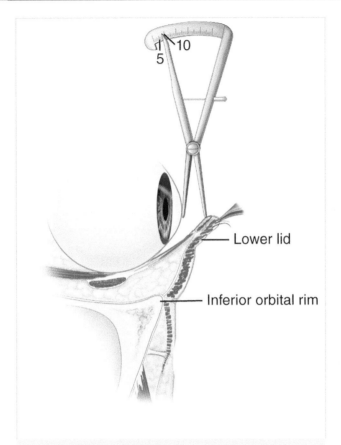

Fig. 40.2 A skin distraction test is generally considered positive when the lower eye lid skin can be distracted from the globe more than 6 mm, but distraction as little as 2 mm with a delayed "snap back" may require tarsoligamentous tightening. (Reproduced with permission from Nahai F, ed. The Art of Aesthetic Surgery: Principles & Techniques. 2nd ed. New York, NY: Thieme; 2010.)

- Utility of mucosal grafts and spacer grafts to increase length of posterior lamella.
- Close long-term monitoring for maintenance canthoplasty to maintain lid position.

40.4 Technique

Although the subperiosteal cheek lift was initially described to combat the effects of gravity and aging on both the lower lid and malar region, it has been proven useful to recruit healthy tissue into an area of deficient or scarred tissue. Since the patient has a full-thickness injury of the lower eyelid resulting in lid retraction, both anterior and posterior lamella will ultimately require intervention. The goal of the subperiosteal cheek lift in this setting would be soft tissue recruitment, restoration of lid position, and partial resection of the burn scar with attention to the deepest/full-thickness areas without overresection/excess tension.

The subperiosteal midface lift relies on the creation of a musculoligamentous carrier encompassing the superficial musculoaponeurotic system, orbicularis, and periosteum to elevate the midface and, in this case, resect scar tissue. This musculoligamentous carrier will allow a firm attachment of the midface to its new superior location and minimize subsequent descent and lid retraction.

The approach to the subperiosteal midface lift first involves a subciliary approach with a skin muscle flap. The incision is made elevation of a skin/muscle flap with continued dissection in the subperiosteal plane to mobilize the midface. The arcus marginalis and orbitomalar ligament are released. Adequate subperiosteal dissection, to "recruit" soft tissue and skin, involves freeing the superior and inferior periosteum around the infraorbital nerve with medial limit of nasolabial fold, inferior limit at the edge of malar eminence, and lateral limit of the medial third of zygomatic arch, as demonstrated in ▶Fig. 40.3.

Once the midface is mobilized, a muscle flap is developed by separating the skin, in this case the scar, from the muscle. The muscles are then secured to the temporal fascia to suspend the midface. Typically, three sutures are placed to hold the tissues in place and to support the lid (▶Fig. 40.4).

Once the musculoligamentous flap has been properly secured, attention can now be turned to the scar excision. With recruited full-thickness tissue to the area of scar, conservative excision can now be completed with decreased risk of lid retraction. There is a temptation in this patient to excise the scar in its entirety, but its broad extension would undoubtedly result in significant lid retraction. The focus therefore should be excision of the full-thickness skin injury of the delicate lower lid skin. ▶Fig. 40.5 should be used as a guide for skin excision in an attempt to avoid lid retraction.

As discussed above, any resection of lower lid skin should prompt completion of a lid distraction test to determine need for further horizontal skin excision to allow proper lid margin adherence to the globe. Although some partial-thickness injury remained due to surface area of initial injury, the result was appropriate lid position and avoidance of initial skin graft, which would have resulted in both further scar contraction and noticeable skin color/texture changes.

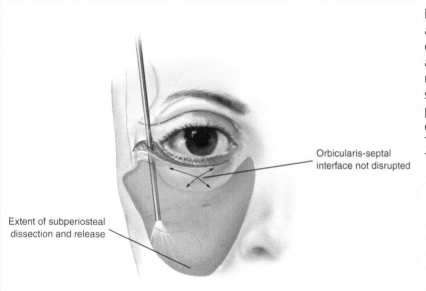

Orbicularis-septal interface not disrupted

Extent of subperiosteal dissection and release

Fig. 40.3 Although the endoscopic approach was not utilized in this case, the image demonstrates the area of undermining (subperiosteal) required to advance the midface superiorly. (Reproduced with permission from Nahai F, ed. The Art of Aesthetic Surgery: Principles & Techniques. 2nd ed. New York, NY: Thieme; 2010.)

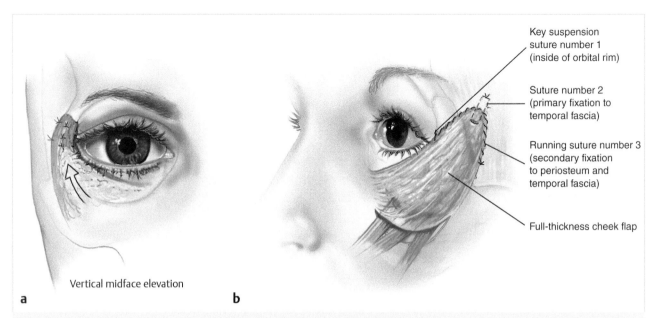

Fig. 40.4 (a,b) Mobilization of the muscle flap with lateral and superior vector of pull. This muscle flap should be secured to the temporal fascia with three sutures. (Reproduced with permission from Nahai F, ed. The Art of Aesthetic Surgery: Principles & Techniques. 2nd ed. New York, NY: Thieme; 2010.)

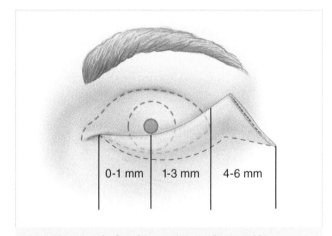

Fig. 40.5 Guide for skin excision after midface lift: medial canthus to pupil, 0–1 mm; pupil to lateral canthus, 1–3 mm; lateral to lateral canthus, 4–6 mm. (Reproduced with permission from Nahai F, ed. The Art of Aesthetic Surgery: Principles & Techniques. 2nd ed. New York, NY: Thieme; 2010.)

The patient continued to maintain adequate lid position, but given remnant partial-thickness injury of the anterior lamella, she required repeat canthoplasty to correct ectropion and maintain lid position. Over the course of 2 years, the patient maintained lower lid position with minimal irritation of globe, which allowed time for mild development of skin laxity that resulted in repeat subperiosteal cheek lift and further scar excision. The remaining scar was then excised a year later and replaced with a small full-thickness skin graft when compared to initial defect. Lastly, a mucosal skin graft and AlloDerm spacer graft were utilized to add length to the posterior lamella after skin graft correction of the anterior lamella.

40.5 Postoperative Photographs and Critical Evaluation of the Results

This patient has minimal evidence of scarring to both the lower eyelid and malar region. She does not currently complain of dry eye or vision changes. The lid has been maintained in a youthful position despite serial skin excisions of the lower eyelid and malar region. Additionally, the final skin graft was sufficiently small, which minimizes detection of subtle color changes of the graft. The patient reports she is very pleased with the results, although they require constant monitoring. The final result is a testament to both patient and serial small excisions combined with persistent maintenance of lid position to minimize the adverse effects of an unfortunate injury (▶Fig. 40.6).

40.6 Teaching Points

- Resurfacing is not without its complications.
- Severe lid retraction and skin fibrosis may require several procedures to adequately correct.
- Stabilizing lid position with multiple procedures in the acute and chronic setting is required to counteract contraction of scar.
- The subperiosteal midface lift is a very useful technique for recruiting skin and soft tissue to correct lid retraction, and in most patients, it obviates the need for skin grafts.

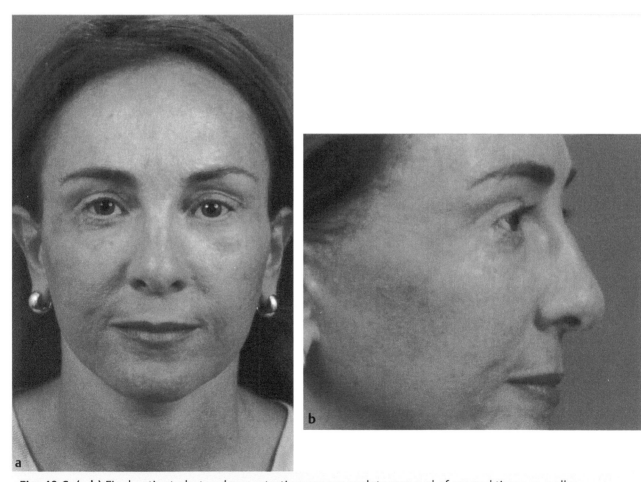

Fig. 40.6 (a,b) Final patient photos demonstrating near-complete removal of scarred tissue as well as appropriate lower lid position with no scleral show.

Acknowledgment

We thank Dr. McCord for his contribution to the patient's care.

Suggested Reading

[1] Hester TR, Jr, Codner MA, McCord CD, Nahai F, Giannopoulos A. Evolution of technique of the direct transblepharoplasty approach for the correction of lower lid and midfacial aging: maximizing results and minimizing complications in a 5-year experience. Plast Reconstr Surg. 2000; 105(1):393–406, discussion 407–408

[2] Nahai F. The Art of Aesthetic Surgery. 2nd ed. Vol. I. St. Louis, MO: Quality Medical Publishing, Inc; 201140.6 Teaching Points

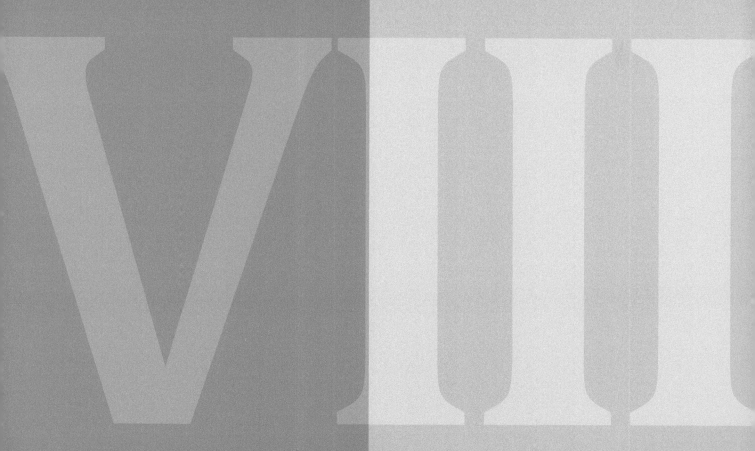

Part VIII

Epiphora

41 Epiphora: Clinical Overview

Ted H. Wojno

Tearing is one of the commonest complaints encountered in the ophthalmologist's office. It is very bothersome to patients and a source of significant visual disturbance. Key for the physician is to be able to distinguish true epiphora, actual excess lacrimation, from other complaints that are often mislabeled as "tearing" by the patient. Symptoms of ocular irritation, foreign body sensation, eye strain (asthenopia), and conjunctival edema are often reported as "tearing." When true epiphora is present, the cause is often elusive even to those whose practice is solely oculoplastics. Eyelid and periorbital surgical procedures may alter the physiology of the tear film causing symptoms of dryness, tearing, and sometimes both. A thorough history and careful examination is necessary. Often, I find that it is useful to directly query patients as to exactly what "tearing" means to them. The answers are often surprising and may save the physician considerable diagnostic time and effort and spare the patient additional and sometimes expensive testing.

42 Epiphora

Ted H. Wojno

Summary
Epiphora is a common complaint in the ophthalmologist's office. This chapter details the common causes of this disorder with special emphasis on evaluation and treatment of the tearing patient after eyelid surgery.

Keywords: epiphora, lagophthalmos, chemosis, ectropion, lacrimal pump

42.1 Patient History Leading to the Specific Problem

The patient is a 68-year-old white woman who had a four-eyelid blepharoplasty 1 month ago. She complains of bothersome tearing from both eyes since the surgery. She has tried over-the-counter artificial tear supplements and a prescription ophthalmic steroid eye drop with no relief. She says that her vision is blurry but does improve when she wipes her eyes. The swelling and discomfort from her surgery has mostly resolved. She is concerned that she has "pink eye" and wants to know if an antibiotic eye drop is needed (▶ Fig. 42.1).

42.2 Anatomic Description of the Patient's Current Status

On examination, the patient still has a slight amount of eyelid edema from her surgery. The eyelids are in good position with no ectropion. There is no sign of lagophthalmos on passive closure. A small amount of conjunctival edema is noted along the lower eyelid margins and the conjunctiva of both eyes is slightly injected. There is no obvious tearing on exam.

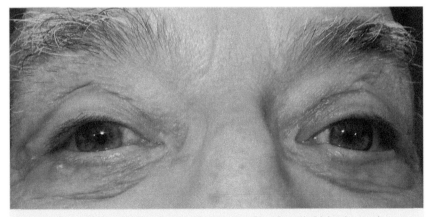

Fig. 42.1 A 68-year-old woman 1 month after four-lid blepharoplasty with persistent edema and erythema of the eyelids.

42.3 Recommended Solution to the Problem

- Determine if there is any conjunctival discharge or conjunctival edema.
- Look for evidence of eyelid malposition and lagophthalmos.
- Check to see if the patient appears to be blinking normally.

42.4 Technique

Closely inspect the eyes to see if there is any evidence of conjunctival discharge. Increased tearing is common after any eye or eyelid surgery. The tear fluid is normally clear but is often thicker after surgery due to increased mucus secretion, a normal response to ocular irritation. Mucus in the tear film is typically white and stringy, while true bacterial conjunctivitis is characterized by a yellow discharge indicative of pus. If there is any doubt, a conjunctival culture will differentiate and suggest appropriate antibiotic therapy if indicated.

Determine if there is any conjunctival edema (chemosis) along the lower eyelid margin (▶Fig. 42.2). Chemosis is quite common after lower eyelid surgery and can disrupt the normal flow of tears across the surface of the eye to the punctum. This is most common in the lateral canthus. Such patients will also complain of a foreign body sensation generated by the swollen conjunctiva and often report that they see a "blister" or "water pocket" on the surface of the eye. Older patients may even have redundant conjunctiva across the entire lower lid margin (conjunctivochalasis) preoperatively and are even more likely to develop postoperative chemosis (▶Fig. 42.3).

Check for any evidence of ectropion of the lower eyelid. If the punctum is displaced outward from its position against the globe, it cannot drain the tears away from the eye and epiphora results. Even the slightest amount of punctual ectropion will lead to tearing (▶Fig. 42.4).

Ask the patient to gently close the eyes to determine if there is any lagophthalmos (▶Fig. 42.5). Even 1 mm of lagophthalmos can lead to significant corneal exposure and complaints of ocular irritation and tearing. It

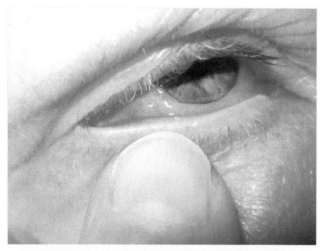

Fig. 42.2 Chemosis (conjunctival edema) of the right eye.

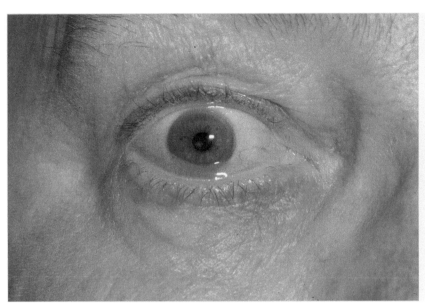

Fig. 42.3 Conjunctivochalasis (redundant conjunctiva) of the right eye.

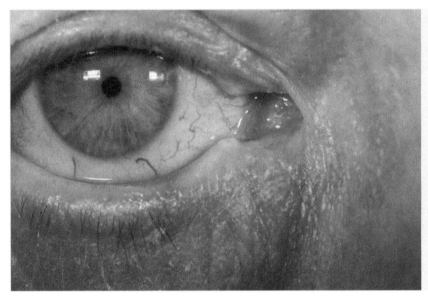

Fig. 42.4 Punctal ectropion of the left lower eyelid.

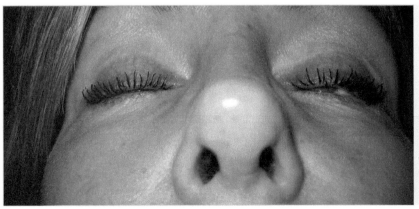

Fig. 42.5 Lagophthalmos of both eyes, worse on the left, in a patient 3 months after four-lid blepharoplasty.

may be necessary to ask the patient's spouse to observe for any signs of nocturnal lagophthalmos since subtle weakness of closure may not be obvious in the examination room. This entity is covered in another chapter in this book.

Evaluate the patient's blinking ability. Is there any sign of the seventh cranial nerve weakness that could have resulted from the surgery? Do the lids appear to blink normally or do they appear to function slower than normal? The tear film is intimately related to and dependent on normal eyelid integrity and mechanics. The eyelids are the "pump" for pushing tears into the lacrimal sac and down the nasolacrimal duct. Any disruption of their ability to do so results in tearing.

42.5 Postoperative Photographs and Critical Evaluation of Results

Next to visual disturbance, tearing is probably the second most common patient complaint after eyelid and ocular surgery. It is important to establish if there is true epiphora characterized by an increase in the tears that literally run down the patient's face or if the eyes simply feel irritated or abnormal to the patient, which too is often reported as "tearing." Likewise, patients who visualize conjunctival edema in the mirror often report this as "tearing" to the physician. Complicating this evaluation is the fact that patients who undergo eyelid surgery are in the age group that commonly also carry a diagnosis of "dry eye" or "blepharitis" and have already been placed on a plethora of over-the-counter and prescription artificial tear drops and ointments, ophthalmic anti-inflammatories, topical steroids, and topical antibiotics, which they faithfully bring in a bag to the physician's office for inspection. Certainly, all of the aforementioned medications contain preservatives that can lead to significant side effects and toxicity. I often believe that the most therapeutic thing I do for some of my patients is to have them stop using all of their topical medications and re-evaluate them in a week to establish a baseline. It is not uncommon for such patients to report that their symptoms have miraculously cleared upon discontinuance of their medicine cabinet full of drops and ointments.

Conjunctival edema (chemosis) will virtually always clear with the passage of time, usually 1 to 2 months, but may be as long as 6 months in rare cases. Persistent cases seem to induce tremendous anxiety in patients but they can be assured that this will resolve. Typically, the last-tried treatment that coincides with spontaneous resolution is credited to be the "cure." Such treatments include topical steroid drops and ointments, nonsteroidal anti-inflammatory drops, mast cell inhibitors, hypertonic saline drops, topical vasoconstrictors, cold compresses, warm compresses, temporary lateral tarsorrhaphy, lymphatic drainage massage, injection of hyaluronidase, and direct incision or excision of the offending conjunctiva. Again, calm reassurance may have the greatest therapeutic value.

Punctal ectropion can result from excess skin excision, failure to correct existing excess horizontal lid laxity, or failure to recognize its presence preoperatively. Punctal ectropion can also manifest after surgery due to chemosis that will push the lower lid margin away from the ocular surface. Fortunately, punctal ectropion often resolves as swelling decreases and eyelid mechanics normalize. If not, surgical correction is needed.

As stated above, the lacrimal pump is inherently dependent on normal eyelid movement for proper function. Given that the eyelids have been

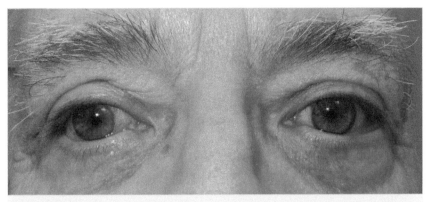

Fig. 42.6 The same patient shown in ▶ Fig. 42.1 2 months later with resolution of symptoms of epiphora.

surgically tightened and manipulated and are now swollen to some degree, it is not surprising that lid function is compromised. When lid surgery is combined with other facial surgery, there may be additional effects on the seventh nerve integrity that are typically temporary but occasionally permanent. All of these alterations to the normal anatomy and physiology affect the lacrimal pump, leading to tearing in the postoperative period. Again, the vast majority of these problems resolve without surgical intervention and the patient can be safely assured that the bothersome symptoms will pass.

This patient experienced resolution of her symptoms within the next 2 months without any additional therapy (▶ Fig. 42.6). It is likely that her symptoms of epiphora were due to slight conjunctival edema combined with a mildly decreased blink secondary to lid edema and the horizontal lid tightening at surgery.

42.6 Teaching Points

- Epiphora is a common complaint in the postoperative period of eyelid surgery.
- Most epiphora in the postoperative period is due to a variety of mechanical alterations with the eyelids and conjunctiva.
- Most complaints of epiphora can be easily diagnosed and resolve with time and no special treatment.

Suggested Reading

[1] Bosniak SL. Advances in Ophthalmic Plastic and Reconstructive Surgery. The Lacrimal System. New York, NY: Pergamon; 1984
[2] Fleming JC, Avakian A. Pseudoepiphora: dry eye causing tearing. In: Mauriello JA, ed. Unfavorable Results of Eyelid and Lacrimal Surgery. Prevention and Management. New York, NY: Butterworth Heinemann; 2000:401–420
[3] Hugh WL. Conjunctivochalasis. Am J Ophthalmol. 1942; 25:48
[4] Liu D. Conjunctivochalasis. A cause of tearing and its management. Ophthal Plast Reconstr Surg. 1986; 2(1):25–28
[5] Meller D, Tseng SCG. Conjunctivochalasis: literature review and possible pathophysiology. Surv Ophthalmol. 1998; 43(3):225–232

Index

Note: Page numbers set in **bold** or *italic* indicate headings or figures, respectively.

N

Nitropaste 288

O

Ocular motility disorders
- after blepharoplasty **5**
- anatomy in **38**, *39*
- forced duction testing in 41, *42*
- history in **38**
- ocular alignment exam in 40, *41*
- ocular motility exam in 40, *41*, *42*
- outcomes in **42**
- vision exam in 39
Ophthalmic artery, in blindness after blepharoplasty and injectables 32, *33*
Optic nerve ischemia, in blindness after blepharoplasty and injectables *26*
Optic neuritis, in blindness after blepharoplasty and injectables *26*
Orbicularis wedge 90
Orbital apex syndrome, in blindness after blepharoplasty and injectables *26*
Orbital decompression, in blindness after blepharoplasty and injectables 34
Orbital fat transposition, in overresection of upper lid 103
Orbital pseudotumor 23, *24*
Orbital vector analysis **209**, *210*
Orbitotomy, anterior, in periocular infection **21**
Osmotic expander insertion, for lower lid retraction **216**, *217*
Overresection, in blepharoplasty *102*, *107*
- anatomy in **101**, **107**
- bipolar coagulation in 102
- fat grafting in 103, *104*, *105*, **108**, *109*
- fat preservation in 102
- history in **101**, **107**
- outcomes in **104**, *105*, **109**, *110*
- volume replacement in **103**

P

Palpebral artery, large 43
PBLER 308. *See* Postblepharoplasty lower eyelid retraction (PBLER)
Peels 308. *See also* Resurfacing
Penlight, in dry eye 144, *146*
Peptic ulcer disease (PUD), in blindness after blepharoplasty and injectables *26*
Periocular infection 308. *See also* Infection
Phlebitis, in blindness after blepharoplasty and injectables *26*
Photography, preoperative 89
Postblepharoplasty lower eyelid retraction (PBLER) *164*
- anatomy in **164**
- anterior lamellar shortage in 240, *241*
- assessment of *165*, 166
- background in **239**
- distraction test in *241*
- eyelid laxity in 240, *241*
- eyelid vector in 240, *241*
- factors in 239
- filler treatment for **240**, *242*
- forced traction test in 240
- history in **164**
- internal eyelid scar in 240, **245**, *246*, *247*
- measurement of 239, *240*
- minimally invasive orbicularis-sparing lower lid recession in **242**, *243*, *244*, *245*
- orbicularis strength in *240*, *242*, *243*, *244*, *245*
- outcomes in *169*, *170*
- physical examination in **239**, *240*
- skin grafting for *167*, *168*
- volume deficit in 240, *241*, *242*
Posterior ciliary artery, in blindness after blepharoplasty and injectables 32
Preoperative photography 89
Pseudotumor, orbital 23, *24*
Ptosis
- after blepharoptosis correction
-- anatomy in *83*
-- history in **83**
-- outcomes with **86**, *87*
-- resection for **84**, *85*
- age-related 48, *49*
- as filler complication **280**, *282*
- congenital vs. acquired 47, 48, *49*
- postblepharoplasty
-- anatomy in **76**, *78*
-- brow **91**, *92*
-- brow stability and **90**
-- case example **92**
-- crease symmetry and **93**
-- hematoma in 90
-- history in **76**, *77*
-- intraoperative prevention of **89**
-- levator advancement for **77**, *79*
-- management of **91**
-- Müllerectomy for **80**, *81*
-- outcomes with **80**, *82*
-- preoperative evaluation and 76, **88**
-- preoperative photography and 89
-- prevention of **88**
-- transient 76
- with botulinum toxin injection **280**, *282*
Pull-away test 139

R

Raynaud's syndrome, in blindness after blepharoplasty and injectables *26*
Resurfacing
- botulinum toxin injection and 279
- combining surgery with 293
- filler injections and 279
- for scars 54
- laser, burns in *294*, *296*, *297*, *298*, *299*
Retinal ischemia, in blindness after blepharoplasty and injectables *26*
Retinal nerve ischemia, in blindness after blepharoplasty and injectables *26*
Retrobulbar hematoma, after blepharoplasty 4
Retrobulbar hemorrhage
- anatomy in **15**
- canthotomy in *15*, *16*, *17*
- compartment syndrome in 15
- in blindness after blepharoplasty and injectables *26*
- outcomes with **18**
- patient history in **14**
- suture release in 15
Rosacea 147
Round eye deformity *172*
- anatomy in *172*, *173*
- correction of **174**, *175*, *176*, *177*
- defined 171
- history in **171**
- outcomes in **175**, *178*, *179*

S

Scars
- donor site 231, *232*
- in postblepharoplasty lower eyelid retraction 240, **245**, *246*, *247*
- upper eyelid
-- 5-fluorouracil for 53, **54**, *55*
-- anatomy in **52**
-- causes of 52
-- crease malposition and *68*
-- history in **51**
-- lagophthalmos and *68*
-- outcomes with **54**, *55*
-- silicone gel dressings for 53
-- triamcinolone acetonide for 53, **54**
Schirmer tear strip *146*, *147*
Secretion tear test 144
Silicone gel dressings, for upper eyelid scarring 53
Slit-lamp biomicroscope 139
Snap back test 139, *140*
Spacer grafts 96, 222, *223*
Staphylococcus aureus, in periorbital infection 22
Steroids, in blindness after blepharoplasty and injectables 34
Streptococcus, in periorbital infection 22

Supraorbital artery, filler injection into 32
Supratrochlear artery, filler injection into *32*

T

TAC 308. *See* Triamcinolone acetonide (TAC)
Tarsoligamentous sling 138
Tarsorrhaphy, in blindness after blepharoplasty and injectables 34
Tear film 143
Tear trough deformity 156, *159*
Tenon's capsule, in chemosis *126*, *127*
Tensor fascia lata (TFL) graft, in recurrent ectropion 222, *226*, *227*, *228*
TFL 308. *See* Tensor fascia lata (TFL) graft
Thrombocytopenia, in blindness after blepharoplasty and injectables 26
Thyroid eye disease 23, *141*, **197**, 308. *See also* Blepharoptosis
Triamcinolone acetonide (TAC), for upper eyelid scarring 53, **54**
Trichloroacetic acid (TCA) 293
Two-finger test 139, *140*, *141*

U

Underresection, in blepharoplasty *111*
- anatomy in **111**
- history in **111**
- outcomes in *116*
- persistent lower eyelid fat in **113**, **114**, *115*
- persistent upper eyelid fat in **112**, **114**, *115*
- persistent upper eyelid skin in **112**, **113**, *114*
Upper eyelid
- anatomy *47*
- crease 49
-- anatomy in **57**, *58*
-- correction **58**, *59*, *60*, *61*, *62*, *63*
-- history in **57**
-- malposition
--- beveled approach for 69, *70*, *71*, *72*, *73*, *74*
---- clinical findings in *67*
--- high **66**
--- scarring and *68*
-- outcomes with **64**
-- symmetry **93**
- overresection of, in blepharoplasty *102*, *107*
-- anatomy in **101**, **107**
-- bipolar coagulation in 102
-- fat grafting in 103, *104*, *105*, **108**, *109*
-- fat preservation in 102
-- history in **101**, **107**
-- outcomes in **104**, *105*, **109**, *110*
-- volume replacement in **103**
- persistent fat of, in underresection in blepharoplasty **112**, **114**, *115*
- persistent skin of, in underresection in blepharoplasty **112**, **113**, *114*
- ptosis
- age-related 48, *49*
-- congenital vs. acquired 47, 48, *49*
- scars
-- 5-fluorouracil for 53, **54**, *55*
-- anatomy in **52**
-- causes of 52
-- crease malposition and *68*
-- history in **51**
-- outcomes with **54**, *55*
-- silicone gel dressings for 53
-- triamcinolone acetonide for 53, **54**

V

Visual loss 308. *See also* Blindness
Volume replacement, in overresection **103**

Z

Zygomaticomaxillary complex fracture, in blindness after blepharoplasty and injectables *26*